Natural Health
COMPLETE
GUIDE *to*
MEDICINAL
HERBS

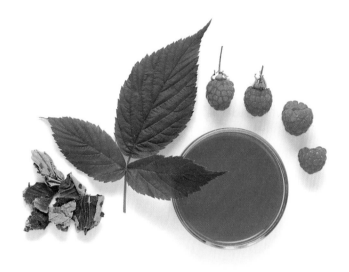

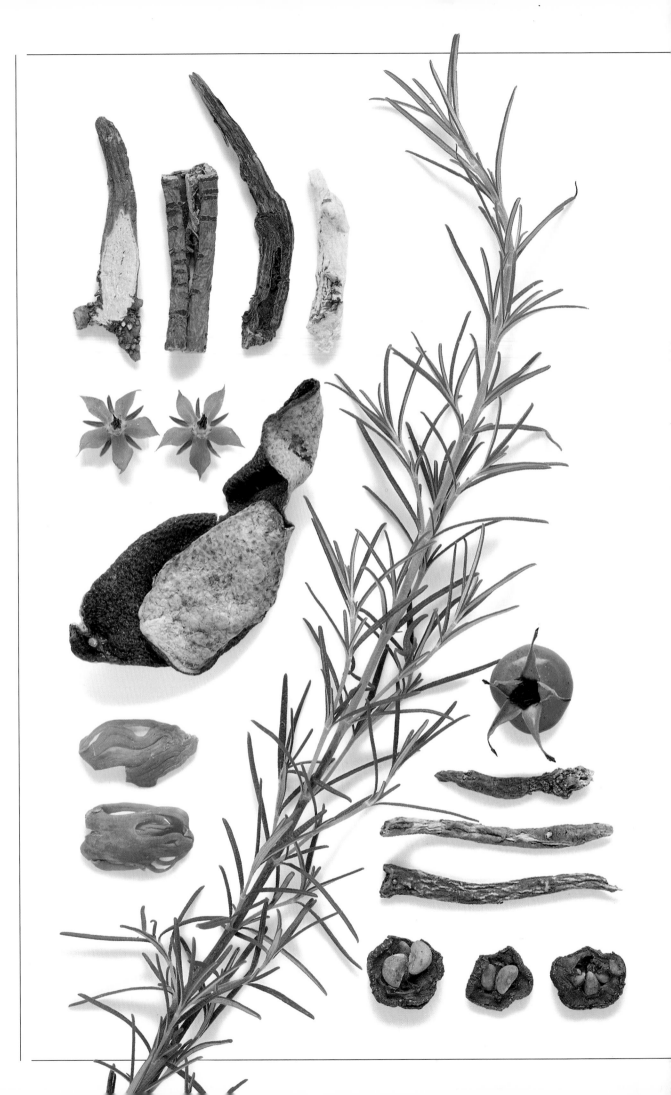

Natural Health
COMPLETE GUIDE *to* MEDICINAL HERBS

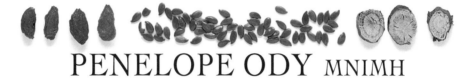

PENELOPE ODY MNIMH

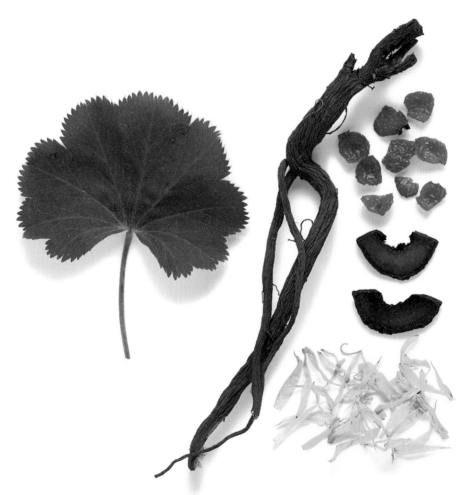

A Dorling Kindersley Book

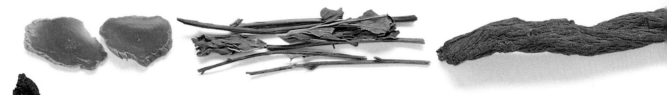

Dorling **DK** Kindersley

LONDON, NEW YORK, SYDNEY, DELHI, PARIS, MUNICH and JOHANNESBURG

Natural Health magazine is the leading publication in the field of natural self-care.
For subscription information call 800-526-8440 or visit www.naturalhealthmag.com.
Natural Health® is a registered trademark of Weider Publications, Inc.

Project editor Molly Perham • *Art editor* Karen Sawyer
Senior editor Jude Garlick • *Senior art editor* Dawn Terrey
US project editor Barbara Minton • *Assistant editor* Jane Perlmutter
Senior managing editor Krystyna Mayer • *Deputy art director* Carole Ash
Production manager Sarah Coltman
Main photographer Steve Gorton

FIRST EDITION
Project editor Tanya Hines • *Assistant editor* Blanche Sibbald
Art editor Tina Hill • *Assistant designer* Kate Sarluis
Senior managing editor Daphne Razazan • *Managing art editor* Carole Ash
Production manager Maryann Rogers
Main photographer Steve Gorton

IMPORTANT NOTICE

The recommendations and information in this book are appropriate in most cases. However, the advice this book contains is general, not specific to individuals and their particular circumstances. Any plant substance, whether used as food or medicine, externally or internally, can cause an allergic reaction in some people. Neither the author nor the publishers can be held responsible for any injury, damage or otherwise resulting from the use of herbal medicines. Do not try self-diagnosis or attempt self-treatment for serious or long-term problems without consulting a medical professional or qualified practitioner. Do not undertake any self-treatment while undergoing a prescribed course of medical treatment without first seeking professional advice. Always seek medical advice if symptoms persist.

First American edition 1993
Second American edition 2000
2 4 6 8 10 9 7 5 3 1

Published in the United States
by Dorling Kindersley, Inc., 232 Madison Avenue
New York, New York 10016

Copyright © 1993, 2000 Dorling Kindersley Limited, London
Text copyright © 1993, 2000 Penelope Ody
Foreword © 1993 Mark Blumenthal

All rights reserved under International and Pan-American Copyright Conventions. No part of this publication may be reproduced, stored in a retrieval system, or transmitted in any form or by any means, electronic, mechanical, photocopying, recording, or otherwise, without the prior written permission of the copyright owner.
Published in Great Britain by Dorling Kindersley Limited.

Library of Congress Cataloging-in-Publication Data
Ody, Penelope.
    Complete guide to medicinal herbs / Penelope Ody.--U.S. ed.
        p. cm.
    Includes index.
    ISBN 0-7894-6785-2 (alk. paper)
        1. Herbs–Therapeutic use. I. Title.
RM666.H33 038   2000
615'.321–dc21   00-025779

GUIDE TO MEASUREMENTS
2 cups = 500 milliliters (ml)
1 cup = 250 ml
½ cup = 125 ml

Reproduced in Singapore by Colourscan
Printed in China by Sun Fung

see our complete
catalog at
www.dk.com

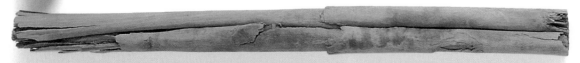

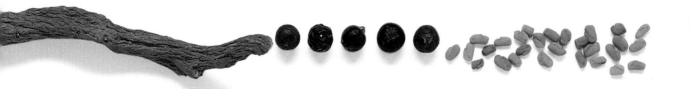

CONTENTS

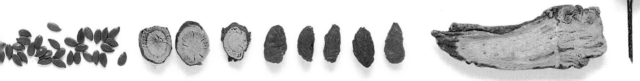

FOREWORD

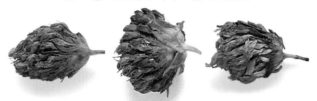

The use of herbs and medicinal plants as the first medicines is a universal phenomenon. Every culture on Earth, through written or oral tradition, has relied on the vast variety of natural chemistry found in healing plants for their therapeutic properties.

The majority of herb books and "herbals" available today in the US focus on one cultural tradition or another. Most medicinal plant manuals are derived from the rich European herbal tradition, which is a synthesis of herbal wisdom created from Celtic, Roman, Greek, and Arabic cultures. Recent books have begun to educate Westerners about the fertile knowledge of Traditional Chinese Medicine (TCM) and from Ayurveda, the traditional healing system of ancient India. Few books, however, offer a comprehensive integration of both Eastern and Western herbal traditions into one volume in order to develop a more "ecumenical" herbalism.

In *The Complete Medicinal Herbal*, Penelope Ody has synthesized some of the material of European, Chinese, and Ayurvedic herbalism, but also presents some of the theoretical basis for understanding the human body, its physiological processes, and how herbs are applied accordingly.

Written from the perspective of the practitioner, the book is a practical how-to manual, offering detailed advice on the preparation of herbal remedies, plus information on their dosage and use that is seldom found in contemporary herbals. The result is an eclectic blend of authoritative recipes, formulas, recommendations, and cautions that embody several traditions of herbalism and some related modalities.

No doubt the author's statements and recommendations will raise a few eyebrows among conventionally trained pharmacists or physicians. The inclusion of homeopathic remedies that include standard homeopathic products mixed with the relatively recent "flower essences" (reportedly designed to affect physiological and emotional states) will provide a real "stretch" for most health professionals. Yet, as herbs and other "alternative" forms of "natural" healing are increasingly sought after by an interested lay public, it becomes incumbent upon health professionals to approach new and old therapies with an open mind.

This is not an invitation to quackery. To the contrary, the author represents a new breed of herbalist who draws from a variety of cultural traditions, as well as from the scientific literature itself. Information is included about the chemical makeup of the herbs she recommends, plus considerable cautions about their potential for misuse. In a number of cases she recommends supervision by an experienced herbalist or other qualified health practitioner, and where cases warrant, she prudently advises the reader to seek appropriate medical advice.

The author is aware that if herbalists expect to have their craft accepted by mainstream medicine and public, they must be willing to rely on information from scientific and medical domains. Accordingly, as the public demand more natural forms of healthcare and as healthcare costs continue to spiral out of control, mainstream health practitioners and policy makers might also become more willing to reconsider some of the practices associated with herbalism, with both its scientifically confirmed and its less scientific yet hard-to-dismiss, empirical treatments.

MARK BLUMENTHAL

INTRODUCTION

ONE OF THE EARLIEST Chinese herbals – Shen Nung's *Classic of Materia Medica* dating from the first or second centuries A.D. – listed 365 healing remedies, most of them plants but including a few mineral and animal extracts. The Greek physician Dioscorides, writing in the first century A.D., mentioned about 400 herbs. Today, the list of plants with known medicinal properties is rather longer: about 5,800 in the Chinese *Materia Medica*, 2,500 in India, at least 800 regularly collected from the tropical forests of Africa, almost 300 currently detailed for the medical profession in Germany (so far the only Western country with official herbal monographs), and many thousands more known only to traditional healers in the more remote corners of the world. To produce a truly complete medicinal herbal would fill many volumes and be the work of several lifetimes. Yet, despite this bewildering array of healing plants, the average Western herbalist generally finds that a working knowledge of 150 to 200 plants is more than enough to cope with most human ailments.

Herbs may be defined as any plants that can be put to culinary or medicinal use and include those we associate with conventional drugs, such as foxglove and opium poppy, as well as everyday plants, such as garlic or sage. The herbs in this book are a representative cross section of these potent plants, ranging from exotic Eastern herbs such as *ma huang* and ginseng to more mundane apples and cabbages.

Interest in herbal remedies has grown steadily in the past decade. In the years since 1993, when the first edition of this book appeared, there has been a significant increase in sales of ready-made herbal remedies and more interest from the conventional medical profession in using herbal extracts as an alternative to powerful and potentially hazardous drugs. That interest has been fueled by concerns over the growing numbers of antibiotic-resistant microorganisms. In the West, people often cite the risk of side effects from powerful conventional drugs as a reason for turning to gentler plant medicines. In the developing world, a lack of hard currency to pay for imported pharmaceuticals is encouraging a reappraisal of traditional folk remedies.

This trend toward more natural medicine has gained added impetus from our growing concern with environmental issues, such as the destruction of the rain forests and the loss of rare species. Although the therapeutic effects of many herbs have not been

scientifically proven, research continues to identify the active ingredients that may one day form the basis of drugs to fight cancer or AIDS.

And yet, in extracting these chemicals and seeking to turn herbal remedies designed to help the body heal itself into powerful drugs to obliterate symptoms, we forget one of the basic tenets of traditional healing: a belief that the cause of disharmonies and "disease" should be treated rather than the effects. We forget, too, that traditional health care has as much to do with preventing disease as with curing it.

The use of simple herbal remedies can encourage us once again to take responsibility for our own health. Instead of trying to obliterate symptoms when they become severe, we need to be sufficiently in tune with our bodies to recognize those symptoms as they develop and treat likely causes – whether physical, emotional, or spiritual – to restore balance.

In this book I do not simply aim to give a wealth of detail about a limited number of plants or provide cure-all lists of remedies that can be taken to alleviate symptoms. I have tried instead to look at how some herbs have been used by the traditional healers of many cultures, and I have suggested a therapeutic approach for ailments that focuses on healing the whole person. For some, these suggesions may represent an effective solution. For others, they will only be the starting point for a wider exploration of the healing power of herbs.

Penelope Ody

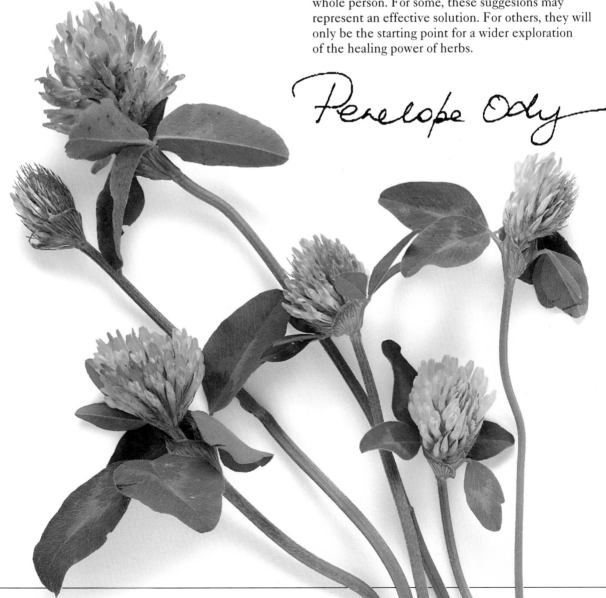

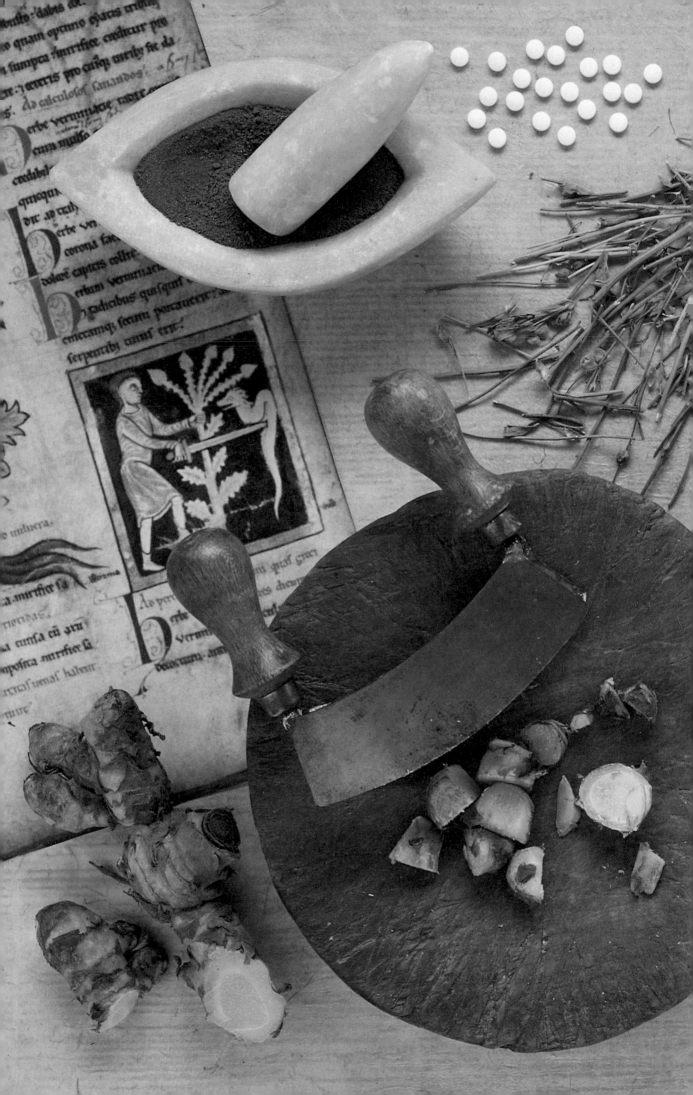

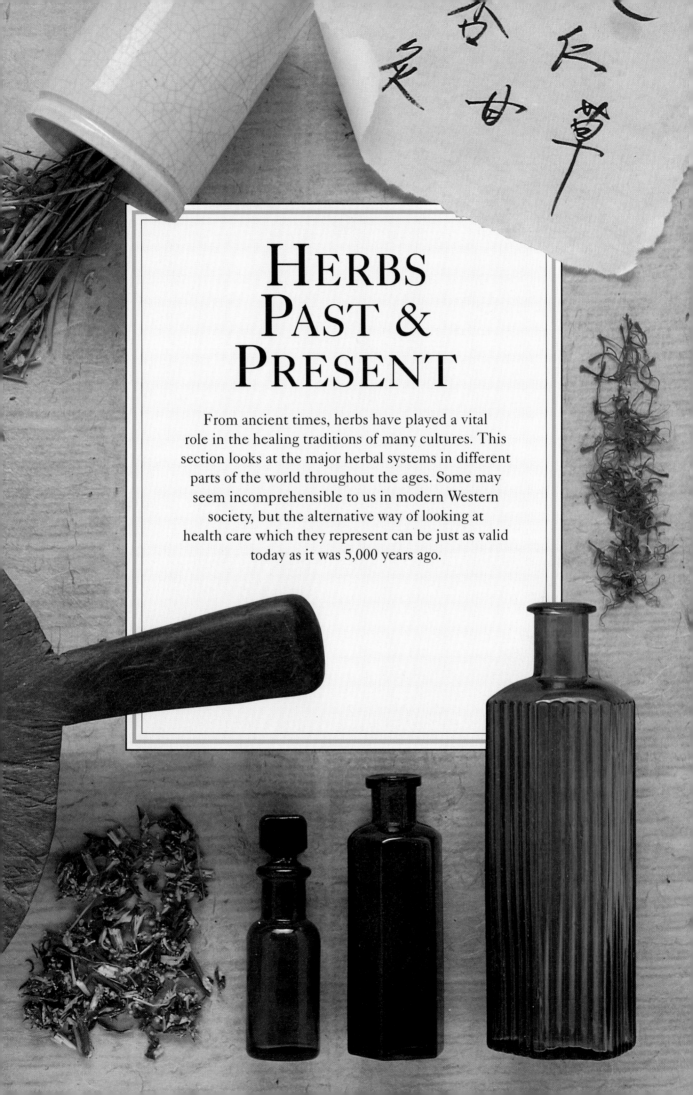

HERBS PAST & PRESENT

From ancient times, herbs have played a vital role in the healing traditions of many cultures. This section looks at the major herbal systems in different parts of the world throughout the ages. Some may seem incomprehensible to us in modern Western society, but the alternative way of looking at health care which they represent can be just as valid today as it was 5,000 years ago.

ORIGINS OF WESTERN HERBALISM

HIPPOCRATES MAY BE KNOWN today as the father of medicine, but for centuries medieval Europe followed the teachings of Galen, a 2nd-century physician, who wrote extensively about the body's four "humors" – blood, phlegm, black bile, and yellow bile – and classified herbs by their essential qualities: as hot or cold, dry, or damp.

These theories were later expanded by 7th-century Arab physicians, such as Avicenna, and today Galenical theories continue to dominate *Unani* medicine, practiced in the Muslim world and India. Galen's descriptions of herbs as, for example, "hot in the third degree" or "cold in the second," were still being used well into the 18th century.

Ancient Civilizations

HERBS IN PAPYRI
Surviving Egyptian papyri dating back to about 1700 B.C. record that many common herbs, such as garlic and juniper, have been used medicinally for about 4,000 years. In the days of Rameses III, hemp was used for eye problems just as it may be prescribed for glaucoma today, while poppy extracts were used to quiet crying children.

THE GREEK CONTRIBUTION
By the time of Hippocrates (468-377 B.C.), European herbal tradition had already absorbed ideas from Assyria and India, with Eastern herbs such as basil and ginger among the most highly prized, and the complex theory of humors and essential body fluids had begun to be formulated. Hippocrates categorized all foods and herbs by fundamental qualities – hot, cold, dry, or damp. Good health was maintained by keeping qualities in balance, as well as taking plenty of exercise and fresh air.

Pedanius Dioscorides wrote his classic text *De Materia Medica* in about A.D. 60, and this remained the standard textbook for 1,500 years. Dioscorides was reputed to have been either the physician to

The Greek model
Early Greeks saw the world as composed of four elements: earth, air, fire, and water. These elements were related to the seasons, to four fundamental qualities, to four bodily fluids or humors, and to four temperaments. In almost all individuals, one humor was thought to dominate, affecting both personality and the likely health problems that would be suffered.

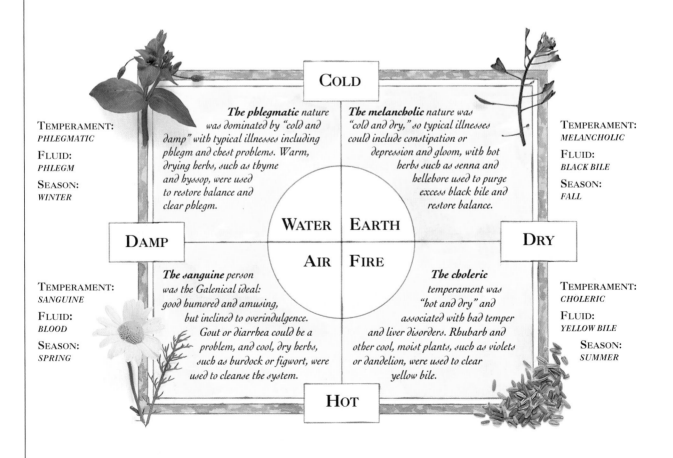

COLD

The phlegmatic nature was dominated by "cold and damp" with typical illnesses including phlegm and chest problems. Warm, drying herbs, such as thyme and hyssop, were used to restore balance and clear phlegm.

The melancholic nature was "cold and dry," so typical illnesses could include constipation or depression and gloom, with hot herbs such as senna and hellebore used to purge excess black bile and restore balance.

TEMPERAMENT:
PHLEGMATIC

FLUID:
PHLEGM

SEASON:
WINTER

TEMPERAMENT:
MELANCHOLIC

FLUID:
BLACK BILE

SEASON:
FALL

WATER **EARTH**

DAMP

AIR **FIRE**

DRY

The sanguine person was the Galenical ideal: good humored and amusing, but inclined to overindulgence. Gout or diarrhea could be a problem, and cool, dry herbs, such as burdock or figwort, were used to cleanse the system.

The choleric temperament was "hot and dry" and associated with bad temper and liver disorders. Rhubarb and other cool, moist plants, such as violets or dandelion, were used to clear yellow bile.

TEMPERAMENT:
SANGUINE

FLUID:
BLOOD

SEASON:
SPRING

TEMPERAMENT:
CHOLERIC

FLUID:
YELLOW BILE

SEASON:
SUMMER

HOT

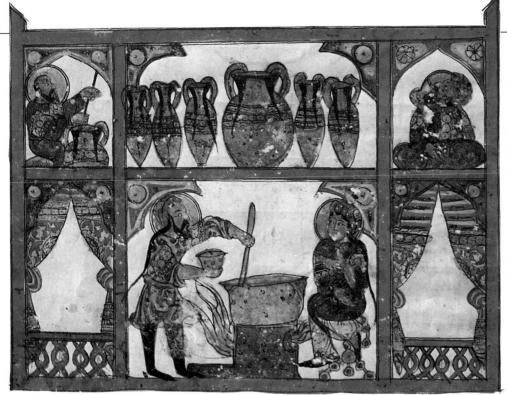

Classification of herbs
Dioscorides' herbal covers about 600 "medicinal trees." These were grouped by character – aromatics or "herbs with a sharp quality" – and by appearance or part used – "roots," "herbs," and "ground trees" (herbaceous plants with treelike leaves). In this 13th-century version of Dioscorides' herbal, an Islamic herbalist is seen preparing his remedies.

Antony and Cleopatra or an army surgeon during the reign of the Emperor Nero. Many of the actions Dioscorides describes are familiar today: parsley as a diuretic, fennel to promote milk flow, and white horehound mixed with honey as an expectorant.

ROMAN REMEDIES
The Greek theories of medicine reached Rome about 100 B.C. As time passed, they became more mechanistic, presenting a view of the body as a machine to be actively repaired, rather than following the Hippocratic dictum of allowing most diseases to cure themselves. Medicine became a lucrative business with complex, highly priced herbal remedies.

Opposing this practice was Claudius Galenus (A.D. 131-199), who was born in Pergamon in Asia Minor and was a court physician to the Emperor Marcus Aurelius. Galen reworked many of the old Hippocratic ideas and formalized the theories of humors. His books soon became the standard medical texts not only of Romans, but also of later Arab and medieval physicians, and his theories still survive in *Unani* medicine today.

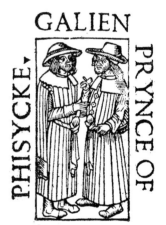

The "Prynce of Phisycke"
Galen's writings were influential for centuries; this woodcut dates from 1542.

Islamic Influences

THE ARAB WORLD
With the fall of Rome in the 5th century, the center of Classical learning shifted East and the study of Galenical medicine was focused in Constantinople and Persia. Galenism was adopted with enthusiasm by the Arabs and merged with both folk beliefs and surviving Egyptian learning. It was this mixture of herbal ideas, practice, and traditions that was reimported into Europe with the invading Arab armies.

Probably the most important work of the time was the *Kitab al-Qanun*, or *Canon of Medicine*, by Avicenna. This was based firmly on Galenical principles and by the 12th century had been translated into Latin and brought back to the West to become one of the leading textbooks in Western medical schools.

Eastern spices
The Arabs were great traders and introduced many herbs and spices from the East, such as nutmeg, cloves, saffron, and senna, to the materia medica of Dioscorides and Galen. Here, a Cairo street trader displays his wares.

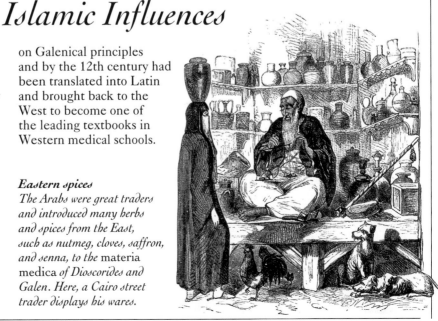

A SCIENCE OF LIFE

THE TERM AYURVEDA comes from two Indian words: *ayur*, or life, and *veda*, or knowledge. Ayurvedic medicine is thus described as a "knowledge of how to live," emphasizing that good health is the responsibility of the individual. In Ayurvedic medicine, illness is seen in terms of imbalance, with herbs and dietary controls used to restore equilibrium. The earliest Ayurvedic texts date from about 2500 B.C. with successive invaders adding new herbal traditions: the Persians in 500 B.C.; the Moguls in the 14th century, bringing the medicine of Galen and Avicenna (known as *Unani*); and the British, who closed down the Ayurvedic schools in 1833 but luckily did not obliterate the ancient learning altogether. Tibetan medicine has much in common with Ayurveda but can be vastly more complicated, having 15 subdivisions for the humors and placing strong emphasis on the effect of past lives – *karma* – on present health.

The Way of the Ayurveda

A WORLDVIEW
As in Ancient Greek and traditional Chinese medicine, the Ayurvedic model links the microcosm of the individual with the cosmos. At the heart of the system are three primal forces: *prana*, the breath of life; *agni*, the spirit of light or fire; and *soma*, a manifestation of harmony, cohesiveness, and love. There are also five elements comprising all matter: earth, water, fire, air, and ether (a nebulous nothingness that fills all space and was also known to the Ancient Greeks).

BALANCING THE HUMORS
The five universal elements are converted by *agni*, the digestive fire, into three humors, which influence individual health and temperament and are sometimes called waste products of digestion. If digestion were perfect there would be no humoral imbalance, but because it is not, imbalance and ill health can follow. Air and ether yield *vata* (wind), fire produces the humor *pitta* (fire or bile), while earth and water combine to give *kapha* (phlegm). The dominant humor is seen as controlling the character of the individual: a *vata*-type roughly conforms to Galen's melancholic personality, *pitta* matches the choleric type, and a *kapha* person is reminiscent of the phlegmatic. Food, drink, sensual gratification, light, fresh air, and spiritual activities are used to "feed" the digestive fire and produce the correct mix of humors.

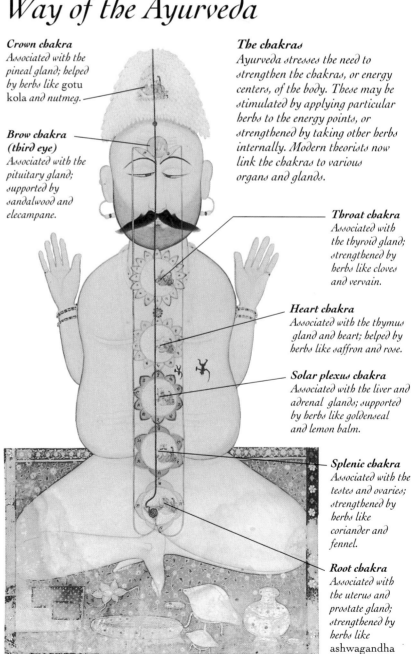

Crown chakra
Associated with the pineal gland; helped by herbs like gotu kola *and* nutmeg.

Brow chakra (third eye)
Associated with the pituitary gland; supported by sandalwood *and* elecampane.

The chakras
Ayurveda stresses the need to strengthen the chakras, or energy centers, of the body. These may be stimulated by applying particular herbs to the energy points, or strengthened by taking other herbs internally. Modern theorists now link the chakras to various organs and glands.

Throat chakra
Associated with the thyroid gland; strengthened by herbs like cloves and vervain.

Heart chakra
Associated with the thymus gland and heart; helped by herbs like saffron and rose.

Solar plexus chakra
Associated with the liver and adrenal glands; supported by herbs like goldenseal and lemon balm.

Splenic chakra
Associated with the testes and ovaries; strengthened by herbs like coriander and fennel.

Root chakra
Associated with the uterus and prostate gland; strengthened by herbs like ashwagandha *or* haritaki.

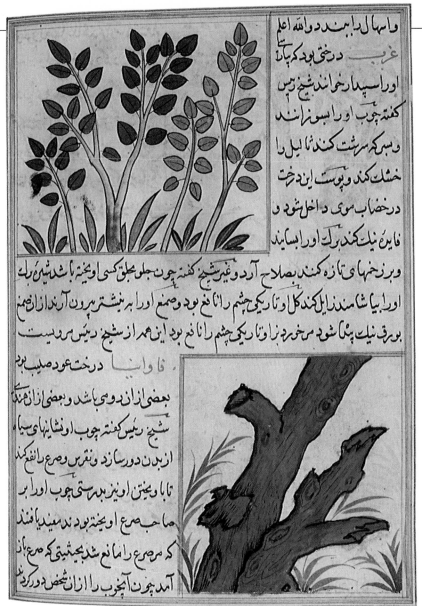

Indian herbal
In Mogul India, Ayurvedic traditions were less valued than Greek or Arab ideas. This herbal is written in Persian.

such as *gotu kola*, *gugguli*, or myrrh, all designed to dry excess water or phlegm. In Ayurvedic theory, taste is important: pungent, bitter, and astringent tastes can help reduce *kapha*, so the diet would favor these over sweet, salty, or sour flavors. Treatment might also include massage with warm herbal oils, such as eucalyptus; burning pungent incense, such as frankincense; and encouraging the sufferer to wear bright, hot reds and yellows, instead of cold blues or white.

OTHER PRINCIPLES

Ayurvedic medicine emphasizes a "holistic" approach, treating the whole person with appropriate remedies for the mind, body, and spirit. This can include meditation, physical exercises, or herbs that are focused at some particular aspect of being. Problems of the heart, for example, are considered as much a spiritual issue as pathology since the heart is the seat of the *atman* or divine self. Suitable herbs might include *arjuna*, used as a heart tonic, with sandalwood oil as a sedating massage oil to calm and uplift the spirits and encourage joy.

The essential energy of the body (*ojas*, like the Chinese *qi*) can be strengthened with tonic herbs, such as *ashwagandha*, *shatavari*, or *guduchi*. Like the Chinese *wei qi*, *ojas* is associated with the immune system, and herbs to strengthen it tend to be immunostimulants.

A health problem associated with excess phlegm, such as mucus, edema, or water retention, for example, would be treated with warm, light, dry foods, fasting, and avoiding cold drinks that would increase *kapha*. Herbal remedies might include hot spices, such as cayenne, *pippali*, and cinnamon; bitters, such as aloe or turmeric; pungent tonics, such as saffron; and stimulating, mind-clearing herbs,

Tibetan Herbalism

RITUAL & RELIGION

Before the Chinese invasion of 1959, medicine in Tibet was largely under the control of the lamas and closely linked with religion. Medical students memorized four complex "tantras," which explained the cause and progression of disease with the aid of "illustrated trees of medicine." Physicians used meditation and mantras to "energize" the medicine and increase its efficacy, and harvesting of herbs was also carefully timed to use any helpful astrological influences.

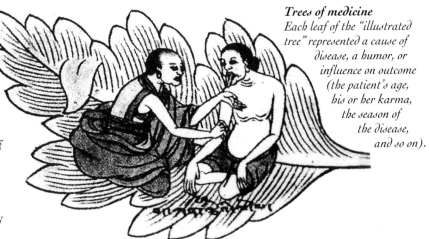

Trees of medicine
Each leaf of the "illustrated tree" represented a cause of disease, a humor, or influence on outcome (the patient's age, his or her karma, the season of the disease, and so on).

CHINESE HERBAL MEDICINE

TRADITIONAL CHINESE MEDICINE is an ancient system of healing that can be traced back to about 2500 B.C. The texts produced at that time are still studied and followed by practitioners, and while much has been added to the basic philosophy, very little has been taken out. In Chinese medicine, illness is seen as a sign of disharmony within the whole person, so the task of the traditional Chinese practitioner is always to restore harmony and balance, thus enabling the body's natural healing mechanisms to work more efficiently. Herbs are central to treatment, aided by other therapies, such as acupuncture or specialist massage. In the past few years, Chinese herbal traditions have become more familiar in the West and are now used by many qualified practitioners.

The Principles of Chinese Medicine

THE THEORY OF ELEMENTS
As with early Greek philosophy, the Chinese tradition is based on a theory of elements (in this model five, rather than the Greek four), which is used to explain every interaction between people and their environment. These elements, namely, wood, fire, earth, metal, and water, are seen to be related, with wood encouraging fire, fire resolving to earth, earth yielding up metal, metal producing water (seen as condensation on a cold metal surface), and water giving birth to wood by encouraging the growth of vegetation.

Each element has a number of associations, ranging from emotions and parts of the body to human sounds, the seasons, colors and tastes, all underpinned by a simple logic. Wood, for example, relates to spring and the color green; fire to summer; and water to the kidneys. For good health to prevail, the elements need to be in harmony; if one element becomes too dominant, illness may result.

Chinese practitioners often look for the cause of illness in a related element: weakness in the liver (wood), for example, may be due to deficiencies in the kidneys (water). A weak stomach (earth) might be caused by overexuberant wood (liver) failing to be controlled by deficient metal (lungs).

The five elements
The elements form a network of relationships: the red arrows in the diagram show how one element gives rise to another; the gray arrows indicate how one element controls another. Herbs can be linked to the model in various ways. The taste of the herb, for example, can suggest the bodily organ that the plant might influence.

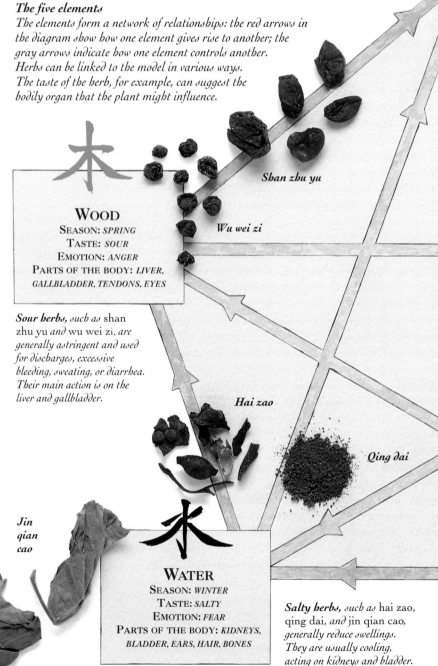

Shan zhu yu

WOOD
SEASON: *SPRING*
TASTE: *SOUR*
EMOTION: *ANGER*
PARTS OF THE BODY: *LIVER, GALLBLADDER, TENDONS, EYES*

Wu wei zi

Qing dai

Sour herbs, such as shan zhu yu *and* wu wei zi, *are generally astringent and used for discharges, excessive bleeding, sweating, or diarrhea. Their main action is on the liver and gallbladder.*

Hai zao

Jin qian cao

WATER
SEASON: *WINTER*
TASTE: *SALTY*
EMOTION: *FEAR*
PARTS OF THE BODY: *KIDNEYS, BLADDER, EARS, HAIR, BONES*

Salty herbs, such as hai zao, qing dai, *and* jin qian cao, *generally reduce swellings. They are usually cooling, acting on kidneys and bladder.*

YIN, YANG, & QI

Complementing the basic model of the five elements is the Chinese theory of opposites – *yin* and *yang*. According to this, everything in the cosmos both contains and is balanced by its own polar opposite. *Yin* is seen as female, dark and cold, while *yang* is characterized as male, light and hot.

In traditional Chinese medicine, *yin* and *yang* need to be in balance to maintain health, and many ills can be attributed to a deficiency or excess of either factor.

Different parts of the body are also described as predominantly *yin* or *yang*: body fluids and blood are mainly *yin*, for example, while *qi*, the vital energy, tends to be *yang*. *Qi* is regarded as flowing in a network of channels, or meridians, through the body and can be stimulated using acupuncture.

ANCIENT CHINESE MEDICINE

The origins of Chinese herbalism are shrouded in myth. There are legendary figures, such as Shen Nung, the "divine cultivator," who "invented" agriculture and identified many medicinal plants. Shen Nung was said to have "tasted the flavor of hundreds of herbs and drank the water from many springs and wells so that people might know which were sweet and which were bitter." He supposedly discovered tea drinking, too, when some leaves fell from a tea bush into a bowl of water boiling nearby. An important Chinese herbal from about 200 B.C. is named after Shen Nung.

The founding father of Chinese medical theory is the Yellow Emperor, who is reputed to have lived around 2500 B.C. However, the classic text that bears his name, the *Huang Ti Nei Ching Su Wên* or *Yellow Emperor's Canon of Internal Medicine*, is generally dated to about 1000 B.C. It could well represent an older verbal tradition. As in the West, medicine at that time was inseparable from philosophy and religion, and the *Nei Ching* is an important Taoist text, rich in spiritual wisdom.

Historically, there were many different medical philosophies and techniques in China, with a mix of itinerant physicians, village herbalists, or native shamans. There were also the Taoist philosopher-doctors, who produced the classic medical texts and who would have been the first choice, in sickness, for the aristocracy.

MODERN CHINESE MEDICINE

By the 19th century, Western mission hospitals had begun to represent a real alternative to the old practices. Chinese medicine survived but became a national, standard medical system only in the 1960s when Mao Tse-tung founded five colleges of traditional Chinese medicine.

Today, older regional healing styles persist among traditional Korean, Vietnamese, and Japanese practitioners; classic styles are also followed by surviving Chinese medical families, many of whom have emigrated to Hong Kong, Singapore, and San Francisco.

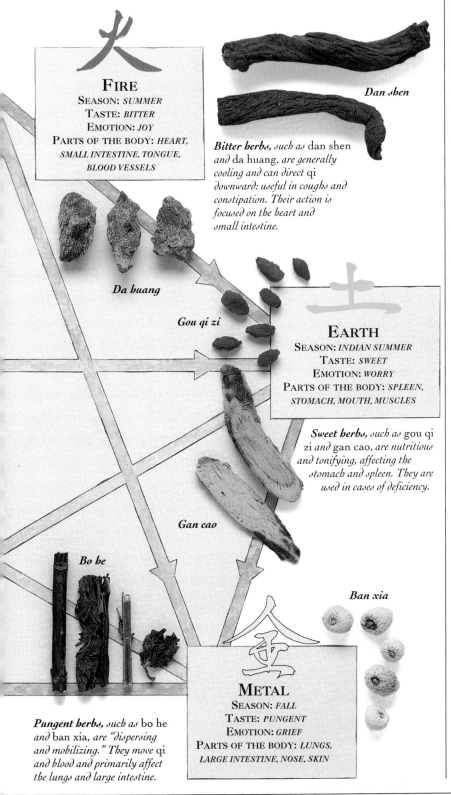

FIRE
SEASON: *SUMMER*
TASTE: *BITTER*
EMOTION: *JOY*
PARTS OF THE BODY: *HEART, SMALL INTESTINE, TONGUE, BLOOD VESSELS*

Dan shen

Bitter herbs, such as dan shen and da huang, are generally cooling and can direct qi downward: useful in coughs and constipation. Their action is focused on the heart and small intestine.

Da huang

Gou qi zi

EARTH
SEASON: *INDIAN SUMMER*
TASTE: *SWEET*
EMOTION: *WORRY*
PARTS OF THE BODY: *SPLEEN, STOMACH, MOUTH, MUSCLES*

Sweet herbs, such as gou qi zi and gan cao, are nutritious and tonifying, affecting the stomach and spleen. They are used in cases of deficiency.

Gan cao

Bo he

Ban xia

METAL
SEASON: *FALL*
TASTE: *PUNGENT*
EMOTION: *GRIEF*
PARTS OF THE BODY: *LUNGS, LARGE INTESTINE, NOSE, SKIN*

Pungent herbs, such as bo he and ban xia, are "dispersing and mobilizing." They move qi and blood and primarily affect the lungs and large intestine.

The Practice of Chinese Medicine

HEATING VERSUS COOLING

Chinese medicine also identifies five tastes that can be characterized as hot or cold: pungent and sweet tastes are both deemed to be heating, while sour, bitter, and salty tastes are more cooling. Some herbs combine several different flavors: the name *wu wei zi* (schisandra berries) literally means "five-taste fruit."

These characteristics also influence which part of the body the herb will affect. Hot things rise or float, for example, so pungent and sweet herbs tend to affect the upper and exterior parts of the body. Cold things sink, so the sour, bitter, and salty herbs are more effective for the lower half or interior of the body. In the treatment of arthritis, for example, the Chinese will often add *qiang huo* to the mixture if the pain is in the shoulders or arms, while *du huo* is preferred if hips or knees are affected. Both of these herbs would be used if the entire body were affected.

Pungent tastes are also stimulating, sour ones cause contraction, sweet are tonifying, bitter are used to send *qi* downward, while salty tastes are softening.

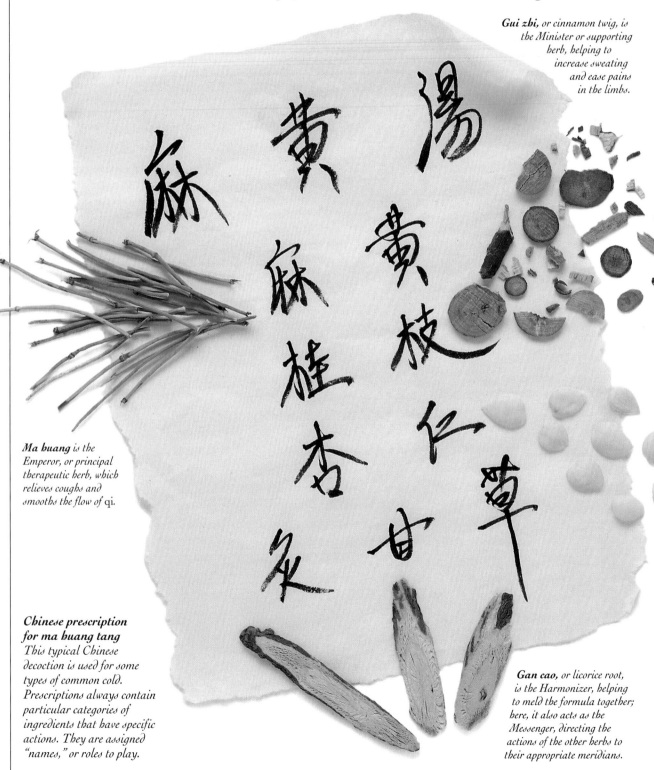

Gui zhi, or cinnamon twig, is the Minister or supporting herb, helping to increase sweating and ease pains in the limbs.

Ma huang is the Emperor, or principal therapeutic herb, which relieves coughs and smooths the flow of qi.

Chinese prescription for ma huang tang
This typical Chinese decoction is used for some types of common cold. Prescriptions always contain particular categories of ingredients that have specific actions. They are assigned "names," or roles to play.

Gan cao, or licorice root, is the Harmonizer, helping to meld the formula together; here, it also acts as the Messenger, directing the actions of the other herbs to their appropriate meridians.

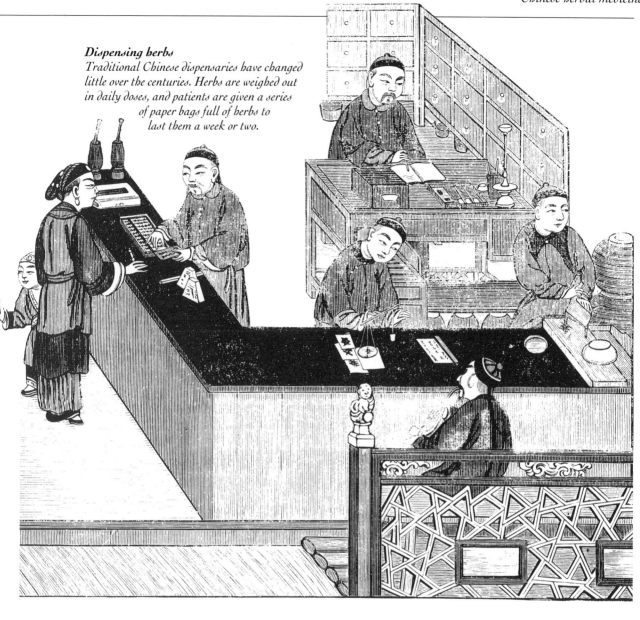

Dispensing herbs
Traditional Chinese dispensaries have changed little over the centuries. Herbs are weighed out in daily doses, and patients are given a series of paper bags full of herbs to last them a week or two.

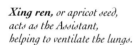

Xing ren, *or apricot seed, acts as the Assistant, helping to ventilate the lungs.*

HOW HERBS ARE PRESCRIBED

The Chinese usually prescribe herbs in standard formulas (there are several thousand in regular use), and these may be adjusted slightly depending on the specific condition affecting the patient. The formulas might include just two herbs or as many as twenty, and the interaction between the different plants is just as significant as their individual properties. The result is often a potent brew that can have a dramatic, therapeutic effect, but generally defies any rational scientific explanation.

Herbs are generally given as pills, powders, or, most commonly, in the form of decoctions, or "soups," which patients brew up at home for an hour or so in special earthenware crocks kept for the purpose. Sometimes the herbs may be cooked with rice to produce a cereal-like therapeutic meal.

HERBS IN HERBALS

In traditional Chinese herbals, the characteristics of a plant always include taste, dominant temperature, and generally an indication of the organ and meridians that it affects. These are sometimes obviously related: Chinese gold thread (*huang lian*), for example, is a very bitter herb; it is cold and linked to the heart – characteristics that can be traced directly to the five-element model. It may be used in conditions associated with too much heat in the heart, which in traditional Chinese medicine would lead to insomnia, palpitations, and hot flashes.

Bai shao yao is sour and widely used for liver problems – both of which are aspects of the element wood – while many nutritious herbs, such as rice or oats, and major tonics, such as ginseng, are characterized as sweet and are good for the stomach and spleen.

OUT OF THE DARK AGES

AFTER THE FALL OF ROME, European herbal traditions were not completely submerged by the ensuing Dark Ages. The "barbarians" brought with them their own herbal healing customs to add to the Roman practices that survived and, with the spread of Christianity, there was considerable exchange of both actual medicines and tried-and-tested remedies. Throughout the Middle Ages, the Church played a significant role both in cultivating "physic gardens" and in introducing new herbs. With the advent of the printing press, Classical knowledge spread from the confines of the cloister to complement the folk medicine and household herbal remedies passed through the generations.

The Growth of European Herbalism

ANGLO-SAXON HERBALS
Europe's oldest surviving herbal written in the vernacular, *The Leech Book of Bald*, dates from the first half of the 10th century and includes remedies sent by the Patriarch of Jerusalem to King Alfred. Numerous treatments are described for ailments caused by "flying venom" and "elfshot," thought to be responsible for a wide range of sudden or wasting illnesses. Among the most popular herbs in Saxon times were wood betony, vervain, mugwort, plantain, and yarrow, taken in many internal remedies but more often worn as amulets to ward off the evil eye.

Although medical schools spread through Europe (the most famous, at Salerno, was founded in the early 10th century and taught the Hippocratic principles of good diet, exercise, and fresh air), healing and herbalism were largely in the hands of the Church, with all monasteries growing medicinal herbs and tending the sick as part of Christian duty. Healing was as much a matter of prayer as medicine, and early herbals frequently combine religious incantations with infusions, concluding that with "God's help" the patient would be cured.

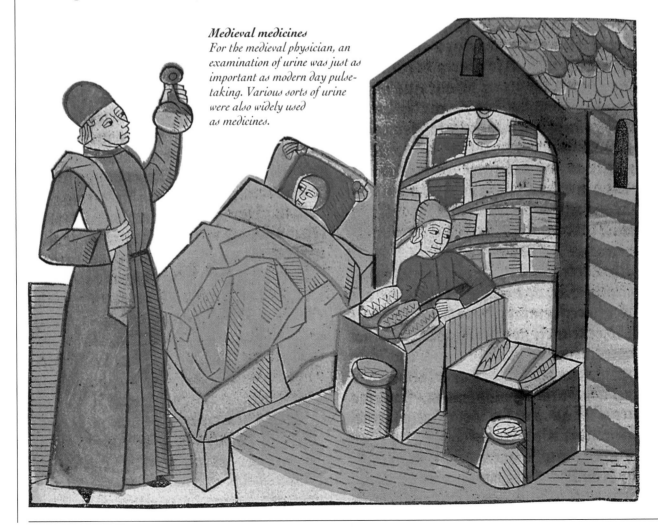

Medieval medicines
For the medieval physician, an examination of urine was just as important as modern day pulse-taking. Various sorts of urine were also widely used as medicines.

PARACELSUS

As learning moved away from the cloister, emphasis was gradually again given to the healing skills and disciplines once taught at the Salerno school. By the 1530s, Paracelsus (born Philippus Theophrastus Bombastus von Hohenheim, near Zürich in 1493) was revolutionizing European attitudes toward health care. As much an alchemist as a physician, he insisted on lecturing in German instead of the usual Latin. He regarded most apothecaries and physicians as crooked conspirators intent upon milking the public. Condemning the complex and often lethal purgatives and emetics they prescribed, he urged a return to simpler medicines inspired by the Doctrine of Signatures.

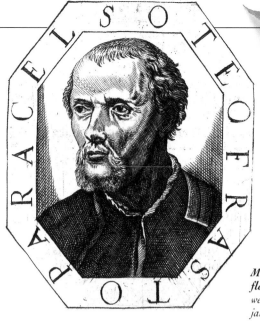

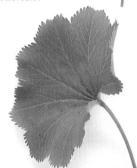

The leaves of lungwort were said to resemble diseased lungs, so the plant was used for bronchitis and tuberculosis.

Doctrine of Signatures
Paracelsus was a supporter of the Doctrine of Signatures, which maintained that the outward appearance of a plant gave an indication of the ailments it would cure. At times the theory was surprisingly accurate. Similar theories still prevail in Africa.

Many yellow-flowered plants were linked with jaundice, so toadflax, greater celandine, and dandelion were used for liver disorders.

The tiny oil sacs in St. John's wort leaves look like holes, while extracts from the plant are blood-red: signs that it will be good for wounds.

Nutmeg and walnuts were compared to the brain and thought helpful for strengthening mental activity.

The round leaves of lady's mantle were compared to the cervix.

Illustrated Herbals

HERBAL WARFARE

Paracelsus was followed by physicians such as William Turner, who wrote in English so that "the apothecaries and old wives that gather herbs" would understand which plants physicians really meant by their Latin prescriptions and would not put "many a good man by ignorance in jeopardy of his life." Nicholas Culpeper (1616-1654) was later to adopt a similar view, earning the wrath of the newly formed College of Physicians by translating their *Pharmacopeia* into English so that ordinary people could find herbal medicines in the hedgerows instead of paying vastly inflated apothecaries' bills.

The battles between physicians, apothecaries, and "herb wives" raged through the 17th and 18th centuries as medicine came more and more under the control of the academic physicians, with their university training, while dispensing was strictly regulated by the apothecaries. The emphasis was on expensive and complex nostrums using ingredients such as the metals mercury and antimony.

REMEDIES FROM AFAR

By the time that the great herbals of Gerard (1597), Parkinson (1640), and Culpeper (1653) appeared, numerous new herbs were starting to be imported from the East Indies and North America. Plants such as yucca, nasturtium, and nutmeg began to appear in the herbals, often accompanied by imaginative applications and claims for their medicinal properties. Tea is a classic example: proclaimed as a cure-all in the 17th century, it is now regarded by many as no more than a popular drink.

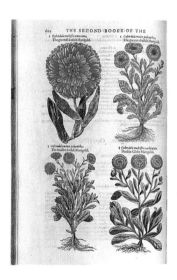

Medicinal marigolds
Gerard describes ten types of marigold, including the "double globe marigold." He recommended marigold conserve as a preventative "in time of plague."

NORTH AMERICAN TRADITIONS

THE FIRST EUROPEAN SETTLERS arriving in North America brought with them the familiar healing plants from home: heartsease and plantain, also known as "white man's foot" because it was soon found growing wherever the settlers penetrated. They also absorbed some Native American healing traditions, discovering new herbs, such as boneset, echinacea, goldenseal, and pleurisy root. Several of the American tribes also made great use of saunalike sweat houses, and the idea of heat as a healing technique was adopted by Samuel Thomson (see below). This melding of traditions bore fruit in the Physiomedical and Eclectic schools, which were later imported to Europe and had a lasting influence on European herbal practices.

Ritual Herbalism

MAGIC & MEDICINE

Native American herbalism was shamanistic – it centered on the activities of the medicine man, or shaman. Through the use of drums and rattles and the smoking of mixtures of tobacco or peyote, the shaman would enter a trancelike state that enabled him to "spirit-travel" and seek out the soul of the sick person in order to rescue and heal it. Today, shamans in South America still use extracts taken from a particular vine – known in Colombia as *yage* and in Peru and Ecuador as *ayahuasca* – in the same way Siberian shamans were once able to "travel" by taking fly agaric toadstool or European witches to "fly" with the help of deadly nightshade, henbane, thorn-apple, or mandrake.

The Native Americans also made ritual use of the medicine wheel and assigned animal totems to the four cardinal directions. They equated these with different personality types, spiritual energies, diseases, and plant medicine. Typically, for example, the South was symbolized by the coyote and the energies of growth and compassion, while the eagle and the powers of wisdom and enlightenment were symbols of the East.

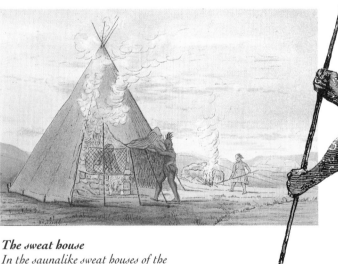

The sweat house
In the saunalike sweat houses of the Native Americans, the ill person was encouraged to perspire to rid the body of toxins and bacteria.

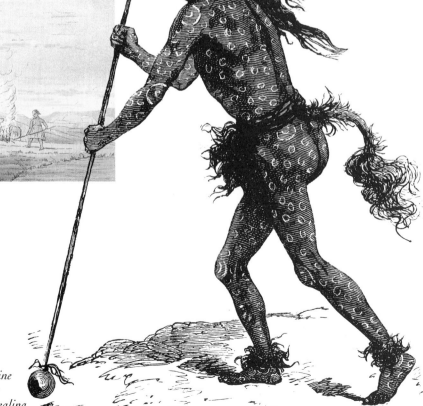

The shaman
The medicine man, or shaman, would "spirit-travel" in the symbolic directions of the medicine wheel to seek the soul of the sick person and find spirit help for healing.

Merging of Practices

PHYSIOMEDICALISM

Before land battles with the Plains tribes decimated the indigenous population, the early pioneers and Native Americans shared much of their herbal lore with each other. An early enthusiast was Samuel Thomson, who founded the Physiomedical movement. Born in New Hampshire in 1769, Thomson learned his craft as a child from Widow Benton, a "root and herb doctor" who combined Native American skills with the traditional role of "herb wife."

Thomson believed that parents were responsible for both their own and their children's health and patented "Thomson's Improved System of Botanic Practice of Medicine," a mixture of handbooks and patent remedies that swept America in the early 19th century. Thomson's principal theory was that "all disease is caused by cold," which in the bitter New England winters may well have been accurate. By the late 1830s, he claimed three million followers.

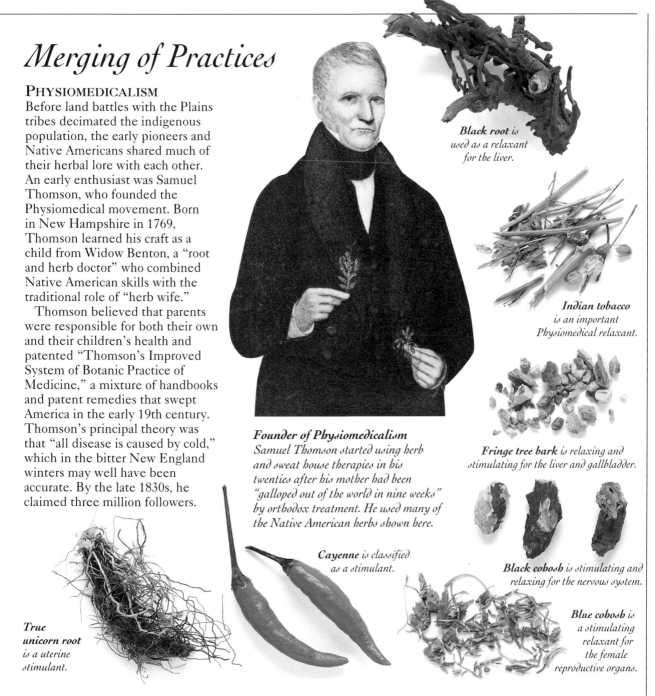

Black root *is used as a relaxant for the liver.*

Indian tobacco *is an important Physiomedical relaxant.*

Fringe tree bark *is relaxing and stimulating for the liver and gallbladder.*

Black cohosh *is stimulating and relaxing for the nervous system.*

Blue cohosh *is a stimulating relaxant for the female reproductive organs.*

Founder of Physiomedicalism
Samuel Thomson started using herb and sweat house therapies in his twenties after his mother had been "galloped out of the world in nine weeks" by orthodox treatment. He used many of the Native American herbs shown here.

Cayenne *is classified as a stimulant.*

True unicorn root *is a uterine stimulant.*

MAINTAINING BALANCE

Central to the Physiomedical view was the belief that it is possible to strengthen the body's "vital force" by keeping both tissues and nervous state in balance. The key therapeutic treatment involved relaxing or tightening tissues, and then stimulating or sedating nerves. Suitable herbs, classified as either stimulating or sedating, relaxing, or astringent, were used to achieve this balance. Irritable bowel syndrome, for example, might be treated with chamomile to sedate the nervous system and relax the digestive tissues, followed by an astringent, such as agrimony, and a stimulant, such as ginger, in order to encourage the vital force and internal energy levels.

ECLECTICISM

Other "botanic" systems followed, among them the Eclectic school founded by Dr. Wooster Beech in the 1830s. Like the Thomsonians, the Eclectics also used herbal remedies and Native American healing practices, but combined these with more orthodox medical techniques in their analysis of disease. At its peak, Eclecticism claimed more than 20,000 qualified practitioners in the United States and was a serious rival to regular medicine. The challenge ended only in 1907 when, following a review of medical training schools, philanthropists Andrew Carnegie and John D. Rockefeller decided to give financial support solely to the orthodox medical schools.

THE MOVEMENT IN EUROPE

Thomsonian Physiomedicalism was brought to Britain in 1838 by Dr. Albert Isaiah Coffin, who set up a similar "system" of patent remedies and do-it-yourself guides to diagnosis. Wooster Beech followed in the 1850s to preach his Eclectic message, and the movement took hold in working-class areas of the country, remaining popular, especially in the North, until well into the 1930s.

In 1864, the various groups merged to form the National Association of Medical Herbalists. The association continues to thrive today as the National Institute of Medical Herbalists – the oldest formalized body of specialist herbal practitioners in Europe.

FROM PLANTS TO PILLS

ALTHOUGH EXTRACTS, such as essential oils, have been prepared from various plants for centuries, traditional herbalism has always combined herbs to modify effects, viewing the whole as greater than the parts. The move to identify the individual active ingredients and use these as single drugs began in the 18th century, and many thousands are now known. These chemicals display quite different properties from the original herbs.

Initially, these drugs could only be obtained from plant extracts but later the chemical structures of many extracts were identified and the drugs are now made synthetically. In the transition from the use of crude plants to clinical pills, modern medicine has lost the art of combining herbs to modify toxicity and of using whole plants, which themselves contain chemical ingredients that can reduce the risk of side effects.

Herbs in Modern Medicine

THE FOXGLOVE CURE

According to tradition, a physician, William Withering, persistently failed to bring about an improvement in a patient suffering from severe dropsy caused by heart failure. Suddenly, the patient started to recover. His relatives admitted administering an herbal brew based on an old family recipe and, in 1775, Dr. Withering began experimenting with the various herbs it contained, identifying foxglove as the most significant. In 1785, he published his *Account of the Foxglove and Some of Its Medical Uses.* This detailed 200 cases of dropsy and heart failure that he had successfully treated with the herb, along with research notes on the parts of the plant producing the strongest effects and when to harvest it to achieve these effects.

Withering also realized that the therapeutic dose of foxglove is very close to the quantity at which toxic side effects develop, so great care was needed in its administration. Further analysis followed, and the cardiac glycosides digoxin and digitoxin were eventually extracted. They are still used in treating heart conditions today.

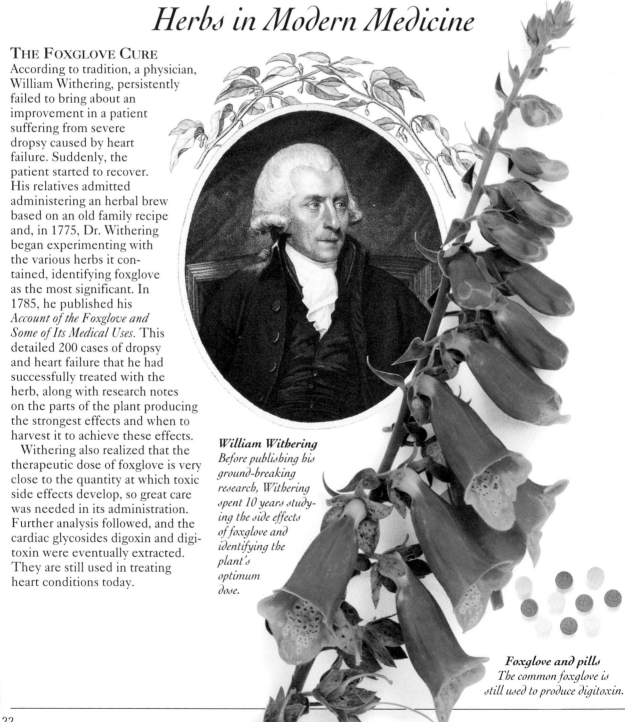

William Withering
Before publishing his ground-breaking research, Withering spent 10 years studying the side effects of foxglove and identifying the plant's optimum dose.

Foxglove and pills
The common foxglove is still used to produce digitoxin.

DRUGS FROM PLANTS

One of the first modern drugs to be isolated from a plant was morphine, first identified in 1803 by Friedrich Serturner in Germany. He extracted white crystals from crude opium poppy. Similar techniques soon produced aconitine from monkshood, emetine from ipecacuanha, atropine from deadly nightshade, and quinine from Peruvian bark. All of these compounds, categorized as alkaloids, are extremely potent and could only be obtained from the raw plants until scientists were able to synthesize them.

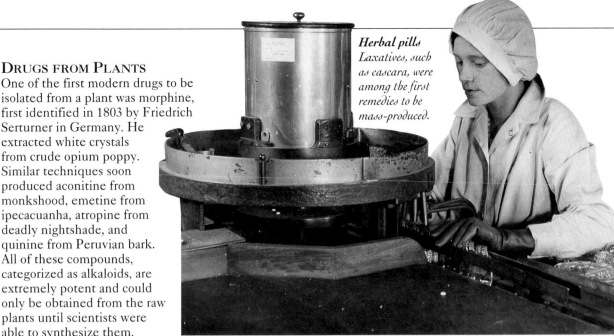

Herbal pills
Laxatives, such as cascara, were among the first remedies to be mass-produced.

SYNTHESIZED SUBSTANCES

The breakthrough came in 1852 when salicin, identified as one of the active ingredients in willow bark, was artificially synthesized for the first time. This was later modified to be less of an irritant on the stomach, and acetylsalicylic acid was launched as aspirin, in 1899, by the drug company Bayer.

In less than 100 years, plant extracts have filled pharmacists' shelves. There are many ephedrine preparations from *ma huang*, for example, both prescription and over-the-counter, which are mainly used for coughs, phlegm, hay fever, or asthma. Pilocarpine, obtained from jaborandi, is used for treating glaucoma; vincristine, from the Madagascar periwinkle, is used for leukemia; while strophanthin from *Strophanthus kombé* (found in tropical Africa and used to tip poison arrows) is taken for severe heart problems.

CHEMICAL POWER

Extracted chemicals can often be extremely potent and can cause effects that were unknown when the whole plant was used. Indian snakeroot, *Rauwolfia serpentina*, for example, has been used for centuries in Ayurvedic medicine for a range of ailments including snakebites, anxiety, headaches, fevers, and abdominal pains. Mahatma Gandhi reputedly drank snakeroot tea at night if he felt overstimulated. In the West, snakeroot was valued as a potent tranquilizer and was used for high blood pressure; it was also prescribed in the treatment of schizophrenia and psychosis.

In 1947, CIBA extracted the alkaloid reserpine from snakeroot and began marketing the drug Serpasil as a cure for hypertension. However, resperine has unfortunate side effects that include severe depression and abnormal slowing of the heartbeat. A new tranquilizer drug was developed from the herb in the 1950s. It has always been restricted to the status of prescription-only in the United States. To this day, however, snakeroot continues to be widely used in other parts of Europe and Asia, taken by many as a soothing tranquilizer.

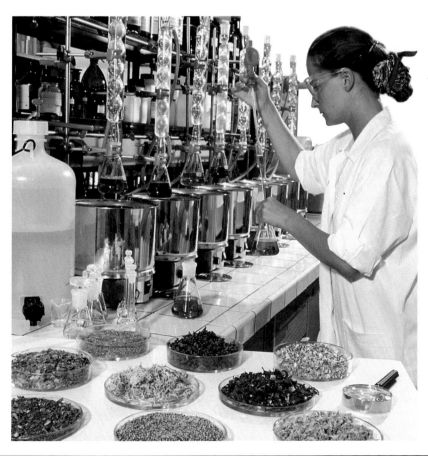

High-tech herbalism
In mainland Europe, herbal remedies are widely used in conventional medicine. Production is as streamlined and clinical as in any modern pharmaceutical plant.

MEDICINAL MEALS

TODAY'S CATEGORIZATION OF PLANTS as herbs, vegetables, fruits, and even "weeds" is a recent invention. To the 17th-century cook, cabbage, carrots, and cucumbers were all "kitchen herbs" just as marigolds or marjoram were. We often forget, too, that the active constituents, such as alkaloids or saponins, in "herbs" are not confined to the plants we label as such; fruits and vegetables can also be both therapeutic or, in excess, damaging. Past cultures have classified foods by temperature or taste, matched to the body's needs to maintain balance: Hippocrates noted that fresh foods "give more strength" because they are more alive, while Tibetan medicine regards frozen foods as colder and more mucus-forming than their fresh originals.

Galenical Menu-making

"One good old fashion is not yet left off, viz to boil fennel with fish: for it consumes that phlegmatic humor which fish most plentifully afford and annoy the body with, though few that use it know wherefore they do it."
Nicholas Culpeper, 1653.

Classifications of foods
Hippocrates first classified foods into hot, cold, dry, or damp categories in about 420 B.C. (Some examples are shown below.) Galen and others later expanded these ideas into a complex classification in which many foods were considered to belong to more than one category: apples, for example, were both cold and damp.

THERAPEUTIC FOODS
Galen and his followers labeled not only what we term "herbs" as hot or cold, dry or damp, but "foods" as well. In the Galenical system, meat tended to be heating, fish was damp, fresh beans and apples cold and moist, wheat generally hot, and moist, and so on.

Food intake was considered to have a direct action on the four humors: blood, phlegm, yellow bile, and black bile. For example, eating too many cold, moist foods would encourage the phlegmatic humor, and this could lead to mucus. Too many hot, dry foods, on the other hand, encouraged the choleric humor (yellow bile), with resulting liver or skin problems.

The medieval housewife would automatically balance the character of different ingredients, cooking fish with "hot and dry" fennel, or adding pepper to "cold and moist" beans, and she would have been quite appalled at the thought of serving strawberries in the middle of winter, as we are able to do now: this cold fruit would inevitably lead to stomach chills if eaten at such a time. Today we have lost sight of this sense of balance, eating foods regardless of climate.

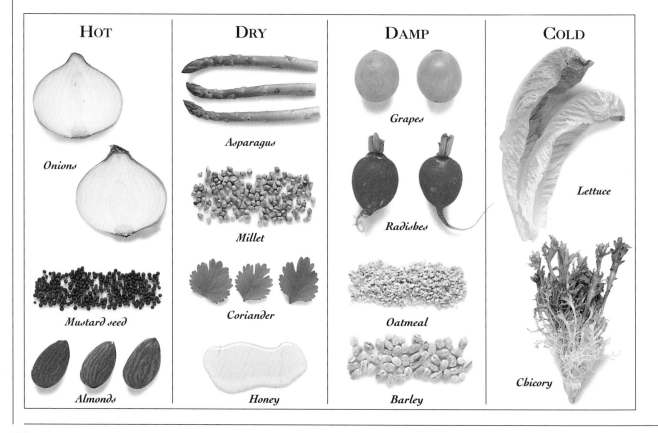

HOT	DRY	DAMP	COLD
Onions	Asparagus	Grapes	Lettuce
Mustard seed	Millet	Radishes	Chicory
Almonds	Coriander	Oatmeal	
	Honey	Barley	

The Taste of Health

"From food are born all creatures, which live upon food and after death return to food. Food is the chief of all things. It is therefore said to be the medicine of all diseases of the body."
The Upanishads, c. 500 B.C.

The six tastes
In Ayurveda, all foods and herbs can be classified in terms of the six tastes. Selected examples for each of the categories are shown below.

BALANCING TASTES
In Ayurvedic medicine, taste is all-important and different foods can be categorized according to the six defined tastes. These are believed to act on the body to increase or decrease the three humors: *kapha* (water or phlegm), *pitta* (fire or bile), and *vata* (air or wind).

The humors are regarded as the waste products of digestion – consequently, if food intake is too heavily biased toward one or another of the humors, imbalance and illness can follow. A healthful diet has to contain a good mixture of the six tastes, while in ill health, particular tastes can be emphasized to restore balance. The correct combination of tastes is also considered so essential for growth and normal development that special herbal pills containing all six tastes are regularly given to children.

SWEET

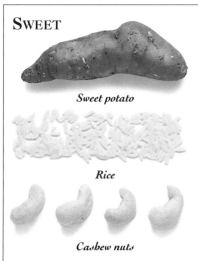

Sweet potato

Rice

Cashew nuts

Sweet, or madhura, *tastes increase body secretions, particularly milk or semen, and reduce pitta-related problems, such as toxins. Sweet tastes should be avoided where there is an excess of* kapha, *such as in colds, chills, and some rheumatic complaints.*

SOUR

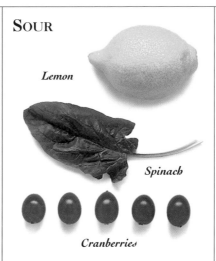

Lemon

Spinach

Cranberries

Sour, or amla, *tastes reduce vata, while increasing kapha and pitta. Such foods stimulate the digestion and are often used for debility. An excess leads to muscle weakness and illnesses related to excess pitta, such as ulcers and liver disorders.*

SALTY

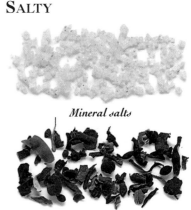

Mineral salts

Seaweed

Salty, or lavana, *tastes increase pitta and kapha. They help to retain fluids and clean the body's ducts by attracting water and thus loosening toxins. Salty foods are used as expectorants. Excess can lead to premature aging, impotence, or skin problems.*

PUNGENT

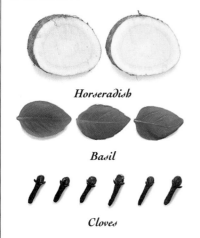

Horseradish

Basil

Cloves

Pungent, or katu, *tastes increase vata and pitta and reduce kapha. Such foods, stimulating and warming, are used for chills, lethargy, or depression; they can also remedy obesity. An excess can lead to burning sensations, thirst, and nervous exhaustion.*

BITTER

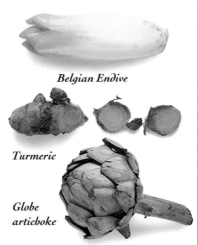

Belgian Endive

Turmeric

Globe artichoke

The bitter, or tikta, *taste is composed of the elements air and ether, so increases vata, while reducing pitta and kapha. Such bitter foods stimulate the digestion to absorb phlegm and can also cleanse "fire toxins" from the body, which is useful for fevers or skin disease.*

ASTRINGENT

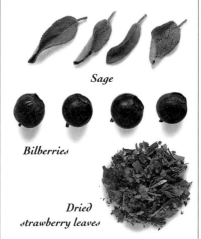

Sage

Bilberries

Dried strawberry leaves

Astringent, or kasaya, *tastes are light, cold and drying, increasing vata but reducing pitta and kapha. Astringent remedies are used for diarrhea or heavy menstruation. Too many astringent foods are overdrying, leading to constipation or stiff joints.*

Balancing Yin and Yang

"To take medicine only when you are sick is like digging a well only when you are thirsty – is it not already too late?"
Ch'i Po, c. 2500 B.C.

HARMONIZING ENERGIES

A balanced diet in Chinese terms is not necessarily one with the right amounts of proteins, vitamins, fats, or sugars, but one that balances the body's energies and ensures that the correct relationship between *yin* and *yang* is maintained.

Foods are classified according to the five-element model (see pp. 14-15), with five flavors – sweet, pungent, sour, bitter, and salty – and five temperatures – hot, cold, warm, cool, and neutral. Many foods are also related to particular organs and acupuncture meridians just as Chinese herbs are. Cool, bitter, and salty foods are more *yin*

in character, while hot, sweet, and pungent foods are more *yang*. Most fruits, for example, are considered very *yin* in character, similar to the "cold and damp" classification in Galenical medicine.

In a hot, dry climate, *yin* can be adversely affected, so eating an adequate quantity of fruit is one way of feeding this type of energy. The tourist from the cold north who heads for the tropics in the depths of winter is a fairly *yin* individual to start with since he or she comes from a cold, damp climate. In the unfamiliar tropical temperatures, such a person may be tempted to "cool off" by eating too many mangoes, papayas, melons, and pomelos, which pushes *yin* energies into excess and results in the cold-moist type of diarrhea that mars so many vacations.

Just as in the Galenical or the Ayurvedic systems, the Chinese may categorize people according to their physical constitution – those who are predominantly hot or cold, dry or damp. For example, a "hot" person, who opens windows and walks around in a T-shirt on a cold autumn day, may be thirsty and prone to boils, acne, hot flashes, or constipation; he or she should eat more cold, bitter foods (such as celery) and avoid pungent foods (such as onions) that tend to be more heating and drying.

The temperature of foods
The Chinese assign foods to the five temperatures, or energies. Hot foods, for example, encourage heat so, while suitable for "cold" individuals, could be contraindicated for those who tend to be "hot" by nature.

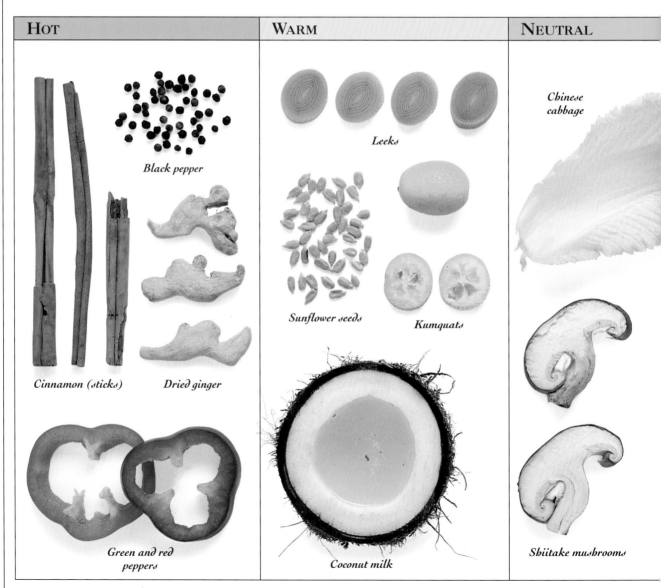

HOT	WARM	NEUTRAL
Black pepper	*Leeks*	*Chinese cabbage*
Cinnamon (sticks) *Dried ginger*	*Sunflower seeds* *Kumquats*	
Green and red peppers	*Coconut milk*	*Shiitake mushrooms*

EATING FOR HEALTH

The idea of hot and cold foods still persists in the traditional cuisine of China, and therapeutic restaurants, where diners are able to select dishes to balance their own particular energy needs, are found throughout the Far East. The emphasis is upon eating particular food types to maintain balance and prevent disease. Foods are not intrinsically "good" or "bad": what matters is how they affect each individual.

In the West, many fashionable "diets" run a great risk of imbalance as the faddists eliminate entire categories of food from their diet, weakening particular aspects of their vital energies and essence. Too little meat, for example, can weaken *yang* energies, while too much can put *yin* under pressure.

Coffee

Bitter *Associated with the heart; cool and drying; used to reduce fevers and dry excess body fluids.*

Lemon

Date

The five tastes
These are linked to the five-element model. Salt, for example, is associated with the kidneys, water, and coldness. Excess increases dampness, while a deficiency leads to dryness and hardening of the tissues. Many foods have more than one taste.

Sour *Associated with the liver; thought to obstruct movement; taken for diarrhea or excessive sweating.*

Sweet *Associated with the stomach; encourages weight gain; slows down and eases acute symptoms.*

Rock salt

Garlic

Salty *Considered stimulant; used to soften hard swellings, such as enlarged lymph nodes or hardened muscles.*

Pungent *Associated with the lungs and skin; used to encourage the circulation of qi (energy) and to increase sweating.*

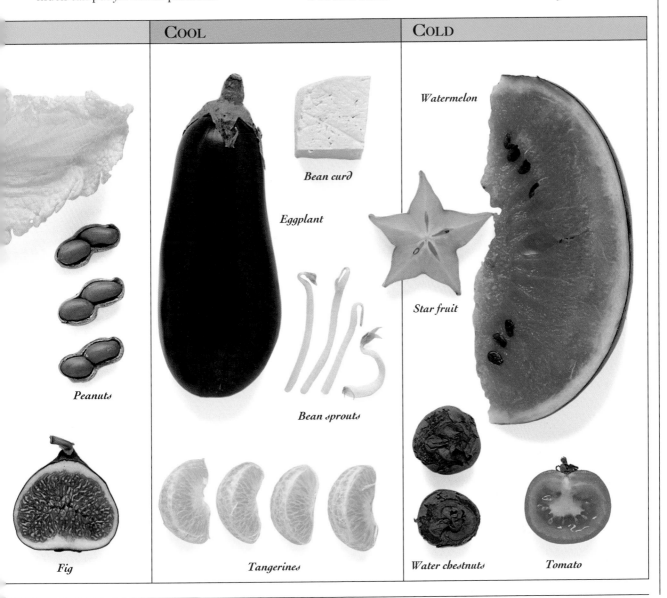

COOL	COLD

Bean curd

Eggplant

Watermelon

Star fruit

Peanuts

Bean sprouts

Fig

Tangerines

Water chestnuts

Tomato

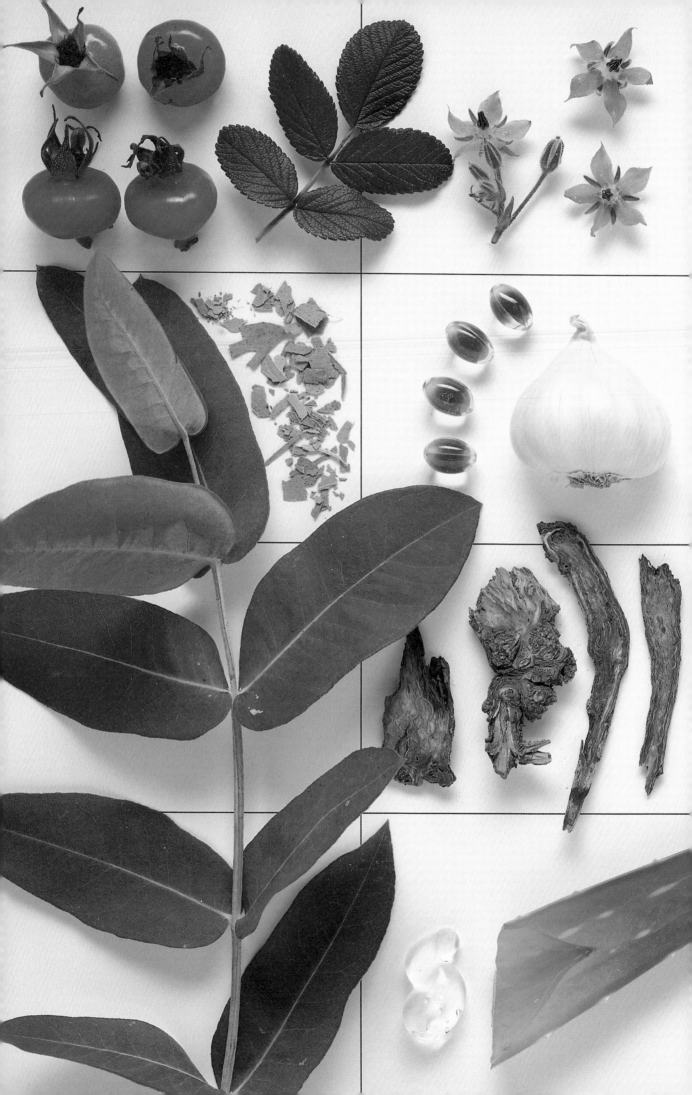

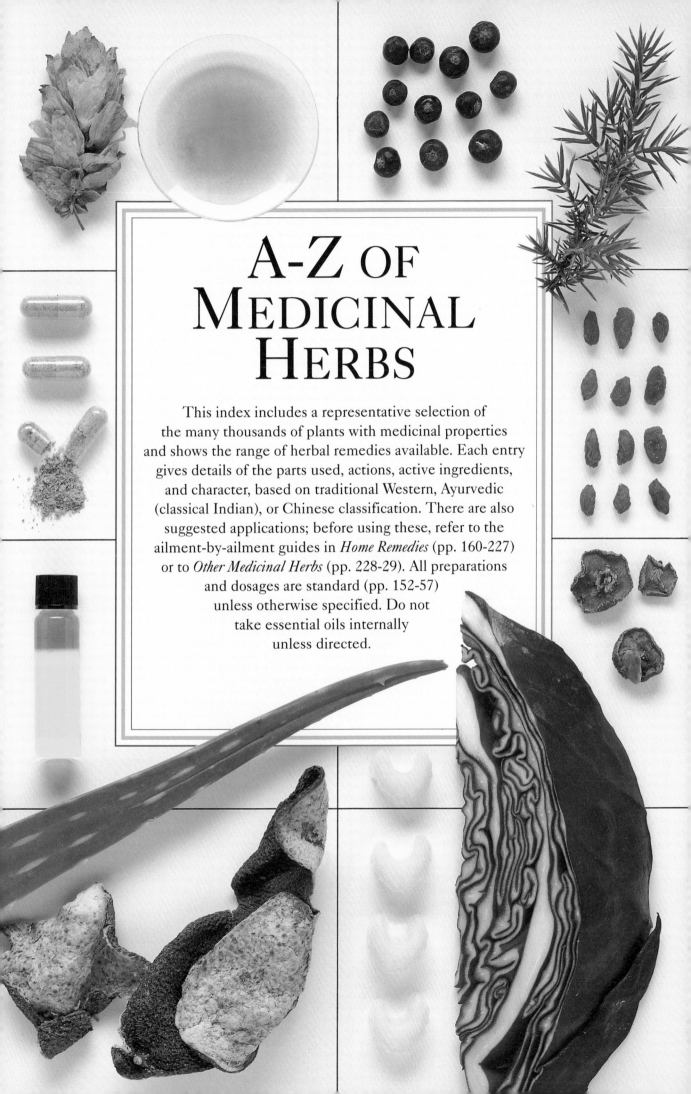

A-Z OF MEDICINAL HERBS

This index includes a representative selection of the many thousands of plants with medicinal properties and shows the range of herbal remedies available. Each entry gives details of the parts used, actions, active ingredients, and character, based on traditional Western, Ayurvedic (classical Indian), or Chinese classification. There are also suggested applications; before using these, refer to the ailment-by-ailment guides in *Home Remedies* (pp. 160-227) or to *Other Medicinal Herbs* (pp. 228-29). All preparations and dosages are standard (pp. 152-57) unless otherwise specified. Do not take essential oils internally unless directed.

Achillea millefolium
YARROW

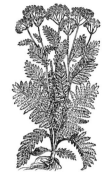

"Most men say, that the leaves chewed, and especially greene, are a remedie for toothach."
John Gerard, 1597.

THE PLANT'S LATIN NAME is derived from the Greek hero Achilles, and during the Trojan wars, yarrow was reputedly used to treat wounds. A folk name, "nosebleed," confirms its traditional first aid use as an emergency styptic to stop bleeding. Today, yarrow is valued mainly for its action in colds and influenza, and also for its effect on the circulatory, digestive, and urinary systems. The plant can usually be found growing in meadows.

Character
Cool, dry; sweet, astringent, slightly bitter taste.
Constituents
Volatile oil (inc. proazulenes), isovalerianic acid, salicylic acid, asparagin, sterols, flavonoids, bitters, tannins, coumarins.
Actions
Aerial parts: astringent, promote sweating, relax peripheral blood vessels, digestive stimulant, restorative for menstrual system, febrifuge.
Essential oil: anti-inflammatory, antiallergenic, antispasmodic.

Parts used

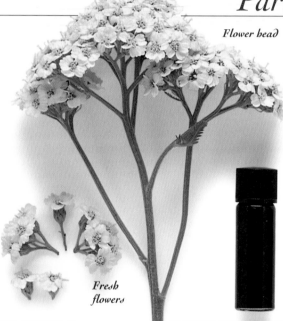

Flower head

Fresh flowers

FLOWERS
Rich in chemicals that are converted by steam into antiallergenic compounds, the flowers are used for various allergic mucus problems, including hay fever. Harvest during summer and fall.

ESSENTIAL OIL
The oil, extracted by steam distillation of the flowers, is generally used as an anti-inflammatory or in chest rubs for colds and influenza. Extracts have also been used as a mosquito repellent.

LEAVES
The leaves encourage clotting, so can be used fresh for nosebleeds. However, inserting a leaf in the nostril may also start a nosebleed; this was once done to relieve migraines. Harvest throughout the growing season.

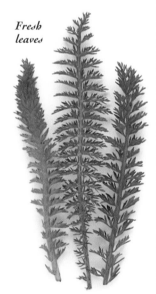

Fresh leaves

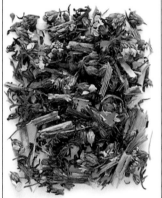

Dried aerial parts

AERIAL PARTS
Used for phlegm conditions, as a bitter digestive tonic to encourage bile flow, and as a diuretic. The aerial parts act as a tonic for the blood, stimulate the circulation, and can be used for high blood pressure. Also useful in menstrual disorders, and as an effective sweating remedy to bring down fevers. Harvest during flowering.

Applications

FLOWERS

INFUSION Drink for upper respiratory phlegm or use externally as a wash for eczema.

INHALATION For hay fever and mild asthma, use fresh in boiling water.

ESSENTIAL OIL

MASSAGE OIL For inflamed joints, dilute 5-10 drops yarrow oil in 25 ml infused St. John's wort oil.

CHEST RUB For chest colds and influenza, combine with eucalyptus, peppermint, hyssop, or thyme oils, diluting a total of 20 drops oil in 25 ml almond or sunflower oil.

LEAVES

FRESH To stop a nosebleed, insert a leaf into the nostril.

POULTICE Wrap washed, fresh leaves on cuts and scrapes.

AERIAL PARTS

INFUSION Use to reduce fevers and as a digestive tonic.

TINCTURE Use for urinary disorders or menstrual problems. Prescribed for cardiovascular complaints.

COMPRESS Soak a pad in the infusion or dilute tincture to soothe varicose veins.

CAUTIONS
• In rare cases, yarrow can cause severe allergic skin rashes; prolonged use can increase the skin's photosensitivity.
• Avoid large doses in pregnancy because the herb is a uterine stimulant.

Agrimonia spp.
AGRIMONY

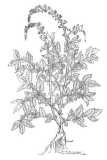

"If it be leyd under mann's heed,
He shal sleepyn as he were deed,
He shal never drede ne wakyn,
Till fro under his heed it be takyn."
Medieval medical manuscript.

MAINLY VALUED TODAY as a healing herb for the mucous membranes and for its astringent properties to stop bleeding, *A. eupatoria* has been used since Saxon times for wounds. In the 15th century, it was the prime ingredient of "arquebusade water," a battlefield remedy for gunshot wounds. This healing power is now attributed to the herb's high silica content. A related variety, *A. pilosa*, known as *xian he cao* in China, is used in a similar way.

Character
Cool, drying; bitter, astringent taste.
Constituents
Tannins, silica, essential oil, bitter principle, flavonoids, minerals, vitamins B, K.
Actions
Astringent, diuretic, tissue healer, stops bleeding, stimulates bile flow, some antiviral activity reported.
A. PILOSA: also antiparasitic and antibacterial.

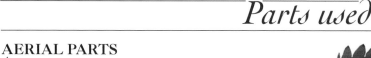

Parts used

AERIAL PARTS
A. EUPATORIA
A cooling astringent, the aerial parts can be used for "hot" conditions, including diarrhea, bronchitis, and urinary infections; to clear inflammations, phlegm, and toxins; and encourage healing. Good for skin inflammations and ulcers, they stem bleeding from cuts. Gather before and during early flowering in summer.

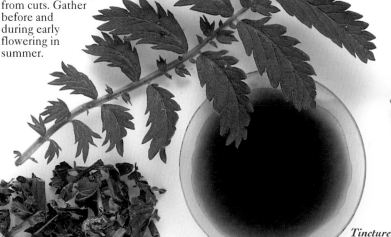

Fresh aerial parts

Dried aerial parts

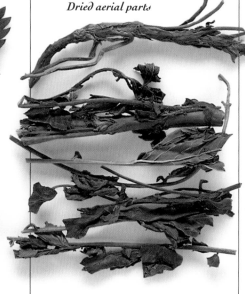

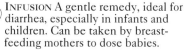

Dried aerial parts

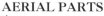
Tincture

AERIAL PARTS
A. PILOSA
As well as stopping bleeding, the Chinese variety has antibacterial and antiparasitic actions and is used for *Trichomonas vaginalis*, tapeworms, dysentery, and malaria.

Applications

AERIAL PARTS/LEAVES
A. EUPATORIA

 INFUSION A gentle remedy, ideal for diarrhea, especially in infants and children. Can be taken by breast-feeding mothers to dose babies.

 TINCTURE More potent and drying than the infusion, and effective if the condition involves excess phlegm or mucus. Use for cystitis, urinary infections, bronchitis, and heavy menstrual bleeding.

 POULTICE Apply a poultice of the leaves for migraines.

WASH Use the infusion for wounds, sores, eczema, and varicose ulcers.

 EYEWASH Use a weak infusion (10 g herb to 2 cups [500 ml] water) for conjunctivitis.

 GARGLE Use the infusion for sore throats and nasal mucus.

AERIAL PARTS
A. PILOSA

 DECOCTION Used in China for heavy uterine bleeding, blood in the urine, dysentery, and digestive parasites.

 COMPRESS Soak a pad in the decoction and use for boils.

 DOUCHE Use the cooled, strained decoction for *Trichomonas vaginalis*.

CAUTION
• Because the herb is astringent, do not take if suffering from constipation.

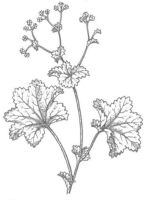

Alchemilla xanthoclora
LADY'S MANTLE

REMINISCENT OF THE VIRGIN'S cloak in medieval paintings, the leaves with scalloped edges are reputed to give lady's mantle its name. Like many herbs with "lady" or "mother" as part of their common name, it is a valuable gynecological herb, specifically for heavy menstrual bleeding and vaginal itching. Highly astringent and rich in tannins, it was one of the most popular wound herbs on the battlefields of the 15th and 16th centuries.

"It is one of the most singular wound herbs and therefore highly prized and praised, used in all wounds, inwards and outwards."
Nicholas Culpeper, 1653.

Character
Cool, dry; bitter, astringent taste.
Constituents
Tannins, salicylic acid, saponins, phytosterols, volatile oil, bitter principle.
Actions
Astringent, menstrual regulator, digestive tonic, anti-inflammatory, heals wounds.

Parts used

AERIAL PARTS
The astringent aerial parts are good for gastroenteritis and diarrhea. As well as helping to control heavy menstruation, they can be used for menstrual pain, to regulate the cycle, and for vaginal discharges. They are cooling, and useful in inflammation and infections. Water extracts have recently been shown to be highly antioxidant. Harvest while flowering in summer.

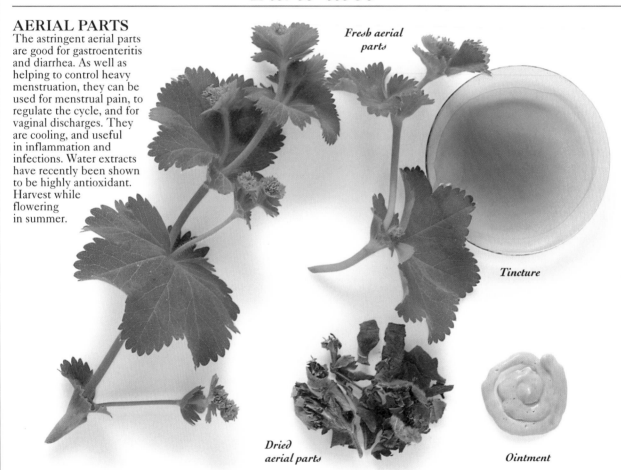

Fresh aerial parts

Tincture

Dried aerial parts

Ointment

Applications

AERIAL PARTS

 INFUSION Use for gastroenteritis or diarrhea: take up to five times daily for acute symptoms.

 TINCTURE Use for menstrual pain and irregularities or for menopausal problems.

 OINTMENT To relieve vaginal itching, combine 50 g ointment base with around 20 ml rosewater and 15 ml of the infusion or tincture, and use night and morning.

 WASH Apply the infusion externally for weeping eczema or sores.

 MOUTHWASH/GARGLE Use the infusion for sore throats, laryngitis, and mouth ulcers.

 DOUCHE Use the infusion for vaginal discharges and itching.

 SUPPOSITORIES Use for vaginal discharges and itching. Combine 20 drops tincture with 20 g cocoa butter to make 12-16 suppositories, depending on mold size.

CAUTIONS
• Avoid the herb in pregnancy as it is a uterine stimulant.
• Seek professional advice for any sudden or abnormal change in uterine bleeding.

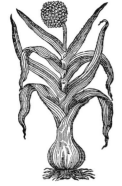

Allium sativum
GARLIC

"...in men oppressed by melancholy it will... send up... many strange visions to the head: therefore, inwardly, let it be taken with great moderation."
Nicholas Culpeper, 1653.

PRIZED FOR AT LEAST 5,000 years, garlic has long been known to reduce cholesterol levels. Even orthodox medicine acknowledges that the plant reduces the risk of further heart attacks in cardiac patients; it is also a stimulant for the immune system and an antibiotic. Garlic's strong odor is largely due to sulphur-containing compounds that account for most of its medicinal properties; deodorized preparations are significantly less effective.

Character
Very hot, dry, pungent.
Constituents
Volatile oil with sulphur-containing compounds (notably allicin, alliin and ajoene); enzymes, B vitamins, minerals, flavonoids.
Actions
Antibiotic, expectorant, promotes sweating, reduces blood pressure, anticoagulant, lowers cholesterol levels, lowers blood sugar levels, antihistaminic, antiparasitic.

Parts used

CLOVES
The cloves are used widely for infections, especially chest problems, digestive disorders, and fungal infections such as yeast infections. They are a good long-term remedy for cardiovascular problems, reducing excessive cholesterol levels, athero-sclerosis, and the risk of thrombosis; they also dilate peripheral blood vessels, lower-ing blood pressure. Garlic also helps regulate blood sugar levels, and so can be helpful in late-onset diabetes, and may act as a preventative for can-cer. Topically, the cloves are effective for skin infections and acne. Best used fresh.

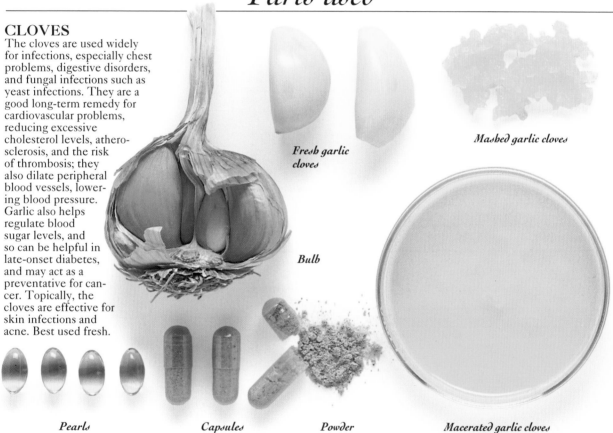

Fresh garlic cloves

Mashed garlic cloves

Bulb

Macerated garlic cloves

Pearls

Capsules

Powder

Applications

CLOVES

FRESH Rub on acne, or mash and use on warts and plantar warts, or to draw corns. Add the cloves regularly to the diet as a prophylac-tic against infection, to reduce high cholesterol levels, to improve the quality of the cardiovascular system, and help lower blood sugar levels. Eat crushed cloves (3-6 daily in acute conditions) for severe digestive disorders (gastroenteritis, dysentery, worms), and infections.

JUICE Drink for digestive disorders and infections, or to combat atherosclerosis.

MACERATION Steep 3-4 garlic cloves in water or milk overnight and drink the liquid the next day for intestinal parasites.

CAPSULES Garlic powder can be made into capsules as an aromatic alternative to commercial "pearls." Clinical trials suggest that 2 g powder in capsules daily can prevent further heart attacks in those who have already suffered one attack. Taking the capsules daily can also combat infections, including yeast infections.

PEARLS Use as an alternative to cap-sules. The more "deodorized" the pearls, the less effective they are.

CAUTIONS
• Garlic is very heating and can irritate the stomach.
• While culinary quantities are generally safe, do not take garlic in therapeutic doses during pregnancy (might promote uterine con-tractions) and lactation; it can cause digestive prob-lems, and babies may dislike the taste in breast milk.
• Garlic's strong aromatic compounds are excreted via the lungs and the skin; eat-ing fresh parsley may elimi-nate odor on the breath.

Aloe vera
ALOE

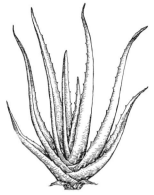

THE ALOE ORIGINATES from tropical Africa, where related species are used as an antidote to poison arrow wounds. It was known to the Greeks and Romans, who also used the gel for wounds; one of Pliny's many recommendations was to rub leaves on "ulcerated male genitals". Aloe was a favorite purgative during the Middle Ages. In China, similar uses developed to those in the West, although only the gel is used; in India, the gel is a highly regarded cooling tonic. Aloe reached the West Indies in the 16th century and is widely cultivated there.

"There are many uses for it, but the chief is to relax the bowels, for it is almost the only laxative that is also a stomach tonic..."
Pliny, AD 77.

Character
Leaves: bitter, hot, moist.
Gel: salty, bitter, cool, moist.
Constituents
Anthraquinone glycosides, resins, polysaccharides, sterols, gelonins, chromones.
Actions
Purgative, promotes bile flow, heals wounds, tonic, demulcent, antifungal, stops bleeding, sedative, expels worms, reputedly rejuvenative and anti-aging, reduces blood sugar and cholesterol levels.

Parts used

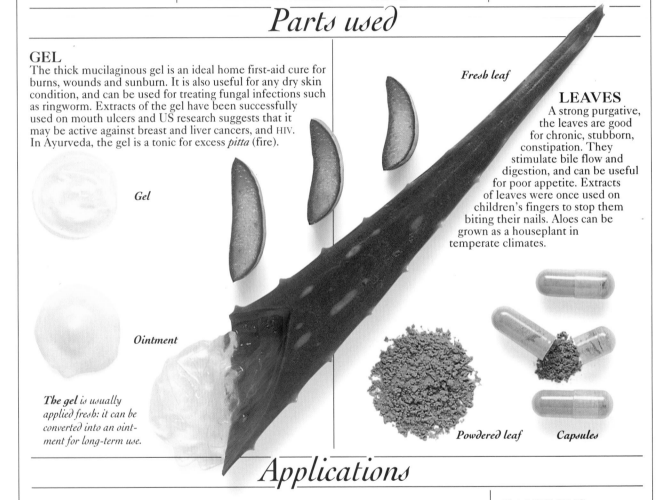

GEL
The thick mucilaginous gel is an ideal home first-aid cure for burns, wounds and sunburn. It is also useful for any dry skin condition, and can be used for treating fungal infections such as ringworm. Extracts of the gel have been successfully used on mouth ulcers and US research suggests that it may be active against breast and liver cancers, and HIV. In Ayurveda, the gel is a tonic for excess *pitta* (fire).

Gel

Ointment

The gel *is usually applied fresh: it can be converted into an oint- ment for long-term use.*

Fresh leaf

LEAVES
A strong purgative, the leaves are good for chronic, stubborn, constipation. They stimulate bile flow and digestion, and can be useful for poor appetite. Extracts of leaves were once used on children's fingers to stop them biting their nails. Aloes can be grown as a houseplant in temperate climates.

Powdered leaf

Capsules

Applications

GEL
 FRESH Apply the split leaf directly to burns, wounds, dry skin, fungal infections and insect bites. Take up to 2 tsp in a glass of water or fruit juice, three times a day, as a tonic.

 OINTMENT Split several leaves to collect a large quantity of gel, and boil it down to a thick paste. Store in clean jars in a cool place and use as the fresh leaves.

 TONIC WINE Fermented aloe gel with honey and spices is known as kumaryasava in India, and is used as

a tonic for anemia, poor digestive function, and liver disorders.

 INHALATION Use the gel in a steam inhalation for bronchial congestion.

LEAVES
 TINCTURE Use 1-3 ml per dose as an appetite stimulant or for constipation. The taste is unpleasant.

 POWDER Use 100-500 mg per dose or in capsules as a purgative for stubborn constipation and to stimulate bile flow.

CAUTIONS
• Aloe should not be taken internally by children under the age of 12.
• Do not take aloe internally for more than two weeks.
• Avoid in pregnancy as the anthraquinone glycosides are strongly purgative.
• High doses of the leaves can cause vomiting.

Alpinia galanga
GALANGAL

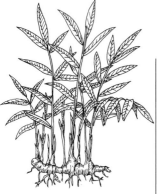

ORIGINALLY FROM SOUTHEAST ASIA, *A. galanga* is an important herb in the traditions of Chinese and Ayurvedic medicine. It is known in Hindi as *kulanjian* and used in India as a popular stomach remedy. The dried rhizomes of this herb were brought to Europe by Arab traders in the 9th century, and were a favorite with the mystic Hildegard of Bingen, who used galangal to treat a wide range of heart disorders. A related variety, lesser galangal (*A. officinarum*), is used similarly to treat digestive disorders in India. It is known as *gao liang jiang* in China.

"... whoever has heart pain and is weak in the heart, should instantly eat enough galangal, and he or she will be well again."
Hildegard of Bingen, 1098-1179.

Character
Pungent, hot, dry.
Constituents
Essential oil (inc. cineole, eugenol, pinene), sesquiterpene lactones (inc. galangol), flavonoids.
Actions
Carminative, digestive tonic, promotes sweating, prevents vomiting, stimulant, antifungal.

Parts used

FRESH RHIZOME
A. GALANGA
In the Middle East and Thailand the fresh rhizome is used in cooking, and is commonly available in Western supermarkets. The root is used in a similar way to fresh ginger – to warm decoctions, treat colds, chills, and motion sickness.

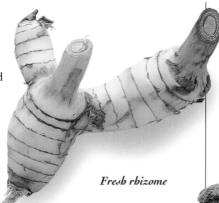

Fresh rhizome

RHIZOME
A. OFFICINARUM
The Chinese use lesser galangal (*gao liang jiang*) as a warming remedy for the stomach and spleen, and to relieve cold and pain. The fresh rhizome can be used in cooking.

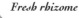

Fresh rhizome

DRIED RHIZOME
A. GALANGA
In India, the dried rhizome is used for digestive and respiratory problems and is classified as an aphrodisiac. German studies based on the work of Hildegard of Bingen have confirmed that the herb is also effective for easing heart pain, dizziness, and fatigue, and can be given for chronic heart disorders such as angina pectoris.

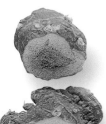

Dried rhizome

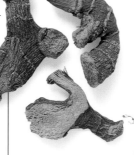

Dried rhizome

Applications

FRESH RHIZOME
A. GALANGA

 DECOCTION Add 1-2 slices per mug for minor digestive problems and chills.

DRIED RHIZOME
A. GALANGA

 CAPSULES Take 1-2 x 200 mg capsules for digestive upsets, stomach cramps, indigestion, and gas.

 TINCTURE Use 10 drops per dose as a circulatory and heart tonic, or 2-3 drops on the tongue as required for attacks of angina pectoris, dizziness, and palpitations.

DRIED RHIZOME
A. OFFICINARUM

 DECOCTION Use for chills, minor stomach pains, and indigestion.

CAPSULES Take 1-2 x 200 mg capsules before traveling to combat motion sickness.

TINCTURE Take 2-10 drops per dose for nausea, stomach chills, or indigestion.

CAUTIONS
• Heart problems such as angina pectoris require professional treatment.
• Do not use the herb to replace prescribed medication without professional guidance.

Althaea officinalis
MARSHMALLOW

TAKING ITS BOTANICAL NAME from a Greek word, *altho*, meaning "to heal", marshmallow has been used since Ancient Egyptian times. The root, rich in sugars, is very mucilaginous and softening for the tissues. The leaves are not as mucilaginous as the root and are used as an expectorant and as a soothing remedy for the urinary system. Both leaves and root have been used as a vegetable. All members of the mallow family have similar properties, with varieties such as garden hollyhocks and common mallow occasionally used medicinally as well.

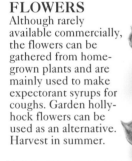

"... whoever swallows daily half a cyathus of the juice of any one of them [the mallows] will be immune to all diseases."
Pliny, AD 77.

Character
Cool, moist, sweet.
Constituents
Flowers: mucilage, flavonoids.
Leaves: mucilage, flavonoids, coumarin, salicylic and other phenolic acids.
Root: mucilage, polysaccharides, asparagin, tannins.
Actions
Flowers: expectorant.
Leaves: expectorant, diuretic, demulcent.
Root: demulcent, expectorant, diuretic, heals wounds.

Parts used

FLOWERS
Although rarely available commercially, the flowers can be gathered from home-grown plants and are mainly used to make expectorant syrups for coughs. Garden holly-hock flowers can be used as an alternative. Harvest in summer.

Fresh flowers

Powdered root

Paste

Dried root

LEAVES
Mainly used to soothe and heal bronchial and urinary disorders, including conditions such as bronchitis, irritating coughs and cystitis. Harvest after flowering in late summer.

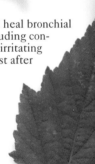

Fresh root

Dried leaf

Fresh leaf

ROOT
Externally, the root is used for wounds, burns, boils, and skin ulceration. Internally, it is taken for inflammations of the mucous membranes: gastritis, esophagitis, enteritis, peptic ulceration, to ease hiatus hernia and for urinary inflammations such as cystitis. Harvest in autumn or winter.

Applications

FLOWERS
 SYRUP Use a syrup made from the infusion as a cough expectorant.

LEAVES
 INFUSION Use for bronchial and urinary disorders.

ROOT
 DECOCTION For inflammations such as esophagitis and cystitis, use 25 g root to 4 cups (1 liter) water, and boil down to about 3 cups (750 ml). This may need further dilution.

 TINCTURE Use for inflammations of the mucous membranes of the digestive and urinary systems.

 POULTICE Use the root or a paste of the powdered root mixed with water for skin inflammations and ulcers.

 OINTMENT For wounds, skin ulceration, or to help draw splinters, melt 50 g anhydrous lanolin, 50 g beeswax, and 300 g soft paraffin together, then heat 100 g powdered marshmallow root in these liquid fats for an hour over a waterbath. When cool, stir in 100 g powdered slippery elm bark.

CAUTION
• If using the tincture for digestive or urinary disorders, use the hot-water method (see p. 125) to reduce the alcohol.

Amni visnaga
KHELLA

SINCE ANCIENT TIMES khella seeds have been used in Arab and Middle Eastern medicine as a smooth muscle relaxant to ease colic and asthma. Pliny reports that the plant was used in a similar way to cumin, and Hippocrates referred to it as "royal cumin" because he believed its effects to be superior to cumin. The use of khella spread to Europe from North Africa with the Moors, and was a popular remedy for whitening teeth in parts of Spain. A close relative, bishopsweed (*A. majus*), is used in similar ways, and was called ameos or ammi in Elizabethan times.

"... The seed of ameos is good to be drunken in wine against the biting of all manner of venomous beasts and hath power against poison or plague."
John Gerard, 1597.

Character
Hot, dry, pungent.
Constituents
Furanochromones and coumarins (inc. khellin), borneol, linalool, flavonoids, sterols.
Actions
Antispasmodic, relaxant, anti-asthmatic, diuretic, relaxes the coronary arteries.

Parts used

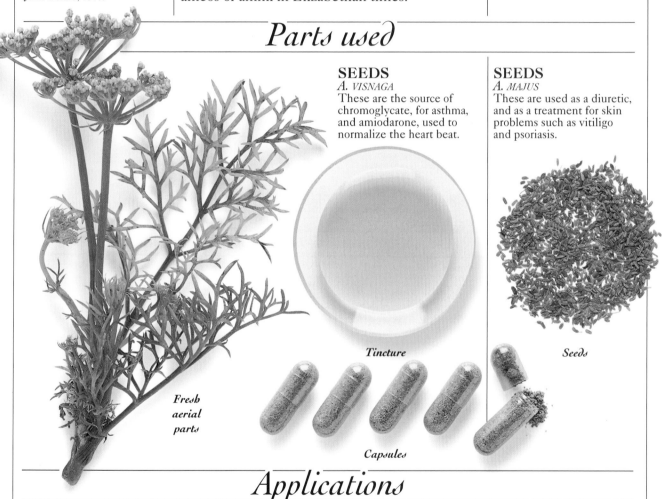

SEEDS
A. VISNAGA
These are the source of chromoglycate, for asthma, and amiodarone, used to normalize the heart beat.

SEEDS
A. MAJUS
These are used as a diuretic, and as a treatment for skin problems such as vitiligo and psoriasis.

Fresh aerial parts

Tincture

Seeds

Capsules

Applications

SEEDS
A. VISNAGA

INFUSION Use a weak infusion for asthma, bronchial spasms or bronchitis.

TINCTURE Use 20 drops per dose in a little water to relieve colic, urinary spasms and gall bladder pain. The same mixture can also help asthma.

STEAM INHALANT Put 1 teaspoon of seeds into a basin of boiling water and use as a steam inhalant to relieve mild asthma attacks, hay fever, bronchial spasms, and colic.

CAPSULES Use 1-2 x 200 mg capsules up to three times daily to combat mild asthma attacks, or to improve the blood supply to the heart in angina pectoris.

SYRUP Use a syrup made from the infusion for bronchitis or whooping cough.

SEEDS
A. MAJUS

CREAM Apply regularly to patches of psoriasis or vitiligo.

CAUTIONS
• The use of khella is restricted in some countries such as Australia.
• Long-term use or high doses of the herb may lead to nausea and insomnia.
• Stop using khella immediately if allergic reactions occur.
• Avoid the herb in diabetes and high blood pressure.

Angelica spp.
ANGELICA

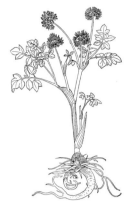

"*A water distilled from the root... eases all pains and torments coming of cold and wind…*"
Nicholas Culpeper, 1653.

THE LIQUEUR BENEDICTINE derives its distinctive flavor from *A. archangelica*, a tall biennial. The candied stalks and roots were traditionally taken as a tonic to combat infection and improve energy levels. Several other species are used in Eastern medicine, including *A. polyphorma var. sinensis (dang gui)*, one of the most important of the great Chinese tonic herbs, used in many patent remedies as a nourishing blood tonic and to regulate the menstrual cycle. Many over-the-counter preparations based on *dang gui* are available in the West.

Character
Sweet, pungent, warm, generally drying.
Constituents
Volatile oil, bitter iridoids, resin, coumarins, valerianic acid, tannins, bergapten; vitamins A and B also reported in Chinese species.
Actions
A. ARCHANGELICA: carminative, antispasmodic, promotes sweating, topical anti-inflammatory, expectorant, diuretic, digestive tonic, anti-rheumatic, uterine stimulant.
A. SINENSIS: blood tonic, circulatory stimulant, laxative.

Parts used

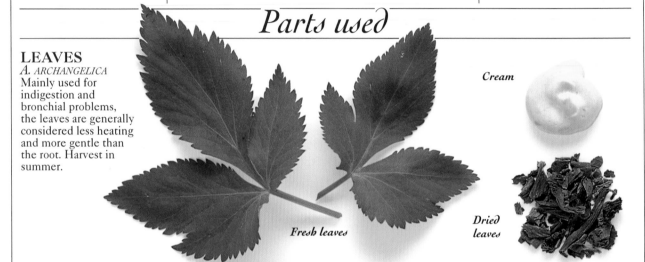

LEAVES
A. ARCHANGELICA
Mainly used for indigestion and bronchial problems, the leaves are generally considered less heating and more gentle than the root. Harvest in summer.

Fresh leaves

Cream

Dried leaves

ROOT
A. ARCHANGELICA
Used for digestive and bronchial problems, to stimulate the appetite and liver, to relieve rheumatism and arthritis, and promote sweating in chills and influenza. As a uterine stimulant, the root has been used in prolonged labor or retention of the placenta. Harvest in the fall of the first year.

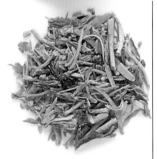

Dried root

ROOT
A. POLYPHORMA VAR. SINENSIS
The root, *dang gui*, is valuable in anemia and menstrual pain, or as a general tonic after childbirth. It clears liver stagnation (of both energy and toxins), has been used to treat liver cirrhosis, and can relieve constipation, especially in the elderly.

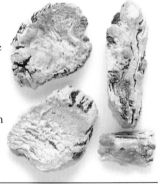

Dried dang gui

Applications

LEAVES
A. ARCHANGELICA

 INFUSION Take in standard doses for indigestion.

 TINCTURE Take up to 3 ml, three times a day, for bronchitis or flatulence.

 CREAM Apply to skin irritations.

ROOT
A. ARCHANGELICA

 TINCTURE Take for bronchial phlegm, chest coughs, digestive disorders, or as a liver stimulant.

 COMPRESS Soak a pad in the hot diluted tincture or decoction and apply to painful rheumatic or arthritic joints.

 MASSAGE OIL Dilute up to 10 drops angelica oil in 25 ml almond or sunflower oil for arthritic or rheumatic pains.

ROOT
A. SINENSIS

 DECOCTION Prescribed for anemia, menstrual irregularities or pains, liver stagnation, or weakness after childbirth.

CAUTIONS
• Avoid regular or large doses in pregnancy, because it is a uterine stimulant, and in diabetes (because of sugar content).
• Angelica is heating, so can be contraindicated in "hot" conditions.
• The oil can increase photosensitivity, so avoid excess exposure to sunshine if using angelica externally.

Apium graveolens
CELERY

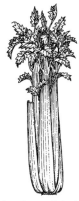

A FAMILIAR AND POPULAR VEGETABLE, celery is also an important medicinal herb. In Eastern medicine, it is categorized as bitter-sweet, making it moist and cooling, and thus good for balancing hot, spicy dishes. The whole plant is gently stimulant, nourishing, and restorative for weak conditions. In the past, celery was grown as a vegetable for winter and early spring; because of its antitoxic properties, it was a cleansing tonic after the stagnation of winter. A homeopathic extract of the seeds is widely used in France to relieve retention of urine.

"The plant is one of the herbs which is eaten in the spring, to sweeten and purify the blood."
Nicholas Culpeper, 1653.

Character
Slightly cool, moist, bitter-sweet.
Constituents
Volatile oil, glycosides, furanocoumarins, flavonoids.
Actions
Antirheumatic, sedative, urinary antiseptic, increases uric acid excretions, carminative, reduces blood pressure, some anti-fungal activity reported.

Parts used

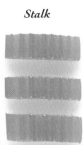

SEEDS
Mainly used as a diuretic, these help clear toxins from the system, so are especially good for gout, where uric acid crystals collect in the joints, and arthritis. Slightly bitter, they act as a mild digestive stimulant. Harvest after the plant flowers in its second year.

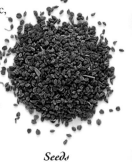

Seeds

ESSENTIAL OIL
Distilled from the seeds, the essential oil is more potent therapeutically. Use with care.

STALK
This shares the medicinal properties of other parts of the plant to a lesser extent. Eating fresh stalks can help stimulate milk flow after childbirth. Although wild celery is more effective, commercially grown varieties can be used.

ROOT
Rarely used today, the root is an effective diuretic and has been taken for urinary stones and gravel. It also acts as a bitter digestive remedy and liver stimulant.

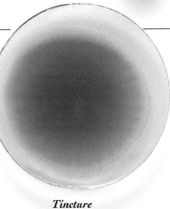

Tincture

Stalk

Applications

SEEDS
 INFUSION For rheumatoid arthritis and gout, combine 2 tsp celery seeds with 1 tsp *lignum vitae*, and add 1/2 tsp to a cup of boiling water.

ESSENTIAL OIL
 OIL For painful gout in the feet or toes, add 15 drops oil to a bowl of warm water, and soak the feet.

 MASSAGE OIL Dilute 5-10 drops celery oil in 20 ml almond or sunflower oil, and massage into arthritic joints.

ROOT
 TINCTURE In the past used mainly as a diuretic in hypertension and urinary disorders, as a component in arthritic remedies, or as a kidney energy stimulant and cleanser.

WHOLE PLANT
 JUICE Liquefy the whole fresh plant (seeds, root, stalks, and leaves) and drink the juice for joint and urinary tract inflammations, such as rheumatoid arthritis, cystitis, or urethritis, for weak conditions, and for nervous exhaustion.

CAUTIONS
• Bergapten in the seeds could increase photosensitivity, so do not apply the essential oil externally in bright sunshine.
• Avoid the oil and large doses of the seeds during pregnancy: they can act as a uterine stimulant.
• Do not buy seeds intended for cultivation, because they are often treated with fungicides.

Arctium lappa
BURDOCK

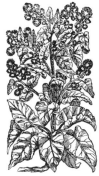

ONCE WIDELY USED in cleansing remedies, burdock is familiar for its hooked burrs, which readily attach themselves to clothing. This property is reflected in the herb's botanical name, from the Greek *arktos*, or bear, suggesting rough-coated fruits, and *lappa*, to seize. Burdock was a traditional blood purifier, often combined in folk brews such as dandelion and burdock wine, and it was once popular for indigestion. In China, the seeds, *niu bang zi*, are used to dispel "wind and heat evils"; they also lower blood sugar levels.

"They are but burs, cousin, thrown upon thee in holiday foolery." As You Like It, William Shakespeare, 1599.

Character
Root/Leaves: cool, drying, bitter; root is slightly sweet.
Seeds: cold, pungent, bitter.
Constituents
Root/Leaves: glycosides, flavonoids, tannins, volatile oil, polyacetylenes, resin, mucilage, inulin, alkaloids, essential oil.
Seeds: essential fatty acids, vitamins A, B₂.
Actions
Root: alterative, mild laxative, diuretic, promotes sweating, antirheumatic, antibiotic.
Leaves: mild laxative, diuretic.
Seeds: prevent fever, anti-inflammatory, antibacterial, reduce blood sugar levels.

Parts used

ROOT
The Japanese use burdock root, which they call *gobo*, as a vegetable. Western herbalists consider it the most important part of the herb, using it as a cleansing, eliminative remedy where a buildup of toxins causes skin problems, digestive sluggishness, or arthritic pains. Also used externally for skin sores and infections. Harvest in fall.

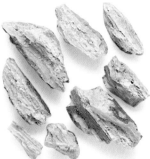

Dried root

SEEDS
American Eclectics (see p. 21) used the seeds for skin diseases and as a diuretic. In China, the seeds are thought suitable for common colds characterized by a sore throat and unproductive cough. Harvest when ripe in late summer.

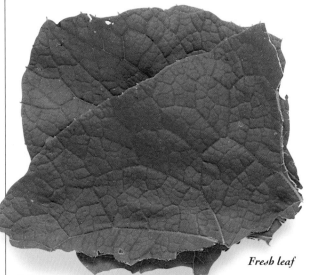

Fresh leaf

LEAVES
Generally less effective than the root, the large leaves can be used in similar ways. They are particularly good for stomach problems including indigestion and general digestive weakness. Harvest before or during early flowering.

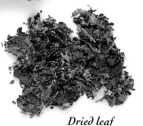

Dried leaf

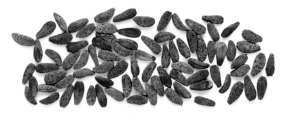

Niu bang zi

Applications

ROOT

 DECOCTION Use for skin disorders, especially persistent boils, sores, and dry, scaling eczema.

 TINCTURE Use in combination with arthritic, digestive herbs such as yellow dock to detoxify the system and stimulate the digestion; also for urinary stones and gravel.

 POULTICE Apply to skin sores and leg ulcers.

 WASH Use the decoction for acne and fungal skin infections such as athlete's foot and ringworm.

LEAVES

 INFUSION Use for indigestion (take in half-cup doses before meals) and as a mild digestive stimulant.

 POULTICE Apply to bruises and skin inflammations, including acne.

 INFUSED OIL Make by the hot infusion method (see p. 154), and use for varicose ulcers.

SEEDS

 DECOCTION Take for feverish colds with sore throat and cough. Use with heartsease for skin eruptions.

Artemisia spp.
WORMWOOD & MUGWORT

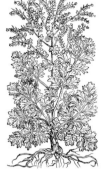

"...eldest of worts... for venom availest, for flying vile things, mighty gainst loathed ones..."
The Lacnunga, 9th century.

THESE TWO RELATED HERBS ARE highly regarded medicinally in both East and West. The Anglo-Saxons listed mugwort as one of the "nine sacred herbs" given to the world by the god Woden. It was also reputedly planted along roadsides by the Romans, who put sprigs in their sandals to prevent aching feet on long journeys. Both herbs are bitter digestive remedies. Extracts of a Chinese variety, *qing hao* (*A. annua*), are increasingly used as a malaria remedy in many parts of the world. As its name implies, wormwood is also used to expel parasitic worms.

Character
Bitter, pungent, drying, quite cold.
Constituents
Volatile oil (inc. sesquiterpene lactones and thujone), bitter principle, flavonoids, tannins, silica, antibiotic polyacetylenes, inulin, hydroxycoumarins.
Actions
A. ABSINTHIUM: bitter digestive tonic, uterine stimulant, expels worms, antibiotic, bile stimulant, carminative, antiseptic.
A. VULGARIS: bitter digestive tonic, uterine stimulant, stimulating nervine, menstrual regulator, antirheumatic.

Parts used

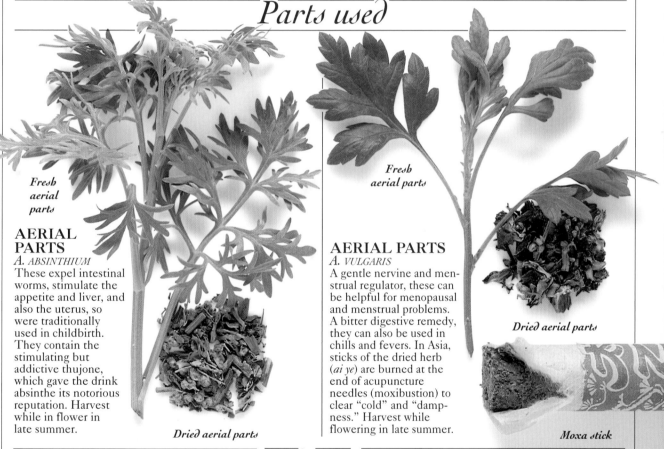

Fresh aerial parts

Fresh aerial parts

AERIAL PARTS
A. ABSINTHIUM
These expel intestinal worms, stimulate the appetite and liver, and also the uterus, so were traditionally used in childbirth. They contain the stimulating but addictive thujone, which gave the drink absinthe its notorious reputation. Harvest while in flower in late summer.

Dried aerial parts

AERIAL PARTS
A. VULGARIS
A gentle nervine and menstrual regulator, these can be helpful for menopausal and menstrual problems. A bitter digestive remedy, they can also be used in chills and fevers. In Asia, sticks of the dried herb (*ai ye*) are burned at the end of acupuncture needles (moxibustion) to clear "cold" and "dampness." Harvest while flowering in late summer.

Dried aerial parts

Moxa stick

Applications

AERIAL PARTS
A. ABSINTHIUM

 INFUSION Take a weak infusion (5-10 g herb to 2 cups [500 ml] water) for sluggish digestion, poor appetite, and gastritis. Prescribed for jaundice and hepatitis, and to expel intestinal worms.

 TINCTURE Use as the infusion, but do not exceed 3 ml daily.

 COMPRESS Soak a pad in the infusion to soothe bruises and bites.

 WASH Use the infusion externally for infestations such as scabies.

AERIAL PARTS
A. VULGARIS

 INFUSION Take for menopausal syndrome or use as a bitter to cool the digestive tract in fever management.

 DECOCTION Combine 5 g with an equal amount of dry ginger to make a warming tea for menstrual pain.

 TINCTURE Take for menstrual pain, scanty menstruation, and prolonged bleeding. Use as a stimulant in liver stagnation and sluggish digestion. In childbirth it is used for prolonged labor and retained placenta.

CAUTIONS
• Avoid both herbs during pregnancy (they are uterine stimulants, and may cause fetal abnormalities) and if breast-feeding (thujone may be passed to the baby in the mother's milk).
• If using the tincture of either herb for liver or digestive disorders, use the hot-water method (see p. 157) to reduce the alcohol.

Asparagus spp.
ASPARAGUS

"...If a man is rubbed with a mixture of pounded asparagus and oil, it is said that he is never stung by bees."
Pliny, *Natural History*, AD 79.

A POPULAR VEGETABLE in the West, asparagus (*A. officinalis*) has also been used as a medicinal herb since ancient times. Pliny calls it "one of the most beneficial foods to the stomach," and says that it "improves the vision, moves the bowels, is aphrodisiac, very useful as a diuretic, and relieves pain in the loins and kidneys." In India, a related species (*A. racemosus*) is used to make an important Ayurvedic tonic, *shatavari*. The name literally means "she who possesses a hundred husbands" because the herb is thought to rejuvenate the female reproductive organs.

Character
Bitter, sweet, cool.
Constituents
Steroidal glycosides (asparagosides), bitters, flavonoids, asparagine.
Actions
A. OFFICINALIS: diuretic, bitter digestive stimulant, mild laxative, sedative, source of folic acid and selenium.
A RACEMOSUS: tonic, demulcent, antibacterial, antitussive, expectorant, antitumor.

Parts used

Shoots

DRIED ROOT
A. RACEMOSUS/ SHATAVARI
In Ayurvedic medicine, *shatavari* is used for debilities associated with the female sexual organs such as infertility, problems in menopause, or after hysterectomy.

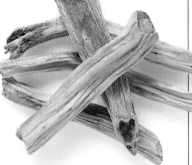

SHOOTS
A. OFFICINALIS
The shoots are less effective as a diuretic than the root, but are useful for mild cases of cystitis, fluid retention during the menstrual cycle, and slight edema. After eating asparagus there is a distinctive smell in the urine caused by the breakdown of asparagine to form methyl mercaptan.

Fresh root

DRIED ROOT
A. RACEMOSUS/TIAN MEN DONG
The Chinese call the roots of both *A. cochinchinensis* and *A. racemosus, tian men dong,* which literally means "lush winter aerial plant." It is used to nourish *yin* and clear heat and is given for symptoms of kidney energy weakness such as night sweats and impotence, in addition to being used to replenish body fluids associated with dry coughs and throats, and constipation.

Applications

FRESH SHOOTS
A. OFFICINALIS

FRESH SHOOTS Eat 3-4 young shoots at meals once or twice a day for cystitis or swollen ankles.

DRIED ROOT
A. RACEMOSUS/SHATAVARI

POWDER Take up to 3 g powder daily in warm milk as a tonic for the female reproductive system.

TINCTURE Add to an equal amount of almond oil and shake well. Use as a rub for stiff joints and muscle spasm.

DRIED ROOT
A. RACEMOSUS/TIAN MEN DONG

DECOCTION Use with ginseng and *sheng di huang* for lingering coughs and debility following influenza.

CAUTION
• Avoid *tian men dong* in cases of diarrhea, and coughs caused by common colds.

Avena sativa
OATS

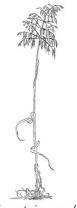

THE TRADITIONAL STAPLE of Northern Europe, oats are a warm, sweet food, ideal in a cold climate. Porridge made from oatmeal (the crushed grain) is a nutritious breakfast. For medicinal purposes the whole plant (known as oatstraw) is generally used, and is gathered when the grains are ripe. The herb is a good restorative nerve tonic, ideal for depression and *qi* (energy) deficiency. Recent research has shown that oatbran, and to a lesser extent oatmeal, can help to reduce abnormally high cholesterol levels.

"...taking oats is a complete body overhaul from the inside to the outside."
Peter Holmes, 1989.

Character
Warm, moist, sweet.
Constituents
Saponins, flavonoids, many minerals, alkaloids, steroidal compounds, vitamins B_1, B_2, D, E, carotene, wheat protein (gluten), starch, fat.
Actions
Oatstraw: antidepressant, restorative nerve tonic, promotes sweating.
Grain: antidepressant, restorative nerve tonic, nutritive.
Oatbran: antithrombotic, reduces cholesterol levels.

Parts used

OATSTRAW
An excellent tonic for the whole system, used for both physical and nervous debility; it is ideal for depression. Oatstraw can also be used for thyroid and estrogen deficiency, for degenerative diseases such as multiple sclerosis, and for colds, especially if recurrent or persistent. The crop is harvested when the grain is ripe, and the whole plant dried and chopped.

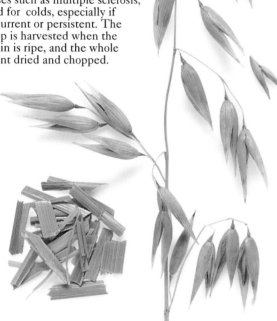
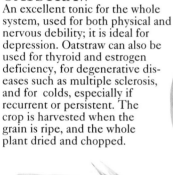

Dried oatstraw

Fresh oats

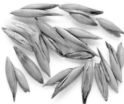

Grain

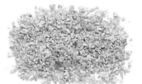

Oatbran is produced from the coarse husks of the grain; it is particularly good at reducing cholesterol levels.

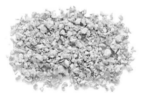

Oatmeal, the ground grains, has a high silica content and can help skin problems if applied externally.

GRAIN
The seeds have very similar properties to the whole plant, and can be used for the same conditions. They are harvested in late summer and milled to produce oatbran and oatmeal.

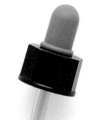

Dr. Bach recommended his Wild Oats flower remedy for times of uncertainty and dissatisfaction.

Applications

OATSTRAW

 FLUID EXTRACT Take doses of 2-3 ml for insomnia, anxiety and depression. (The tincture can be used similarly.) Combines well with vervain. Also makes a nutritive addition to remedies for colds and chills to encourage sweating.

 DECOCTION Make from the whole dried plant, and use for the same ailments as the fluid extract.

 WASH Use the decoction as a healing wash for skin conditions.

GRAIN

 POULTICE Use an oatmeal poultice for skin conditions such as eczema, cold sores, and shingles.

CAUTION
• For those sensitive to gluten (as in celiac disease), allow the decoction or tincture to settle, then decant the clear liquid only for use.

Azadirachta indica
NEEM

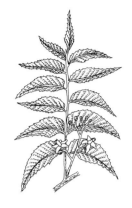

TRADITIONALLY USED AS A COOLING remedy for fevers in Ayurvedic medicine, neem is also highly prized for the insecticidal properties of its wood, which is used for making worm-resistant furniture. In parts of Africa, neem has been introduced into hedges to provide farmers with a natural source of insecticide. Modern studies suggest that the herb has spermicidal properties, and the seed oil is traditionally used as a contraceptive. Neem is also known by the name bead tree, because the hard nuts were used in the past to make rosary beads.

"...It is a powerful febrifuge, effective in malaria and other intermittent and periodic fevers."
David Frawley and
Vasant Lad, 1986.

Character
Bitter, pungent, cooling.
Constituents
Meliacins, triterpenoid bitters, tannins, flavonoids.
Actions
Anti-inflammatory, antifungal, bitter tonic, expels worms, prevents vomiting, cleanses, reduces fevers.

Parts used

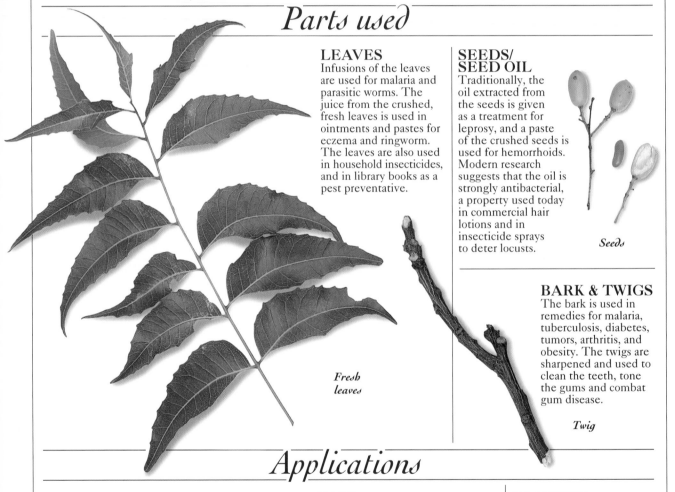

LEAVES
Infusions of the leaves are used for malaria and parasitic worms. The juice from the crushed, fresh leaves is used in ointments and pastes for eczema and ringworm. The leaves are also used in household insecticides, and in library books as a pest preventative.

SEEDS/ SEED OIL
Traditionally, the oil extracted from the seeds is given as a treatment for leprosy, and a paste of the crushed seeds is used for hemorrhoids. Modern research suggests that the oil is strongly antibacterial, a property used today in commercial hair lotions and in insecticide sprays to deter locusts.

Seeds

BARK & TWIGS
The bark is used in remedies for malaria, tuberculosis, diabetes, tumors, arthritis, and obesity. The twigs are sharpened and used to clean the teeth, tone the gums and combat gum disease.

Twig

Fresh leaves

Applications

LEAVES

 HAIR RINSE Add 5-10 drops neem oil to a cup of water and use as a hair rinse for lice and nits.

 POULTICE Crush the leaves and make into a paste or poultice for ringworm or eczema. Alternatively, use a compress soaked in the infusion.

SEED OIL

 LOTION Add 5-10 drops oil to ½ cup (100 ml) distilled witch hazel for ringworm and athlete's foot.

BARK

 WASH Use a strong decoction (50 g bark to 3 cups [750 ml] water) as a wash for skin infestations such as lice and scabies.

 TINCTURE Combine with other anti-inflammatory and cleansing herbs for arthritis and rheumatism.

 DECOCTION Use for feverish conditions.

CAUTION
• Neem should not be given to the very young, elderly or debilitated.

Borago officinalis
BORAGE

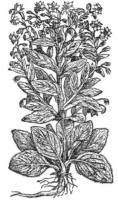

"...of known virtue to revive the hypochondriac and cheer the hard student."
John Evelyn, 1699.

THE GREAT HERBALIST John Gerard, writing in 1597, quotes the old tag *ego borago gaudia semper ago* ("I, borage, always bring courage"). Modern research has given a new slant to the saying, as the plant is now known to stimulate the adrenal glands, encouraging the production of adrenaline, the "fight or flight" hormone that gears the body for action in stressful situations. The pretty blue flowers have been added to salads since Elizabethan times to "make the mind glad", a practice that modern cooks can follow.

Character
Cold, moist, slightly sweet.
Constituents
Leaves/Flowers: saponins, mucilage, tannins, vitamin C, calcium, potassium.
Seeds: essential fatty acids, including *cis*-linoleic and γ-linolenic acids.
Actions
Leaves/Flowers: adrenal stimulants, promote lactation, diuretic, febrifuge, anti-rheumatic, promote sweating, expectorant.
Seeds: relieve eczema, anti-rheumatic, relieve irritable bowel syndrome, regulate menstruation.

Parts used

LEAVES
The fleshy, rather coarse leaves can be used as an adrenal tonic for stress or to counter the lingering effects of steroid therapy. They can also be used for dry, rasping coughs and to stimulate milk flow; they may be prescribed in the early feverish stages of pleurisy or whooping cough. Harvest throughout the growing season.

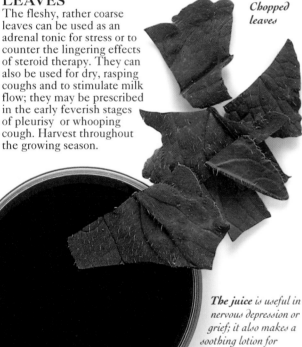

Chopped leaves

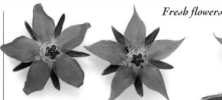

Fresh flowers

FLOWERS
Traditionally, these were added to wine to "maketh men merrie", and were also used in cough syrups.

SEEDS
The oil extracted from the seeds is used as an alternative to evening primrose oil for rheumatic or menstrual disorders, and can be applied externally for eczema. It is also available commercially in capsules.

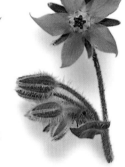

Seeds

The juice is useful in nervous depression or grief; it also makes a soothing lotion for dry, itching skin.

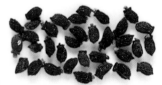

Seed oil and capsules

Applications

LEAVES
 INFUSION Take in the early stages of lung disorders or feverish colds. Lactating mothers may combine it with fennel to stimulate milk.

 TINCTURE Take 10 ml, three times a day, as a tonic following steroid therapy and for stress.

 JUICE Pulp fresh leaves and drink 10 ml of the juice, three times a day, for depression, grief or anxiety.

 LOTION Dilute the juice with an equal volume of water, and use for irritated, dry skin or nervous rashes.

SEEDS
 CAPSULES Take 500 mg oil in capsule form daily as a supplement for eczema or rheumatoid arthritis. The oil is also helpful in some cases of menstrual irregularity, for irritable bowel syndrome, or as emergency first aid for hangovers (take 1 g).

FLOWERS
 SYRUP Take a syrup made from the infusion as an expectorant for coughs. Can be combined with mullein or marshmallow flowers.

CAUTION
• Restricted herb in Australia and New Zealand.

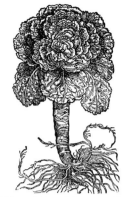

Brassica oleracea
CABBAGE

CULTIVATED IN THE WEST since at least 400 B.C., cabbage is a valuable medicine. It has been used since Dioscorides' time as a digestive remedy, a joint tonic, and for skin problems and fevers; raw cabbage was eaten by overindulgent Romans to prevent drunkenness. Known as colewort in folk medicine, cabbage was a standby for all kinds of family ills.

"The medicine of the poor…"
Dr. Jean Valnet, 1967.

Character
Slightly sweet, salty, drying, cool.
Constituents
Minerals, vitamins A, B_1, B_2, C, amino acids, fats.
Actions
Anti-inflammatory, antibacterial, antirheumatic, heals tissues by encouraging cells to proliferate, liver decongestant.

Parts used

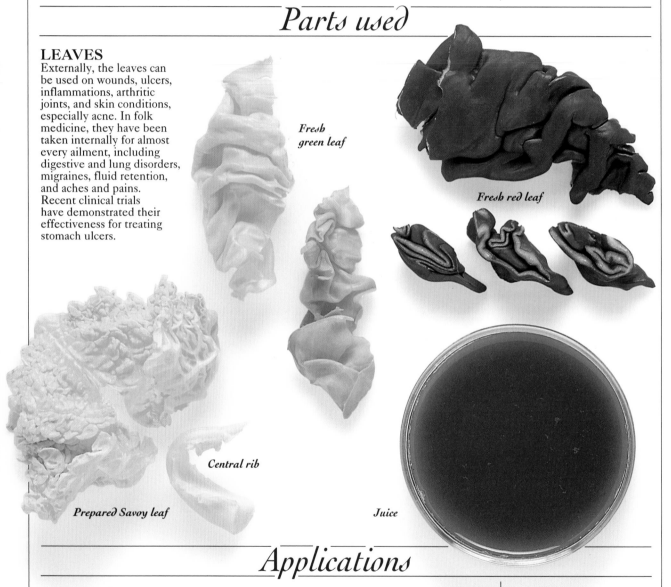

LEAVES
Externally, the leaves can be used on wounds, ulcers, inflammations, arthritic joints, and skin conditions, especially acne. In folk medicine, they have been taken internally for almost every ailment, including digestive and lung disorders, migraines, fluid retention, and aches and pains. Recent clinical trials have demonstrated their effectiveness for treating stomach ulcers.

Fresh green leaf

Fresh red leaf

Central rib

Prepared Savoy leaf

Juice

Applications

LEAVES

 FRESH Use directly on arthritic or sprained joints, varicose ulcers, and wounds. Strip out the central rib of the leaf first, then beat the leaf gently to soften it slightly and bind to the area with a bandage. Place prepared leaves in bra cups for mastitis or engorged breasts.

 DECOCTION For colitis, boil 60 g leaves in 2 cups (500 ml) water for an hour, and drink in half-cup doses.

LOTION For acne, mix 250 g fresh leaves and 1 cup (250 ml) distilled witch hazel in a blender. Strain, and add two drops of lemon juice oil: use night and morning.

 JUICE Prescribed for gastric or duodenal ulceration.

 SYRUP Take a syrup made from the decoction in 10 ml doses for chesty coughs, asthma, and bronchitis.

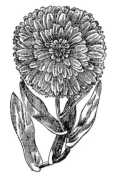

Calendula officinalis
POT MARIGOLD

THE GOLDEN FLOWERS are a favorite among herbalists. Macer's 12th-century herbal recommends simply looking at the plant to improve eyesight, clear the head, and encourage cheerfulness. In Culpeper's day, marigold was taken to "strengthen the heart," and was highly regarded for smallpox and measles. Today, it is widely used in patent homeopathic remedies.

"Somme use it to make theyr here yelow ... not being content with the colour ..."
William Turner, 1551.

Character
Slightly bitter, pungent, drying, gently cooling.
Constituents
Saponins, flavonoids, mucilage, essential oil, bitter principle, resin, steroidal compounds.
Actions
Astringent, antiseptic, antifungal, anti-inflammatory, heals wounds, menstrual regulator, stimulates bile production.

Parts used

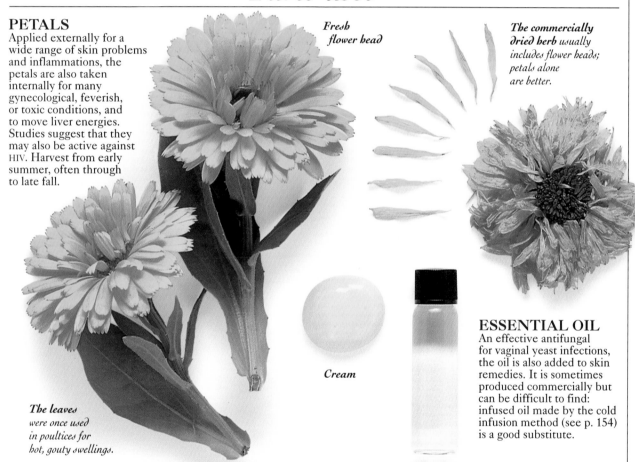

PETALS
Applied externally for a wide range of skin problems and inflammations, the petals are also taken internally for many gynecological, feverish, or toxic conditions, and to move liver energies. Studies suggest that they may also be active against HIV. Harvest from early summer, often through to late fall.

Fresh flower head

The commercially dried herb usually includes flower heads; petals alone are better.

The leaves were once used in poultices for hot, gouty swellings.

Cream

ESSENTIAL OIL
An effective antifungal for vaginal yeast infections, the oil is also added to skin remedies. It is sometimes produced commercially but can be difficult to find: infused oil made by the cold infusion method (see p. 154) is a good substitute.

Applications

PETALS

 INFUSION Take for menopausal problems, period pain, gastritis, and for inflammation of the esophagus.

 TINCTURE Take for stagnant liver problems, including sluggish digestion, and also for menstrual disorders, particularly irregular or painful periods.

 COMPRESS Apply a pad soaked in the infusion to slow-healing wounds or varicose ulcers.

 MOUTHWASH Use the infusion for mouth ulcers and gum disease.

 CREAM Apply for any problem involving inflammation or dry skin: wounds, dry eczema, sore nipples in breast-feeding, scalds, and sunburn.

 INFUSED OIL Use on chilblains, hemorrhoids, and broken capillaries.

ESSENTIAL OIL

 SUPPOSITORIES Use vaginal suppositories containing 2-5 drops each of marigold and tea tree oils, 1-2 times a day, for vaginal yeast infections.

 OIL Add 5-10 drops to bathwater for nervous anxiety or depression.

CAUTION
• Do not confuse this plant or its essential oil with preparations made from the French marigold, *Tagetes patula*, and related species. These are used for warts and also as insecticides or weedkillers.

Camellia sinensis
TEA

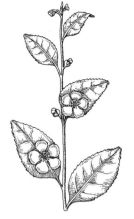

"Better to be deprived of food for three days, than of tea for one."
Ancient Chinese saying.

KNOWN IN CHINA as *cha*, tea has become such a familiar drink that we forget it is also a potent medicinal herb. The Chinese have been drinking tea since around 3000 B.C. and regard it as a good stimulant, an astringent for clearing phlegm, and a digestive remedy. The three types of tea – green, black, and oolong – are made from the leaves of the same species. Far Eastern research shows that some green teas appear to reduce the risk of stomach cancer.

Character
Green/Oolong: bitter-sweet, drying, cooling. **Black:** bitter-sweet, drying, warming.
Constituents
Alkaloids (inc. caffeine and theobromine), tannins (poly-phenols), catechins, volatile oil, fluoride (in some varieties).
Actions
Stimulant, astringent, anti-oxidant, antibacterial, diuretic; some varieties reduce blood cholesterol levels; antitumor properties reported in green tea.

Parts used

LEAVES
The young, fresh leaves and leaf buds are pan-fried, then rolled or dried to make green tea. The fresh leaves are wilted in sunlight, bruised slightly, then partly fermented for oolong tea. Black tea is a fully fermented variety.

GREEN TEA
Rich in fluoride, green tea can reduce the risk of tooth decay. It is also useful for insect bites and to stem bleeding. The tea has been shown to combat stomach and skin cancers, and to boost the immune system.

OOLONG TEA
Some types, such as *Pu erh*, are especially effective at reducing cholesterol levels after a fatty meal. Japanese research suggests that oolong tea can reduce high blood pressure and limit the risk of arterial disease.

BLACK TEA
Widely drunk in Europe, India, and North America, black tea is rich in tannins and is highly astringent, so it is a particularly good remedy for diarrhea.

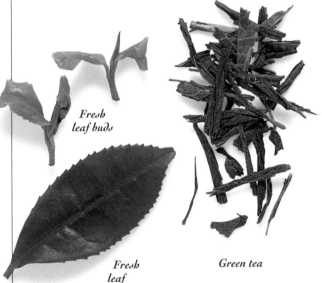
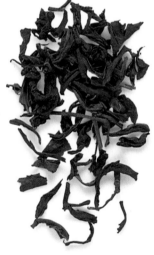
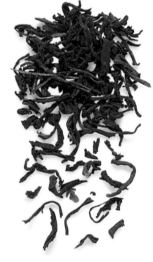

Fresh leaf buds

Fresh leaf

Green tea

Oolong tea

Black tea

Applications

GREEN TEA
 INFUSION Drink after meals to help guard against tooth decay.

 POULTICE Place damp green tea leaves on insect bites to reduce itching and inflammation.

 COMPRESS Use a pad soaked in weak green tea to make an emergency first-aid treatment to ease bleeding from cuts and scrapes.

OOLONG TEA
 INFUSION Drink after fatty meals to reduce cholesterol levels and as a preventative for arterial disease.

BLACK TEA
 INFUSION Take a strong infusion of ordinary tea (2 tsp per cup of boiling water, without milk or sugar) for diarrhea, food poisoning, or dysentery. The infusion is also a traditional Cantonese remedy for hangovers.

 POULTICE Place used tea bags on tired eyes as a poultice. Damp tea leaves can soothe insect bites.

 WASH Use a weak infusion as a cooling wash for sunburn.

CAUTIONS
• Sufferers from an irregular heartbeat, pregnant women, and nursing mothers should limit intake to no more than two cups daily, because high levels of caffeine-like alkaloids can lead to increased heart rate.
• People with stomach ulcers should avoid excessive consumption, because the bitter taste can stimulate gastric acid production.

Capsella bursa-pastoris
SHEPHERD'S PURSE

MORE USUALLY CONSIDERED a weed than a medicinal herb, shepherd's purse has its place in both Eastern and Western practice. The heart-shaped seed pods apparently resemble the leather pouches once carried by shepherds, hence the common name; another is "mothers' hearts," a reminder that this is a useful herb for gynecological conditions. Shepherd's purse is mainly used as a styptic to reduce bleeding; in China, the seeds are said to improve eyesight.

"Few plants possess greater virtues than this, and yet it is utterly disregarded."
Nicholas Culpeper, 1653.

Character
Sweet, dry, cool.
Constituents
Saponins, mustard oil, flavonoids, resin, monoamines, choline, acetylcholine, sitosterol, vitamins A, B, C.
Actions
Astringent, reduces bleeding, urinary antiseptic, circulatory stimulant, reduces blood pressure.

Parts used

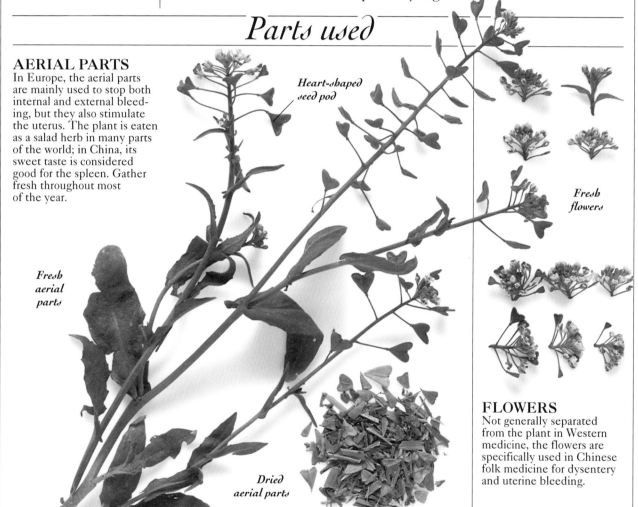

AERIAL PARTS
In Europe, the aerial parts are mainly used to stop both internal and external bleeding, but they also stimulate the uterus. The plant is eaten as a salad herb in many parts of the world; in China, its sweet taste is considered good for the spleen. Gather fresh throughout most of the year.

Heart-shaped seed pod

Fresh flowers

Fresh aerial parts

Dried aerial parts

FLOWERS
Not generally separated from the plant in Western medicine, the flowers are specifically used in Chinese folk medicine for dysentery and uterine bleeding.

Applications

AERIAL PARTS

 INFUSION Take for heavy menstrual bleeding, cystitis, and diarrhea. A strong infusion (twice the standard mix) of fresh or freshly dried herb is best. Sip a hot infusion during labor to stimulate contractions, and after delivery to ease postpartum bleeding.

TINCTURE Take up to 10 ml, three times a day, for heavy menstrual bleeding, cystitis, and diarrhea.

 POULTICE Apply the fresh herb to bleeding wounds.

 COMPRESS Soak a pad in the infusion for cuts. For nosebleeds, soak small cotton swabs in the tincture and insert in the nostril.

CAUTIONS
• Avoid the herb in pregnancy, except during labor, because it stimulates uterine contractions.
• If there is any sudden change in menstrual flow or blood in the urine, seek professional advice before attempting self-medication.

Capsicum frutescens
CAYENNE

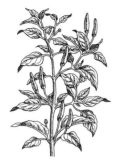

"…it hath in it a malitious qualitie, whereby it is an enemie to the liver and other of the entrails… it killeth dogs."
John Gerard, 1597.

THE HOT RED CAYENNE CHILI arrived in the West from India in 1548, and was known as Ginnie pepper. Gerard describes it as "extreme hot and dry, even in the fourth degree", and recommends it for scrofula, a prevalent lymphatic throat and skin infection commonly known as the King's Evil. Cayenne was popular with the 19th-century Physiomedicalists (see pp. 20-1), who used its warming properties for chills, rheumatism and depression.

Character
Very hot, pungent, drying.
Constituents
Alkaloids, fatty acids, flavonoids, vitamins A, B₁, C, volatile oil, sugars, carotene pigment.
Actions
Circulatory stimulant, promotes sweating, gastric stimulant, carminative, antiseptic, antibacterial, stimulating nerve tonic. Topical: counter-irritant, increases blood flow to an area.

Parts used

FRUIT
A potent stimulant for the whole body, the fruit increases blood flow, tonifies the nervous system, increases the appetite, relieves indigestion, and stimulates *yang* energies (see pp. 14-15). It encourages sweating and is antibacterial, so is ideal for colds and chills. It is also good for throat problems, such as tonsillitis, laryngitis, and hoarseness. Recent research suggests that cayenne creams or lotions can ease the severe pain of shingles and migraine.

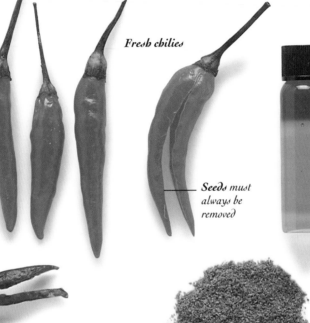

Fresh chilies

Seeds must always be removed

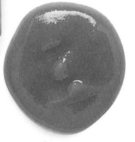

The infused oil and ointment are less burning and irritant to the skin than raw fruits.

Ointment

Dried chilies

Powder

Applications

FRUIT

 INFUSION Add ½ tsp herb to a cup of boiling water, then dilute a tablespoon of this infusion with more hot water to make a cupful, and sip as required. Ideal for colds and chills, cold hands and feet, shock, or depression. Take 2-3 drops of the undiluted infusion to stimulate digestive function.

 TINCTURE Dilute 5-10 drops in half a cup of hot water, and take as a circulatory stimulant and tonic.

 COMPRESS Soak a pad in the infusion, and use for rheumatic pains, sprains, and bruising.

 OINTMENT Use on chilblains, as long as the skin is not broken.

 GARGLE Dilute 5-10 drops of tincture in half a tumbler of warm water, and take for throat problems; this is especially useful in weak and deficient conditions.

 INFUSED OIL Add 25 g powder to 2 cups (500 ml) sunflower oil, and heat over a waterbath for 2 hours. Apply a little to the skin around a varicose ulcer (not on the ulcer) to reduce blood flow to the area.

 MASSAGE OIL Use the infused oil as a warming massage oil for rheumatism, lumbago, and arthritis.

CAUTIONS
• The seeds can be toxic, so do not use them.
• Follow dosages carefully; excessive consumption of cayenne can lead to gastro-enteritis and liver damage.
• Avoid therapeutic doses of cayenne in pregnancy and while breast-feeding.
• Do not leave a compress on the skin for long periods, especially on very sensitive skin, or blistering may occur.
• Avoid touching the eyes or any cuts after handling fresh chilies.

Cimicifuga racemosa
BLACK COHOSH

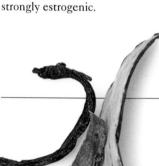

NATIVE AMERICANS used black cohosh, also known as black snakeroot or squaw root, to treat rheumatism, yellow fever, snakebite, kidney disorders and gynecological problems. Early settlers used the herb for smallpox, and by the early 19th century it had entered the European herbal repertoire. Several oriental species (usually *C. foetida* or *C. dahurica*) are used in Chinese medicine as *sheng ma*, primarily regarded as a remedy for colds and measles.

"Unquestionably one of the most valuable of our indigenous medicinal plants."
Dr. A. Clapp, mid-19th century.

Character
Pungent, sweet, slightly bitter, cold.
Constituents
Triterpene glycosides, cinnamic acid derivatives, chromone, isoflavones, tannins, salicylic acid.
Actions
Antispasmodic, antiarthritic, anti-inflammatory, antirheumatic, mild analgesic, relaxing nervine, sedative, relaxes blood vessels, promotes menstruation, diuretic, antitussive, lowers blood sugar levels, reduces blood pressure.

Parts used

FRESH ROOT
C. RACEMOSA
Western herbalists use the herb for a range of ailments including rheumatic problems, respiratory ailments, gynecological disorders, and nervous conditions. Recent German studies confirm that it relieves menopausal symptoms and it is now known to be strongly estrogenic.

Tincture   *Fresh root*

RHIZOME
C. FOETIDA/
C. DAHURICA
In Chinese medicine, *sheng ma* is given for feverish colds, measles, headaches, and mouth ulcers. In very low doses (under 3 g) it can be used for prolapse of the uterus or rectum.

Dried rhizome

Applications

FRESH ROOT
C. RACEMOSA

 DECOCTION Use ½ a cup standard decoction per dose for back pain, facial neuralgia, sciatica, and rheumatic pains. The decoction can be combined with an equal amount of bogbean and valerian.

 TINCTURE Use 20 drops per dose with an equal amount of St. John's wort for relieving hot flashes, night sweats, and emotional upsets during menopause. Can also be used with antirheumatic herbs for low back pain, osteoarthritis, sciatica, and general muscle aches and pains.

 SYRUP Combine with elecampane and licorice for alleviating whooping cough and bronchitis.

 CAPSULES Use 1 x 200 mg, two or three times a day, for back pains and rheumatic problems. Can be combined with devil's claw.

RHIZOME
C. FOETIDA/C. DAHURICA

 DECOCTION Use with red peony (*chi shao yao*), licorice and *ge gen* for measles and feverish chills.

 TINCTURE Use with tonic herbs such as *huang qi*, ginseng and bai zhu to strengthen spleen and stomach *qi*.

CAUTIONS
• Excess black cohosh can cause nausea and vomiting.
• Avoid this herb during pregnancy.

Cinnamomum spp.
CINNAMON

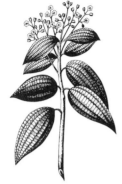

PUNGENT AND WARMING, cinnamon is good for all sorts of "cold" conditions, from the common cold and stomach chills to arthritis and rheumatism. In the West, we generally use the bark of *C. zeylanicum*, which is sold rolled as the familiar cinnamon sticks. The Chinese prefer the native variety, *C. cassia*, and make use of both the bark (*rou gui*) and the twigs (*gui zhi*). Traditionally, the bark was believed best for the torso, the twigs for the fingers and toes. Research has highlighted hypoglycemic properties, useful in diabetes.

"...there is a tale of cinnamon growing around marshes under the protection of a terrible kind of bats ... invented by the natives to raise the price." Pliny, A.D. 77.

Character
Bark: pungent, sweet, very hot.
Twigs: pungent, sweet, less hot.
Constituents
Volatile oil, tannins, mucilage, gum, sugars, coumarins.
Actions
Bark & twigs: carminative, promote sweating, warming digestive remedy, antispasmodic, antiseptic, tonic, uterine stimulant.
Essential oil: potent antibacterial, antifungal, uterine stimulant.

Parts used

BARK
In the West, the inner bark is used mainly for digestive upsets: indigestion, general sluggishness, colic, and diarrhea. Alcoholic extracts have also been used against the *Heliobacter pylorii* bacterium now believed to cause stomach ulcers. In China, *rou gui* is considered very warming and tonifying for the kidneys, a good energizing herb for conditions that can be linked to weak kidney *qi* (energy): asthma and menopausal syndrome, for example. The inner bark promotes sweating and can be used for "cold" conditions.

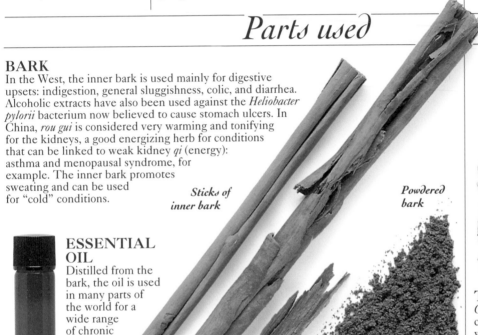

Sticks of inner bark

Powdered bark

Gui zhi

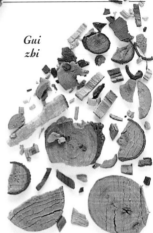

ESSENTIAL OIL
Distilled from the bark, the oil is used in many parts of the world for a wide range of chronic infections.

TWIGS
Gui zhi can be used as a circulatory stimulant to warm cold hands and feet. It also promotes sweating and is ideal for "cold" conditions.

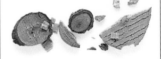

Applications

BARK
 DECOCTION Use for chronic diarrhea or complaints related to weakened kidney *qi* (energy). Can be used for "cold" conditions.

 TINCTURE Dilute up to 5 ml in a little hot water for colds and chills.

 POWDER/CAPSULES Use for "cold" conditions affecting the kidneys and digestion.

ESSENTIAL OIL
 INHALATION Dissolve 5 drops oil in boiling water and inhale the steam for coughs and respiratory irritation.

 MASSAGE OIL Dilute 10 drops cinnamon oil in 25 ml almond or sunflower oil and use for abdominal colic, stomach chills, or diarrhea.

TWIGS
 DECOCTION Take for colds, stomach chills, and as a circulatory stimulant. Combines well with ginger.

 TINCTURE Dilute up to 5 ml in a little hot water and use as the decoction.

 COMPRESS Soak a pad in the decoction or diluted tincture to relieve arthritic and rheumatic pain.

CAUTIONS
• Avoid therapeutic doses of cinnamon in pregnancy, especially the essential oil, because the herb is a potential uterine stimulant.
• Use the herb with care in overheated or feverish conditions.

Citrus spp.
ORANGE

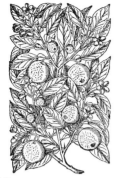

"*The sweet varieties increase bronchial secretion, and the sour promote expectoration. They quench thirst, and are stomachic and carminative.*"
Li Shi Zhen, 16th century.

A VALUABLE MEDICINAL HERB, the orange originated in China, and by the Middle Ages was a favorite with Arabian physicians. In the 16th century, an Italian princess named Anna-Marie de Nerola reputedly discovered an oil extracted from the flowers, which she used to scent her gloves; today neroli oil, as it became known, is prohibitively expensive. The Chinese remain the greatest enthusiasts of medicinal oranges: the bitter Seville orange (*C. aurantium*) and sweeter tangerines and satsumas (*C. reticulata*) are mainly used.

Character
C. AURANTIUM: sour, bitter, slightly cold.
C. RETICULATA: warm, pungent, bitter.
Constituents
Volatile oil, vitamins A, B, C, flavonoids, bitters.
Actions
C. AURANTIUM: carminative, digestive stimulant, nervine, increases blood pressure, diuretic, expectorant, energy tonic.
NEROLI OIL: sedative, tonic, antiseptic, antispasmodic, antidepressant.
C. RETICULATA: diuretic, digestive remedy, expectorant.

Parts used

FRUIT
C. AURANTIUM
In China, both the ripe and unripe fruit are used medicinally, although unripe bitter orange (*zhi shi*) is more potent than ripe (*zhi ke*). The fruit stimulates the digestion, so can help constipation, move stagnant *qi* (energy), and make a cooling expectorant for coughs, especially where the phlegm is thick and yellow. It also calms the nerves, so is useful for insomnia and shock.

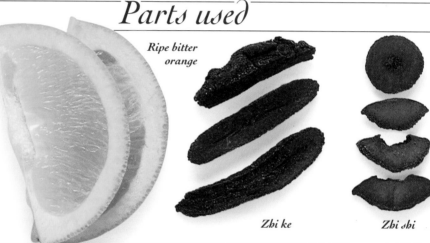

Ripe bitter orange

Zhi ke

Zhi shi

NEROLI OIL
C. AURANTIUM
Extracted from bitter orange blossoms, neroli oil is antidepressant and calming. It can also help chronic diarrhea and will not irritate dry skin or broken veins.

PEEL
C. RETICULATA
The Chinese use two forms: the green (*qing pi*) from unripe fruit and a well-dried type (*chen pi*) from ripe fruit. Both move stagnant *qi* (energy) and help the digestion; *chen pi* is also used as an expectorant for coughs, especially where there is a lot of thin, watery phlegm. Harvest from fresh unripe or ripe fruit, and dry.

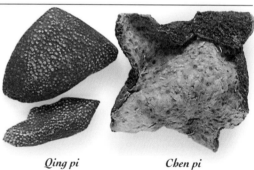

Qing pi

Chen pi

Applications

FRUIT
C. AURANTIUM

 DECOCTION Take for indigestion, constipation, or coughs. Combine with *dang gui* for menstrual pain.

 TINCTURE Use drop doses (see p.120) for uneasiness, shock, or insomnia.

NEROLI OIL
C. AURANTIUM

 CREAM Add 1-2 drops to skin cream and apply to any skin condition.

MASSAGE OIL Add 1-2 drops to 10 ml almond oil for nervous conditions and digestive upsets.

 ORANGE FLOWER WATER A by-product of steam distillation: take as a soothing carminative and for uneasiness, shock, or insomnia. Add 5-10 ml to a baby's bottle for colic or sleeplessness.

PEEL
C. RETICULATA

 DECOCTION Use both types of peel for indigestion and abdominal bloating. Take *chen pi* for coughs.

 SYRUP Take 2-4 ml syrup made from *chen pi* for coughs.

CAUTIONS
• If preparing your own *chen pi* from commercially purchased tangerines, use organic fruit to minimize pesticide contamination.
• Use bitter orange with caution in pregnancy; it can cause contractions.

Commiphora molmol
MYRRH

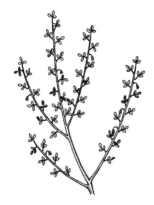

"The marvellous effects that it worketh in newe and greene wounds, were heere to long to set downe..."
John Gerard, 1597.

AN OLEO-GUM RESIN collected from the stems of bushy shrubs growing in Arabia and Somalia, myrrh has been regarded as one of the treasures of the East for millennia. Ancient Egyptian women burned myrrh in pellets to rid their homes of fleas. In folk tradition, myrrh was used for muscular pains and in rheumatic bandages. Called *mo yao* in China, it has been used since the Tang Dynasty (A.D. 600), primarily to heal wounds.

Character
Hot, dry, acrid, bitter.
Constituents
Volatile oil, resin, gums.
Actions
Antifungal, antiseptic, astringent, immune stimulant, bitter, expectorant, circulatory stimulant, reduces phlegm. Recent research suggests extracts may help prevent atherosclerosis.

Parts used

RESIN
The stems are cut, exuding a thick, pale yellow liquid. As it dries, this hardens to a reddish-brown solid, which can be dissolved in tinctures and oils. Astringent, the resin has been used extensively for wounds and is also excellent for sore throats and mouth ulcers. Research suggests that it can lower cholesterol levels. In China, it is taken to "move" blood and relieve painful swellings. Myrrh tastes particularly unpleasant.

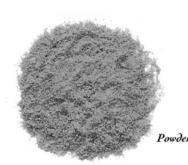

Powder

ESSENTIAL OIL
Distilled from the resin, myrrh oil has been used since Ancient Greek times to heal wounds. It is generally considered *yang* in character but is anti-inflammatory rather than heating. It makes a good expectorant, used in chest rubs for bronchitis and colds with heavy mucus.

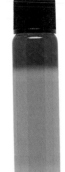

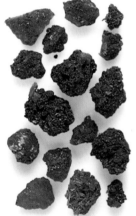

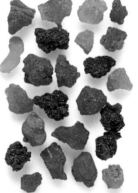

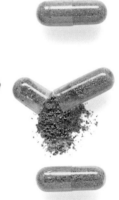

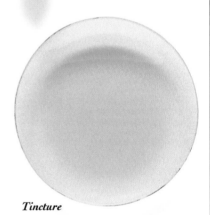

Mo yao   *Solid resin*   *Capsules*   *Tincture*

Applications

RESIN

 TINCTURE Use for infectious, feverish conditions, from head colds to mononucleosis. It is ideal for upper respiratory problems, and can be added to expectorant mixtures. Take up to 5 ml a day in 20-40 drop doses, well diluted with water.

 CAPSULES Use as a more palatable alternative to the tincture; take one 200 mg capsule up to 5 times a day.

 GARGLE/MOUTHWASH Use 20-40 drops tincture in half a cup of water for sore throats and mouth ulcers.

 DOUCHE Use the diluted tincture for vaginal yeast infections.

 POWDER In China, myrrh (3-9 g) is used as an analgesic, powdered with safflowers for abdominal pain associated with blood stagnation, as in menstrual pain.

ESSENTIAL OIL

 OIL Dilute 10 drops in 25 ml water, shake well, and use externally on wounds and chronic ulcers, or in lotions for hemorrhoids.

 CHEST RUB Use 1 ml oil in 15 ml almond or sunflower oil for bronchitis and colds with thick phlegm.

CAUTION
• Avoid in pregnancy, because it is a uterine stimulant.

Crataegus spp.
HAWTHORN

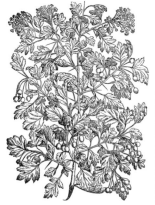

"Crataegus has quickly become one of the most widely used heart remedies."
Rudolf Weiss, 1985.

TRADITIONALLY VALUED for its astringency, hawthorn was used for diarrhea, heavy menstrual bleeding, and in first aid to draw splinters. Over the past century, the plant's considerable tonic action on the heart has been identified; today, it is one of the most popular cardiac herbs. The species generally used in the West are *C. oxycantha* and *C. monogyna*. In China, the berries of *C. pinnatifida* are taken as a digestive and circulatory stimulant.

Character
Flowering tops: cool; astringent taste.
Berries: sour, slightly sweet, warm.
Constituents
Flavonoid glycosides, procyanidins, saponins, tannins, minerals.
Actions
Relaxes peripheral blood vessels, cardiac tonic, astringent.

Parts used

FLOWERING TOPS
C. OXYCANTHA & C. MONOGYNA
The flowers are widely used as a heart tonic. Their precise action is still being researched, but it seems that they improve the coronary circulation, reducing the risk of angina pectoris attacks, and helping to normalize blood pressure. Large doses given by injection have been used successfully for highly irregular heartbeats. Harvest in early summer.

BERRIES
C. OXYCANTHA & C. MONOGYNA
Research suggests that the berries contain fewer cardiac-influencing constituents than the flowers, although both are prescribed by Western herbalists. The berries can also be used for diarrhea. Harvest when ripe in late summer or early fall.

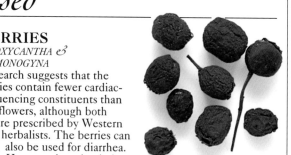
Dried berries

BERRIES
C. PINNATIFIDA
In China, the berries, called *shan zha*, are mainly taken for symptoms of "food stagnation," which can include abdominal bloating, indigestion, and flatulence. They are believed to "move" blood and are used to relieve stagnation, especially after childbirth. Partially charred berries are a standby for diarrhea.

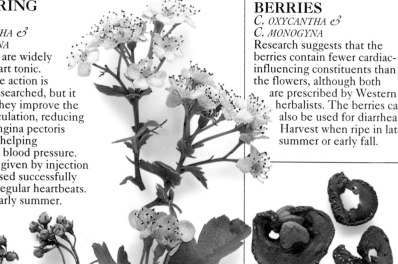

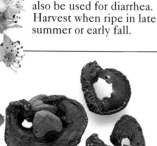
Dried shan zha

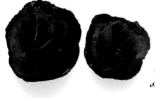
Charred shan zha

Dried flowering tops

Fresh flowering tops

Applications

FLOWERING TOPS
C. OXYCANTHA/C. MONOGYNA

 INFUSION Use to improve poor circulation and as a tonic for heart problems. Combine with yarrow or *ju hua* for hypertension.

 TINCTURE Prescribed with other cardiac herbs for angina, hypertension, and related disorders.

BERRIES
C. OXYCANTHA/C. MONOGYNA

 DECOCTION Use 30 g berries to 2 cups (500 ml) water and decoct for 15 minutes only. Take for diarrhea, or with *ju hua* and *gou qi zi* for hypertension.

 JUICE Use juice from the fresh berries as a cardiac tonic; also for diarrhea, poor digestion, or as a general digestive tonic.

BERRIES
C. PINNATIFIDA

 DECOCTION Use 10-20 g in 2 cups (500 ml) water with *zhi ke* for abdominal bloating, or combine with *dan shen* and *dang gui* for menstrual and postpartum pain.

 CAPSULES Use the powdered berries with *san qi* powder for abdominal pain due to blood stagnation, or for the pain of angina.

Dendranthema x grandiflorum
JU HUA

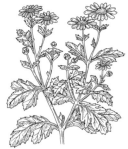

"It mainly treats head wind, head dizziness, and head swelling, and pain with the eyes as if they were fit to burst from their sockets.
Ben Cao Jing, *Shen Nong, c.* 2500 BC.

CHRYSANTHEMUM FLOWERS have been used in Chinese medicine since the days of Emperor Shen Nung (c. 2500 BC) and are associated with liver and eye complaints. The leaves have been used medicinally since around AD 500, and the stems and root are traditionally used in folk medicine. In China, the herb is drunk as a tonic in chrysanthemum wine, and as a popular cooling tea. Chrysanthemums were first introduced into Europe in the 17th century, although it was a 100 years more before they became a familiar ornamental garden plant.

Character
Flowers: pungent, sweet, bitter, cool.
Leaves: hot, wet, neutral.
Constituents
Essential oil (inc. camphor, carvone and borneol), alkaloids (inc. stachydrine and adenine), sesquiterpene lactones, flavonoids.
Actions
Cooling, anti-inflammatory, antimicrobial, reduces fevers, promotes sweating, antiseptic, lowers blood pressure, dilates coronary artery and stimulates blood flow.

Parts used

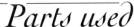

FLOWER HEADS
In China, the flower heads are steamed before drying to reduce bitterness. They are used to cool and calm the liver, clear toxins, soothe eye inflammation, and clear wind and heat. Research has shown that *ju hua* can reduce high blood pressure, especially if associated with headaches and dizziness. Given as a relaxant for the coronary arteries, it may relieve the pain of angina pectoris.

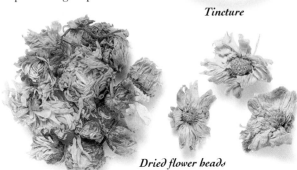

Tincture

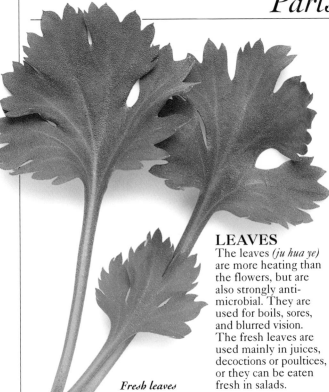

LEAVES
The leaves (*ju hua ye*) are more heating than the flowers, but are also strongly anti-microbial. They are used for boils, sores, and blurred vision. The fresh leaves are used mainly in juices, decoctions or poultices, or they can be eaten fresh in salads.

Fresh leaves

Dried flower heads

Applications

LEAVES

 POULTICE Use the crushed, fresh leaves soaked in a little warm water or alcohol for boils, acne pustules, and skin sores.

 DECOCTION Take a regular decoction of dried leaves to relieve symptoms of vertigo or dizziness.

FLOWER HEADS

 INFUSION Drink regular cups to ease eye strain and headaches associated with overwork, stress, irritability, and emotional upset.

 TINCTURE Use up to 50 drops per dose for headaches and irritability.

 DECOCTION Use with an equal amount of *jin yin hua* in a standard decoction to help reduce high blood pressure. *Ju hua* can also be combined with mulberry leaf, mint and apricot seeds for common colds and coughs.

 POWDER Add 1/2 tsp powder to a small glass of rice wine to relieve vertigo.

 POULTICE Use a few of the infused flowers on gauze as eye pads to relieve the pain of eyestrain, conjunctivitis, and other red or painful eye conditions.

CAUTION
• Avoid *ju hua* if there is diarrhea or debility.

Dioscorea spp.
YAM

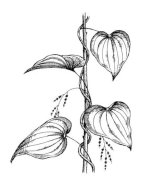

"...wild yams contain diosgenin, a precursor in the synthesis of progesterone."
Rudolf Weiss, 1985.

USED TO MAKE THE ORIGINAL contraceptive pills when synthetic hormone production was not a commercial proposition, Mexican wild yam (*D. villosa*) contains hormonal substances very similar to progesterone. It also relaxes smooth muscle; hence another of its common names, colic root. Many other yams are used as a starter material to produce hydrocortisones for orthodox eczema creams. Several related species are popular in China: *D. hypoglauca* is used for urinary disorders, while *D. opposita* is an important spleen and stomach tonic.

Character
Neutral, generally drying, bitter (most species) or sweet (*D. opposita*).
Constituents
Alkaloids, steroidal saponins, tannins, phytosterols, starch.
Actions
D. VILLOSA: relaxant for smooth muscle, antispasmodic, promotes bile flow, anti-inflammatory, promotes sweating, hormonal action.
D. OPPOSITA: expectorant, digestive stimulant, kidney tonic.
D. HYPOGLAUCA: antibacterial, anti-inflammatory, soothes urinary tract infections.

Parts used

RHIZOME
D. VILLOSA
Mexican wild yam is an important muscle relaxant and antispasmodic, used for colicky pains. It can also be taken for acute rheumatic conditions.

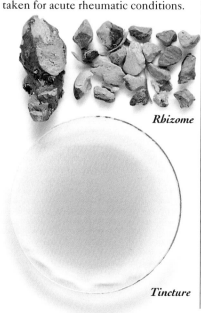

Rhizome

Tincture

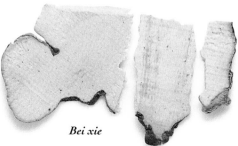

Shan yao

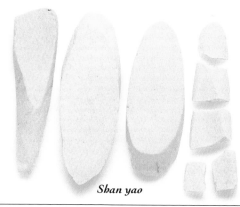

Bei xie

RHIZOME
D. OPPOSITA
The Chinese yam, *shan yao*, is an important tonic herb in Chinese medicine. Its main action is on the kidneys, lungs, and stomach, and it is included in remedies for asthma, menopausal syndrome, urinary disorders, and weak kidney energies.

RHIZOME
D. HYPOGLAUCA
In China, *bei xie* (or "seven-lobed yam") is used mainly for urinary tract infections such as cystitis. Antibacterial and anti-inflammatory, it also relieves rheumatoid arthritis. Extracts of *bei xie* are used in the synthesis of contraceptive pills.

Applications

RHIZOME
D. VILLOSA

DECOCTION Use for the colicky pains associated with irritable bowel syndrome or diverticulosis. Can also be used for period pain, or during labor. Decoct with willow bark for arthritic pains.

TINCTURE Take 5-10 drops as required for labor or postpartum pains. Can be combined with arthritic remedies, such as celery seeds, angelica, meadowsweet, bogbean, or willow, for the acute stages of rheumatoid arthritis.

RHIZOME
D. OPPOSITA

DECOCTION Combine with herbs such as *shu di huang*, *shan zhu yu*, *fu ling*, *gou qi zi* and licorice for menopausal symptoms associated with kidney *yin* deficiency.

TINCTURE Use for dry asthmatic coughs.

RHIZOME
D. HYPOGLAUCA

DECOCTION Use with *huai niu xi* for rheumatic pains.

TINCTURE Take up to 10 ml a day for urinary infections.

CAUTION
• Avoid large doses of *D. villosa* in pregnancy unless under professional guidance; may be taken during labor.

Echinacea spp.
ECHINACEA

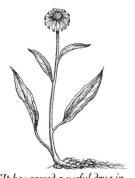

"It has proved a useful drug in improving the body's own resistance in infectious conditions of all kinds..."
Rudolf Weiss, 1985.

THE NATIVE AMERICANS used echinacea to treat snakebite, fevers, and old, stubborn wounds. The early settlers soon adopted the plant as a home remedy for colds and influenza, and it became popular with the 19th-century Eclectics (see pp. 20-21). In the past 50 years, it has achieved worldwide fame for its antiviral, antifungal, and antibacterial properties, and it has also been used in AIDS therapy. Cultivated purple coneflower is usually *E. purpurea*, although *E. angustifolia* is considered more potent by some practitioners.

Character
Cool, dry, mainly pungent.
Constituents
Volatile oil, glycosides, amides, antibiotic polyacetylenes, inulin.
Actions
Antibiotic, immune stimulant, antiallergenic, lymphatic tonic.

Parts used

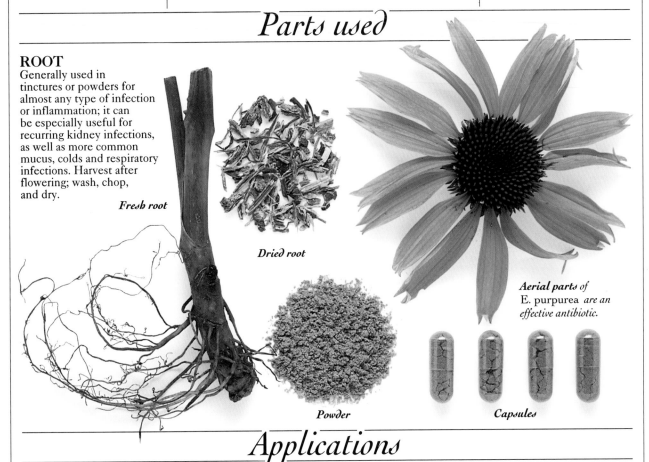

ROOT
Generally used in tinctures or powders for almost any type of infection or inflammation; it can be especially useful for recurring kidney infections, as well as more common mucus, colds and respiratory infections. Harvest after flowering; wash, chop, and dry.

Fresh root

Dried root

Powder

Aerial parts of E. purpurea *are an effective antibiotic.*

Capsules

Applications

ROOT

 DECOCTION Take 10 ml doses every 1-2 hours for the acute stage of infections.

 TINCTURE Take 2-5 ml doses every 2-3 hours for influenza, chills, and urinary tract infections, during the first couple of days of acute symptoms. For more chronic conditions, use standard doses and combine with other suitable herbs, such as buchu and couchgrass for kidney infections, or cleavers for mononucleosis. May be used in 10 ml doses for food poisoning or snakebites.

 WASH Use the decoction or diluted tincture for infected wounds. Bathe the affected area frequently.

 GARGLE Use 10 ml tincture in a glass of warm water for sore throats.

 POWDER Use as a dust for infected skin conditions such as boils (combine with marshmallow) or weeping, infected eczema.

 CAPSULES Take three 200 mg capsules up to three times a day at the onset of acute infections, such as colds, influenza, and kidney or urinary tract infections.

CAUTIONS
• High doses can occasionally cause nausea and dizziness.
• Allergic reaction to echinacea is extremely rare but has been reported.
• Do not take during pregnancy.

Ephedra sinica
MA HUANG

IN CHINA, MA HUANG has been used as an anti-asthmatic for at least 5,000 years. The alkaloid ephedrine, extracted from the plant, was first identified by Chinese scientists in 1924; two years later the pharmaceutical company Merck produced a synthetic version, still used to treat asthma. The Indian variety, *E. gerardiana*, is thought to have been the prime ingredient of *soma*, a potent tonic and elixir of youth.

"As a wise man I have taken soma, the sweet draught that gives strength, lending immortal power and freedom to the gods."
The *Rig Veda*, c. 1000 B.C.

Character
Twigs: pungent, bitter, warm.
Root: pungent, neutral.
Constituents
Alkaloids (inc. ephedrine), saponins, volatile oil.
Actions
Twigs: antispasmodic, febrifuge, promote sweating, diuretic; antibacterial and antiviral properties identified in the essential oil, variable action on blood pressure.
Root: antihydrotic.

Parts used

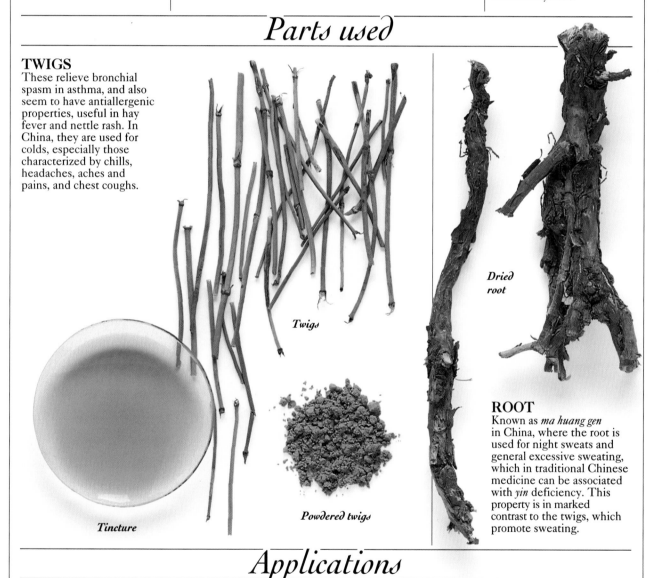

TWIGS
These relieve bronchial spasm in asthma, and also seem to have antiallergenic properties, useful in hay fever and nettle rash. In China, they are used for colds, especially those characterized by chills, headaches, aches and pains, and chest coughs.

Twigs

Dried root

Tincture

Powdered twigs

ROOT
Known as *ma huang gen* in China, where the root is used for night sweats and general excessive sweating, which in traditional Chinese medicine can be associated with *yin* deficiency. This property is in marked contrast to the twigs, which promote sweating.

Applications

TWIGS

TINCTURE Prescribed for asthma, hay fever, or severe chills. Combined with cowslip root and thyme tinctures for bronchial asthma, emphysema, whooping cough, and other severe chest conditions.

DECOCTION Prescribed for common colds, coughs, asthma, and hay fever.

ROOT

DECOCTION The Chinese use the decoction where *yin* or *qi* (energy) weakness leads to uncontrolled sweating.

CAUTIONS
• Do not use in pregnancy.
• Not to be used by patients taking monoamine oxidase inhibitors as antidepressants.
• Avoid in glaucoma, hypertension, and coronary thrombosis; do not combine with other stimulants.
• Possible side effects are: headache, nausea, vomiting, restlessness, tachycardias, and high blood pressure.

Equisetum spp.
HORSETAIL

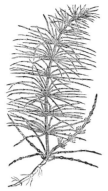

A PREHISTORIC BOTANICAL RELIC, horsetail is a close relative of the trees that grew on earth 270 million years ago in the Carboniferous period, and are the source of our modern coal seams. Its brittle jointed stems are rich in healing silica, and since the time of the Ancient Greeks, horsetail has been used for wounds. It is now considered an invasive weed. The Chinese use *E. hyemale*, or *mu zei*.

"So wonderful is its nature, its mere touch staunches a patient's bleeding."
Pliny, A.D. 77.

Character
Cold, dry, slightly bitter.
Constituents
Silica, alkaloids (inc. nicotine), saponins, flavonoids, bitter principle, minerals (inc. potassium, manganese, magnesium), phytosterols, tannins.
Actions
Astringent, stops bleeding, diuretic, anti-inflammatory, tissue healer.

Parts used

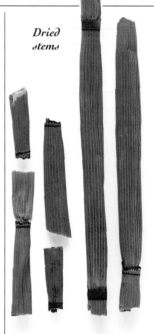

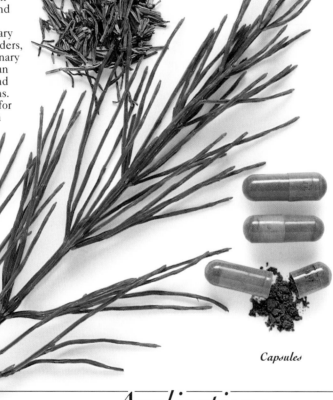

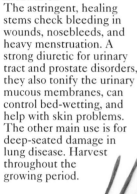

AERIAL PARTS
E. ARVENSE
The astringent, healing stems check bleeding in wounds, nosebleeds, and heavy menstruation. A strong diuretic for urinary tract and prostate disorders, they also tonify the urinary mucous membranes, can control bed-wetting, and help with skin problems. The other main use is for deep-seated damage in lung disease. Harvest throughout the growing period.

Dried aerial parts

Dried stems

Fresh aerial parts

Capsules

AERIAL PARTS
E. HYEMALE
In China, these are mainly used to cool fevers and as a remedy for eye inflammations, such as conjunctivitis and corneal disorders.

Applications

AERIAL PARTS
E. ARVENSE

 DECOCTION Use for heavy menstruation, and skin conditions such as acne and eczema: simmer for at least three hours to extract the main constituents. Prescribed for stomach ulcers, urinary tract inflammations, and prostate and lung disorders.

 POULTICE Make the powder into a paste and use on leg ulcers, wounds, sores, and chilblains.

 MOUTHWASH/GARGLE Dilute the decoction and use for mouth and gum infections or throat inflammations.

 JUICE The liquidized stems are the best form of horsetail: take 5-10 ml, three times a day, for urinary disorders. For nosebleeds, dip a cotton wool swab in a little juice and insert in the nostril. Also prescribed for long-standing lung damage.

 CAPSULES Taking powdered horsetail in capsule form can be more convenient than juices or decoctions; use for the same ailments (excepting nosebleeds).

CAUTIONS
• Seek professional guidance if there is blood in the urine, or for sudden changes in menstrual flow leading to heavy bleeding.
• Though no adverse effects have been reported, horsetail is banned in Canada, except in products where thiaminase-like compounds present in the herb have been removed.

Eucalyptus globulus
EUCALYPTUS

A TRADITIONAL ABORIGINAL fever remedy, eucalyptus was introduced to the West in the 19th century by the director of the Melbourne Botanical Gardens, and cultivation of the tree spread in southern Europe and North America. The properties of oils from different species vary slightly, but all are very antiseptic. Russian research suggests that some species counteract influenza viruses; others are antimalarial or highly active against bacteria.

"For every kind of wound made, father used eucalyptus leaves as taught by the blacks."
May Gilmore, quoted in Bill Wannan, *Folk Medicine*.

Character
Cool, moist, pungent, bitter.
Constituents
Volatile oil, tannins, aldehydes, bitter resin.
Actions
Antiseptic, antispasmodic, stimulant, febrifuge, expectorant, reduces blood sugar levels, expels worms.

Parts used

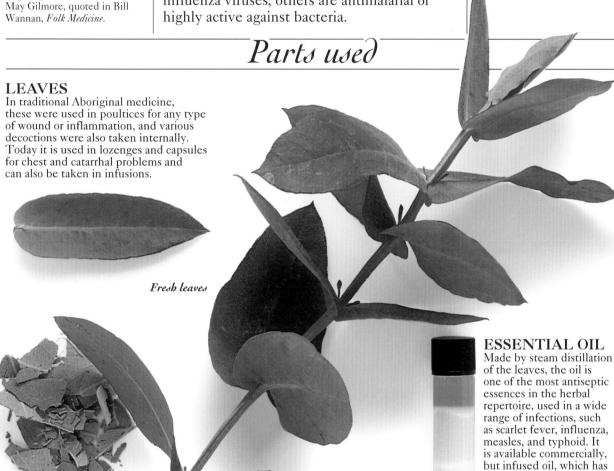

LEAVES
In traditional Aboriginal medicine, these were used in poultices for any type of wound or inflammation, and various decoctions were also taken internally. Today it is used in lozenges and capsules for chest and catarrhal problems and can also be taken in infusions.

Fresh leaves

Dried leaves

ESSENTIAL OIL
Made by steam distillation of the leaves, the oil is one of the most antiseptic essences in the herbal repertoire, used in a wide range of infections, such as scarlet fever, influenza, measles, and typhoid. It is available commercially, but infused oil, which has a similar but less potent action, can be made at home (see p. 154).

Applications

LEAVES

 INHALATION Powdered leaves are available in commercial capsules (200-250 g) for treating respiratory infections and bronchitis.

ESSENTIAL OIL

 COMPRESS Soak a pad in 2 ml oil well dispersed in ½ cup (100 ml) water, and apply to inflammations, painful joints, and burns.

 GARGLE Dilute 5 drops oil in a glass of water, mix well, and gargle for throat infections.

 CHEST RUB Dilute 0.5- 2 ml oil in 25 ml almond oil for colds, bronchitis, asthma, and influenza.

 INHALATION Add 10 drops oil or fresh leaves to hot water, and inhale the steam for chest infections.

 OIL Dilute 2 drops oil in 10 ml sunflower oil or ointment base, and apply to cold sores.

 MASSAGE OIL Combine 10- 20 drops eucalyptus oil with 10- 20 drops rosemary oil in 20 ml infused bladderwrack oil or almond oil for rheumatic or arthritic pain.

CAUTIONS
• In rare cases leads to nausea, vomiting, and diarrhea.
• Use with caution in giving to small children.

Eupatorium spp.
GRAVELROOT

A FAVORITE WITH NATIVE Americans, gravelroot (*E. purpureum*) was known as Joe-Pye weed after a New England medicine man who used it to cure typhus. Boneset (*E. perfoliatum*) was similarly used for "boneset fever"; and is an effective antiviral for influenza. A related European species, hemp agrimony (*E. cannabium*), has undergone a revival because immunostimulant constituents, which increase resistance in viral infections, have been identified in the herb.

"For a cough, bruise hemp agrimony in a mortar and mix the juice with boiling milk, strain and use."
Remedy of the Physicians of Myddfai, Wales, 13th century.

Character
Bitter, pungent, drying; cool or cold depending on species.
Constituents
Tannins, bitter principle, flavonoids, sesquiterpene lactones.
Actions
E. CANNABIUM: febrifuge, diuretic, prevents scurvy, laxative, promotes bile flow and sweating, expectorant, antirheumatic, immune stimulant.
E. PURPUREUM: diuretic, antirheumatic, promotes menstruation.

Parts used

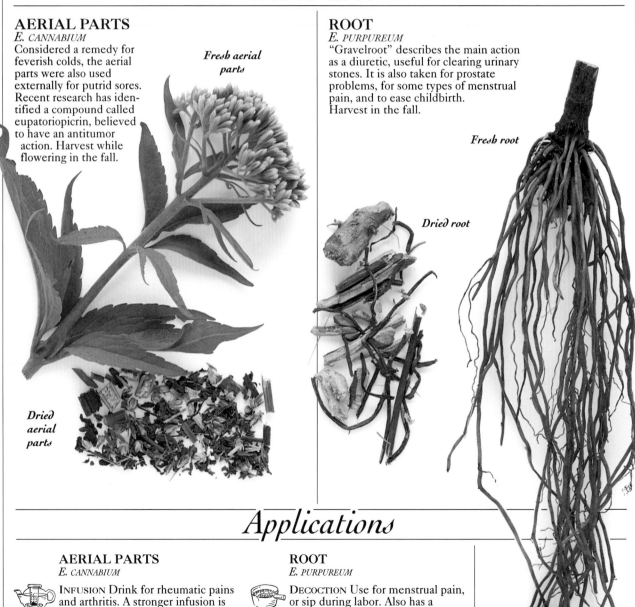

AERIAL PARTS
E. CANNABIUM
Considered a remedy for feverish colds, the aerial parts were also used externally for putrid sores. Recent research has identified a compound called eupatoriopicrin, believed to have an antitumor action. Harvest while flowering in the fall.

Fresh aerial parts

Dried aerial parts

ROOT
E. PURPUREUM
"Gravelroot" describes the main action as a diuretic, useful for clearing urinary stones. It is also taken for prostate problems, for some types of menstrual pain, and to ease childbirth. Harvest in the fall.

Fresh root

Dried root

Applications

AERIAL PARTS
E. CANNABIUM

 INFUSION Drink for rheumatic pains and arthritis. A stronger infusion is purgative for liver stagnation and some types of constipation.

 TINCTURE Take 5 drops as required for feverish colds and influenza. Add to phlegm-reducing mixtures, with herbs such as elderflower and ground ivy.

ROOT
E. PURPUREUM

 DECOCTION Use for menstrual pain, or sip during labor. Also has a cleansing effect for persistent urinary infections.

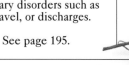 TINCTURE Take 2-3 ml, three times a day, for urinary disorders such as cystitis and gravel, or discharges.

CAUTIONS See page 195.

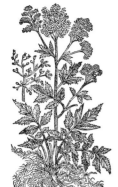

Filipendula ulmaria
MEADOWSWEET

A POPULAR ELIZABETHAN "strewing herb," meadowsweet was also used to ease fever and pains. Anti-inflammatory chemicals called salicylates were first extracted from it in the 1830s. Some 60 years later, the pharmaceutical company Bayer produced acetylsalicylate, a similar substance, artificially. They called this new "wonder drug" aspirin, after *Spiraea ulmaria*, the old botanical name for this herb.

"... the flowers boiled in wine and drunke, do take away the fits of a quartaine fever..."
John Gerard, 1597.

Character
Cold, astringent taste; both moist and drying.
Constituents
Salicylates, flavonoids, tannins, volatile oil, citric acid, mucilage.
Actions
Anti-inflammatory, antirheumatic, soothing digestive remedy, diuretic, promotes sweating.

Parts used

AERIAL PARTS
The cooling aerial parts reduce inflammations and fevers, protect the digestive tract, and modify the action of salicylic acid. Long use of aspirin can lead to gastric ulceration and bleeding, but meadowsweet does not show these side effects, and is actually a gentle digestive remedy for acidity and some types of diarrhea. Harvest while flowering in summer.

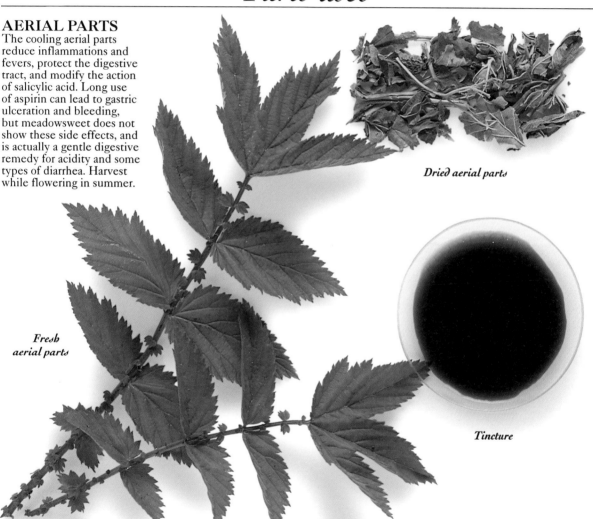

Dried aerial parts

Fresh aerial parts

Tincture

Applications

AERIAL PARTS

INFUSION Take for feverish colds or rheumatic pains. Also soothing for children's stomach upsets.

TINCTURE Generally has a stronger action than the infusion. Add to remedies for gastric ulceration or excess acidity, such as licorice. Use with herbs such as angelica or willow for arthritis.

COMPRESS Soak a pad in the dilute tincture, and apply to painful arthritic and rheumatic joints, or use for neuralgia.

EYEWASH Cool and strain the infusion, and use for conjunctivitis and other eye complaints.

CAUTIONS
• Avoid the herb in cases of salicylate sensitivity.
• If using the tincture for gastric ulceration or excess acidity, use the hot-water method (see p. 157) to reduce the alcohol.

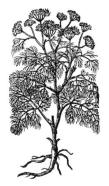

"…both the seeds, leaves and root of our Garden Fennel are much used in drinks and broths for those that are grown fat..."
William Coles, 1650.

Foeniculum officinale
FENNEL

THE ROMANS BELIEVED that serpents sucked the juice of the plant to improve their eyesight, and Pliny recommends the herb for "dimness of human vision." Fennel was also regarded as an early slimming aid, its Greek name *marathron* reputedly derived from a verb meaning "to grow thin." In medieval times, chewing the seeds was a favorite way to stop gastric rumbles during church sermons.

Character
Warming, dry, pungent, sweet.
Constituents
Volatile oil (inc. estragole, anethole), essential fatty acids, flavonoids (inc. rutin), vitamins, minerals.
Actions
Carminative, circulatory stimulant, anti-inflammatory, promotes milk flow, mild expectorant, diuretic.

Parts used

SEEDS
Soothing for the digestion, the seeds also promote milk flow in breast-feeding. When the infusion is taken by nursing mothers, it can also relieve colic in babies. In Chinese medicine, the seeds (*hui xiang*) are thought tonifying for the spleen and kidneys, and are used for urinary and reproductive disharmonies. Harvest in fall when ripe.

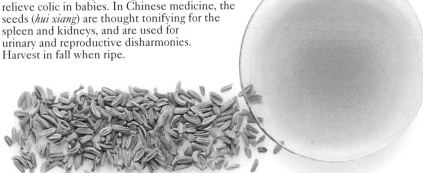

Seeds

Tincture

ESSENTIAL OIL
The oil distilled from the seeds is mainly prescribed for digestive problems and, as a mild expectorant, for coughs and respiratory complaints.

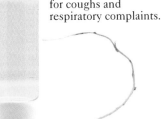

ROOT
Not as effective as the seeds, the root was once used in similar ways. Today it is mainly taken for urinary disorders. Harvest in late fall, when the bulbous stems are collected as a vegetable.

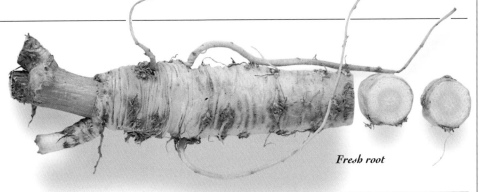

Fresh root

Applications

SEEDS

 INFUSION A useful and palatable digestive remedy: drink after meals for flatulence, indigestion, colic, and other digestive upsets. Can also be taken by nursing mothers to increase milk flow or to relieve a baby's colic.

 DECOCTION Used in Chinese medicine for abdominal pain, colic, and stomach chills.

 TINCTURE Use for digestive problems; combine with laxatives such as rhubarb root or senna to prevent colic.

 MOUTHWASH/GARGLE Use the infusion for gum disorders, loose teeth, laryngitis, or sore throats.

ESSENTIAL OIL

 CHEST RUB Dissolve a total of 25 drops thyme, eucalyptus, and fennel oils in 25 ml sunflower or almond oil for chest complaints.

ROOT

 DECOCTION Prescribed for urinary problems, such as kidney stones, or disorders associated with high uric acid content.

CAUTION
• Fennel is a uterine stimulant, so avoid high doses of the herb in pregnancy; small amounts used in cooking are safe.

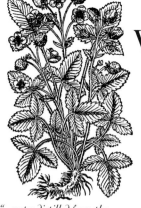

Fragaria vesca
WILD STRAWBERRIES

THE BERRIES, LEAVES, AND ROOT of the wild or "alpine" strawberry have all been used medicinally in the past. The root was once a popular household remedy for diarrhea, and the stalks were used for wounds. The berries were considered cooling; according to Gerard, they "quench thirst, cooleth heate of the stomicke and inflammation of the liver." However, eating them in winter or on a "cold stomicke" was thought to risk an increase in phlegmatic humor and digestive upsets.

"...water distilled from the berries is good for the passions of the heart caused by perturbation of the spirits."
John Parkinson, 1640.

Character
Cool, moist, sweet and sour.
Constituents
Tannins, mucilage, sugars, fruit acids, salicylates, minerals, vitamins B, C, E.
Actions
Astringent, heals wounds, diuretic, laxative, liver tonic, cleansing.

Parts used

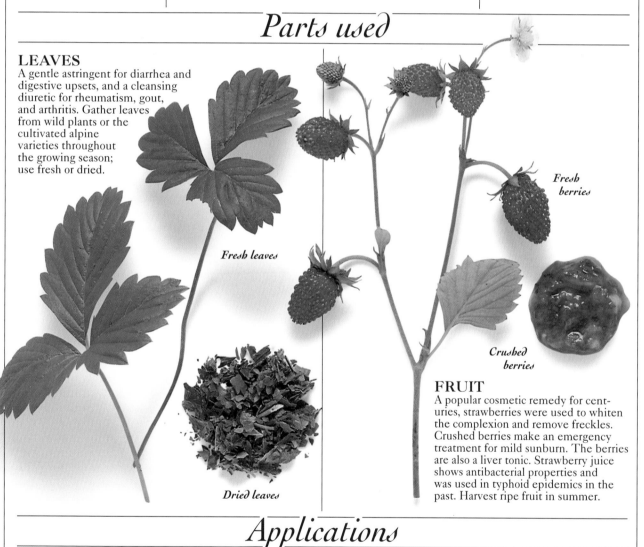

LEAVES
A gentle astringent for diarrhea and digestive upsets, and a cleansing diuretic for rheumatism, gout, and arthritis. Gather leaves from wild plants or the cultivated alpine varieties throughout the growing season; use fresh or dried.

Fresh leaves

Dried leaves

Fresh berries

Crushed berries

FRUIT
A popular cosmetic remedy for centuries, strawberries were used to whiten the complexion and remove freckles. Crushed berries make an emergency treatment for mild sunburn. The berries are also a liver tonic. Strawberry juice shows antibacterial properties and was used in typhoid epidemics in the past. Harvest ripe fruit in summer.

Applications

LEAVES

 INFUSION Take for diarrhea, for gastric inflammations and infections, and for jaundice; use also as an appetite stimulant. Combine with meadowsweet and St. John's wort for mild arthritic pains, or with celery seed for gout.

FRUIT

 FRESH Eat strawberries for gastritis and as a liver tonic: they are good

during convalescence after hepatitis. Also useful in feverish conditions, they are both cooling and unlikely to cause fermentation in the stomach.

 POULTICE Apply crushed berries to areas of sunburn or other skin inflammations.

 TONIC WINE Steep the berries in wine to make a traditional remedy for "reviving the spirits and making the hart merrie."

Fucus vesiculosis
BLADDERWRACK

SEVERAL VARIETIES OF THIS SEAWEED have been used therapeutically. In the 18th century, iodine was isolated by distilling the long ribbons, or thalli, and bladderwrack was this element's main source for more than 50 years. The herb was used extensively to treat goiter, a swelling of the thyroid related to lack of iodine. In the 1860s it was claimed that bladderwrack, as a thyroid stimulant, could counter obesity by increasing the metabolic rate. Since then, it has been featured in numerous slimming remedies.

Character
Salty, cool, moist.
Constituents
Mucilage, iodine and other minerals, mannitol, volatile oil.
Actions
Metabolic stimulant, nutritive, thyroid tonic, antirheumatic, anti-inflammatory.

"...another trial resulted in the cure of some sick horses fed on seaweed, while others fed on oats remained out of health."
Maud Grieve, 1931.

Parts used

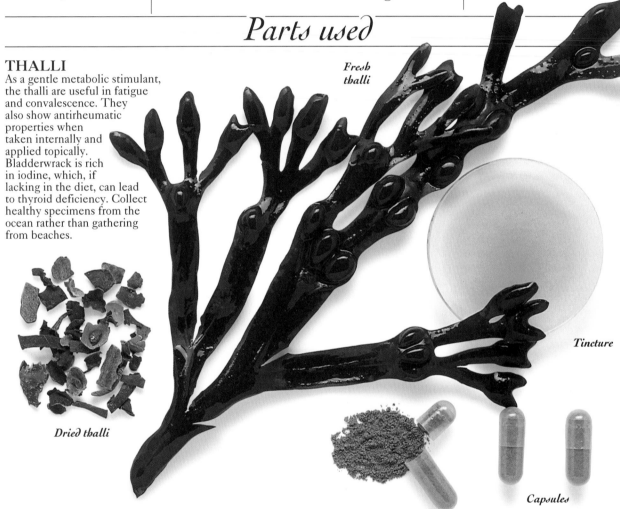

THALLI
As a gentle metabolic stimulant, the thalli are useful in fatigue and convalescence. They also show antirheumatic properties when taken internally and applied topically. Bladderwrack is rich in iodine, which, if lacking in the diet, can lead to thyroid deficiency. Collect healthy specimens from the ocean rather than gathering from beaches.

Fresh thalli

Tincture

Dried thalli

Capsules

Applications

THALLI
 TINCTURE Take for thyroid deficiency, as a gentle metabolic stimulant, or for rheumatic conditions.

 INFUSION Take as the tincture. Can be used as part of a weight-reducing program, especially if obesity is linked to a slow metabolism, but it should not be regarded as an easy method for losing weight.

 PILLS/CAPSULES Take 3-6 a day as a metabolic stimulant. Can help reduce obesity related to thyroid underactivity.

 INFUSED OIL Macerate 500 g dried bladderwrack overnight in 2 cups (500 ml) sunflower oil. Heat in a waterbath for two hours and strain. Use the oil externally for arthritic joint pains or rheumatism.

CAUTIONS
• Like many sea creatures, bladderwrack is at risk from heavy metal pollution. Do not collect where levels of cadmium and mercury are known to be high.
• Avoid if you suffer from hyperthyroidism.

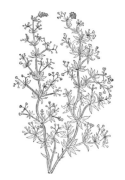

Galium aparine
CLEAVERS

A POPULAR HERB in folk medicine throughout the centuries, cleavers or goosegrass is a vigorously growing weed that twines through hedges or garden shrubberies producing long sticky stems. The young shoots are some of the first weeds to appear in spring and make an excellent cleansing tonic, a remedy widely used in central Europe and the Balkans.

"Women do usually make pottage of clevers... to cause lanknesse and keepe them from fatnes."
John Gerard, 1597.

Character
Cold, slightly dry, salty.
Constituents
Coumarins, tannins, glycosides, citric acid.
Actions
Diuretic, lymphatic cleanser, mild astringent.

Parts used

AERIAL PARTS
Best used fresh, the aerial parts are a potent diuretic and lymphatic cleanser, effective in many cases involving swollen or enlarged lymph glands. Often described as a blood purifier, they are used for skin problems and other conditions where the body is failing to rid itself of toxins. They can also be cooked as a vegetable, gently sweated in the pan like spinach. Harvest from spring to fall.

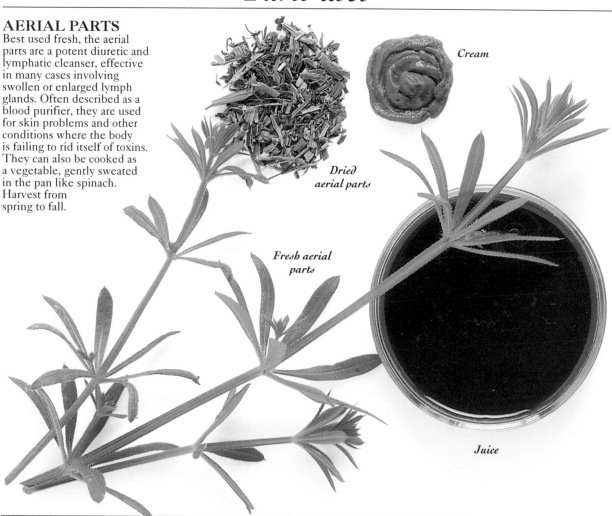

Cream

Dried aerial parts

Fresh aerial parts

Juice

Applications

AERIAL PARTS

 JUICE Liquidize or pulp the fresh plant to make an effective diuretic and lymphatic cleanser for a range of conditions, including glandular fever, tonsillitis, and prostate disorders.

 INFUSION Generally less strong than the juice. Use for urinary problems such as cystitis and gravel; also take as a cooling drink for fevers.

 TINCTURE Use for the same ailments as the infusion. Can be combined with other lymphatic and detoxifying herbs such as dried pokeroot or *lian qiao*.

 COMPRESS Soak a pad in the infusion and use for burns, scrapes, ulcers, and other skin inflammations.

 CREAM Use regularly to relieve psoriasis.

 HAIR RINSE Use the infusion for dandruff or scaling scalp problems.

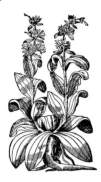

"It is reported to be good for... such as have evill livers and bad stomackes."
John Gerard, 1597.

Gentiana spp.
GENTIAN

THE HERB REPUTEDLY TAKES its name from a king of Illyria who discovered its ability to reduce fevers. In medieval times, gentian was an ingredient of the alchemical brew *theriac*, a cure-all made to a highly secret recipe. *G. lutea* is used in the West, while the Chinese usually use either the large-leaved gentian, *G. macro-phylla* (*qin jiao*), or *G. scabra* (*long dan cao*).

Character
Very bitter, cold, astringent, drying.
Constituents
Bitter glycosides, alkaloids, flavonoids.
Actions
Bitter, tonic, appetite and gastric stimulant, anti-inflammatory, febrifuge.

Parts used

ROOT
G. LUTEA
A strong bitter digestive stimulant, the root is effective for conditions involving poor appetite or sluggish digestion. It is also used in fevers, cooling the system, and maintaining digestive function, so that stomach contents do not stagnate, leading to further health problems. Harvest in late summer and fall.

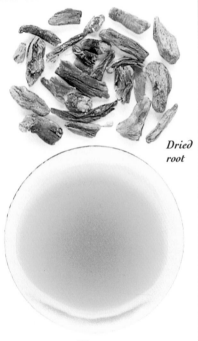

Dried root

Tincture

ROOT
G. MACROPHYLLA & G. SCABRA
Bitter remedies, these roots are used for digestive and feverish conditions. In Chinese medicine, they are usually described as clearing "heat and damp," and may be prescribed for some types of hypertension related to heat in the liver, or for urinary infections and rheumatic disorders.

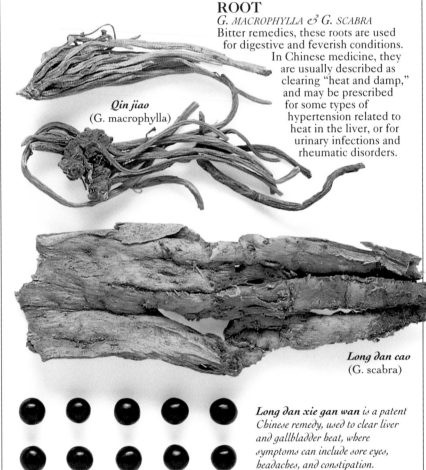

Qin jiao
(G. macrophylla)

Long dan cao
(G. scabra)

Long dan xie gan wan is a patent Chinese remedy, used to clear liver and gallbladder heat, where symptoms can include sore eyes, headaches, and constipation.

Applications

ROOT
G. LUTEA

 DECOCTION Use 10 g herb to 2 cups (500 ml) water and decoct for 20 minutes. Take before meals for fullness and stomach pains.

 TINCTURE Take up to 2 ml three times a day as a digestive stimulant, or in drop doses to allay cravings for sweet foods. Prescribed for liver disease, including hepatitis, gallbladder inflammations, and where jaundice is a symptom.

ROOT
G. MACROPHYLLA

 DECOCTION Use in combination with other herbs, such as *du huo* and cinnamon, for rheumatic pains, fevers, and allergic inflammations.

ROOT
G. SCABRA

 DECOCTION Use in combination with other herbs, such as *chai hu*, *zhi zi* and *huang qin*, for liver disorders, hypertension, and urinary infections.

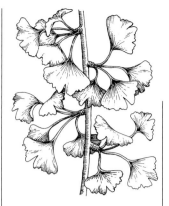

Ginkgo biloba
GINKGO

D ATING BACK AT LEAST 200 million years, the wild maidenhair tree has probably been extinct for centuries, but cultivated trees survived in Far Eastern temple gardens. A deciduous conifer with separate male and female forms, the tree was introduced into Europe in 1730 and became a favorite ornamental. Since the 1980s, Western medical interest in the plant has grown dramatically since its potent actions on the cardiovascular system were identified.

"Significant improvement in mental states, emotional lability, memory, and tendency to tire easily, have been reported..."
Rudolf Weiss, 1985.

Character
Sweet, bitter, astringent, neutral.
Constituents
Leaves: flavone glycosides, bioflavones, lactones, sitosterol, anthocyanin.
Seeds: fatty acids, minerals, bioflavones.
Actions
Leaves: relax blood vessels, circulatory stimulant, anti-inflammatory.
Seeds: astringent, antifungal, antibacterial.

Parts used

LEAVES
Part of the herbal repertoire only since the 1980s, the leaves are used for circulatory diseases; they are particularly good at improving blood flow to the brain. Research has shown that ginkgolide can be as effective as standard pharmaceutical drugs in treating severely irregular heartbeats. The leaves are also used for varicose veins, hemorrhoids, and leg ulcers. Recent studies have suggested that it can help reduce the symptoms of dementia in Alzheimer's disease. Harvest in summer.

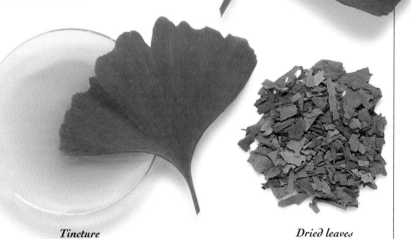

Fresh leaves

SEEDS
In China, the seeds, called *bai gou*, are considered to act on the lung and kidney acupuncture meridians and are traditionally used for asthmatic disorders and chest coughs with thick phlegm. They also have a tonifying effect on the urinary system, so are used for incontinence and excessive urination.

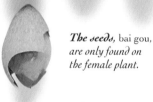

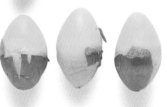

The seeds, bai gou, *are only found on the female plant.*

Tincture

Dried leaves

Applications

LEAVES

 FLUID EXTRACT An extract of the fresh leaves is marketed in Europe for treating cerebral arteriosclerosis in the elderly and for diseases of the peripheral circulation.

TINCTURE Combine with other cardiovascular herbs, such as greater periwinkle and linden, for circulatory problems, or with king's clover for venous disorders.

INFUSION Make with 50 g dried leaves to 2 cups (500 ml) water, and take for arteriosclerosis and varicose conditions. Use as a wash for varicose ulcers or hemorrhoids.

SEEDS

 DECOCTION Combine with herbs such as pill-bearing spurge, elecampane, or mulberry leaves for asthma and persistent coughs: 3-4 seeds are enough for three doses.

CAUTIONS
• Do not exceed the stated dose of the seeds, since this can lead to skin disorders and headaches.
• Cases of contact dermatitis with the fruit pulp (not used medicinally) have been seen.
• Long-term and excessive use may increase bleeding time and cause spontaneous hemorrhage.

Glycyrrhiza spp.
LICORICE

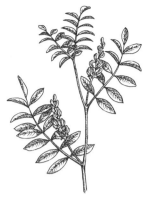

"...it has the property of quenching thirst if one holds it in the mouth..."
Theophrastus of Lesbos, c. 310 BC.

LICORICE HAS BEEN USED medicinally since at least 500 BC, and still features in official pharmacopoeia as a "drug" for stomach ulcers. *G. glabra* originates in the Mediterranean and the Middle East, and has been cultivated in Europe since at least the 16th century. In China, *G. uralensis* or *gan cao* is used; it is called the "great detoxifier", and is thought to drive poisons from the system. It is also an important tonic, often called "the grandfather of herbs".

Character
Very sweet, neutral, moist.
Constituents
Saponins, glycosides (inc. glycyrrhizin), estrogenous substances, coumarins, flavonoids, sterols, choline, asparagine, volatile oil.
Actions
Anti-inflammatory, anti-arthritic, tonic stimulant for adrenal cortex, lowers cholesterol levels, soothes gastric mucous membranes, cooling, expectorant.

Parts used

ROOT
G. GLABRA
Licorice root contains glycyrrhizin, 50 times sweeter than sucrose, which encourages the production of hormones such as hydrocortisone. This helps to explain its anti-inflammatory action and also its role in restimulating the adrenal cortex after steroid therapy. The root can help to heal gastric ulceration and is also a potent expectorant. Harvest in fall.

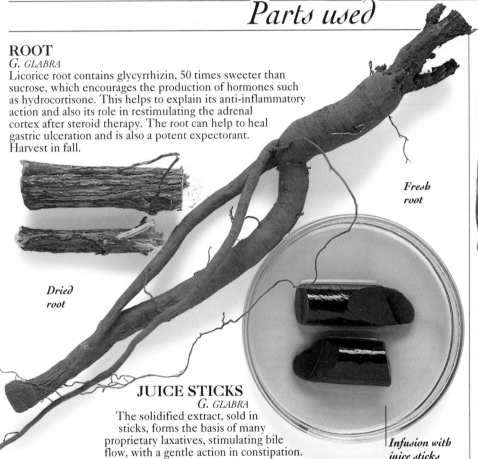
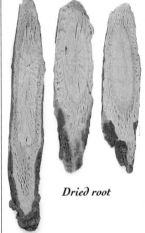

Fresh root

Dried root

Dried root

JUICE STICKS
G. GLABRA
The solidified extract, sold in sticks, forms the basis of many proprietary laxatives, stimulating bile flow, with a gentle action in constipation.

Infusion with juice sticks

ROOT
G. URALENSIS
An energy tonic, particularly for the spleen and stomach, the root is added to many Chinese herbal formulas to balance other herbs. It is also used for asthmatic coughs, as an antispasmodic and ulcer remedy, and to cool "hot" conditions. Dried root can be chewed like candy, and in China is given to children to promote muscle growth.

Applications

ROOT
G. GLABRA

 TINCTURE Use as an anti-inflammatory for arthritic or allergic conditions, as a digestive stimulant or for lung disorders. Prescribed for gastric inflammation or to encourage adrenal function after steroid therapy. Helps to disguise the flavor of other medicines.

 DECOCTION Prescribed to reduce stomach acidity in ulceration.

 SYRUP Take a syrup made from the decoction as a soothing expectorant for asthma and bronchitis.

 INFUSION Let juice sticks dissolve slowly in an equal volume of water to produce a strong extract that can be used as the decoction, tincture, or syrup.

ROOT
G. URALENSIS

 DECOCTION Combine with ginseng as a daily tonic drink.

 TONIC WINE Macerate a piece of root in red or white wine (p. 157) for a few weeks to produce a tonic wine: drink in small doses after meals.

CAUTIONS
• Avoid licorice if you have high blood pressure, as it is believed to cause fluid retention.
• Licorice should not be taken by people on digoxin-based drugs.
• Excessive use of licorice-containing candy and chewing gums has been linked to hypertension and abnormally high potassium levels.

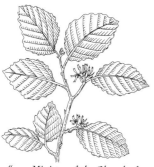

Hamamelis virginianum
WITCH HAZEL

"... a Minister of the Church of England ... saw an allmost total blindness occasioned by a blow cur'd by receiving the Warm Steam of a Decortion of the Bark of this Shrub through a Funnel upon the place ..."
Dr. Cadwallader Colden, 1744.

THE HEALING PROPERTIES of Virginian witch hazel were highly valued by various Native American peoples: the Menominees rubbed a decoction on to their legs to keep them supple during sports, while the Potawatomis added the twigs of the plant to sweat baths to relieve sore muscles. The herb was adopted by settlers and listed in the *US National Formulary* until 1955. Distilled witch hazel is widely available today, and is well known in domestic first aid.

Character
Cool, dry, bitter, pungent, astringent.
Constituents
Tannins, flavonoids (inc. kempferol and quercetin), saponins, bitters, volatile oil (inc. eugenol and safrole), choline, gallic acid.
Actions
Astringent, stops internal and external bleeding, anti-inflammatory.

Parts used

BARK
The bark is used to make commercial tinctures, ointments and fluid extracts. Like the leaf and twig extracts, it is used mainly to stop bleeding, ease irritation and treat varicose veins and hemorrhoids.

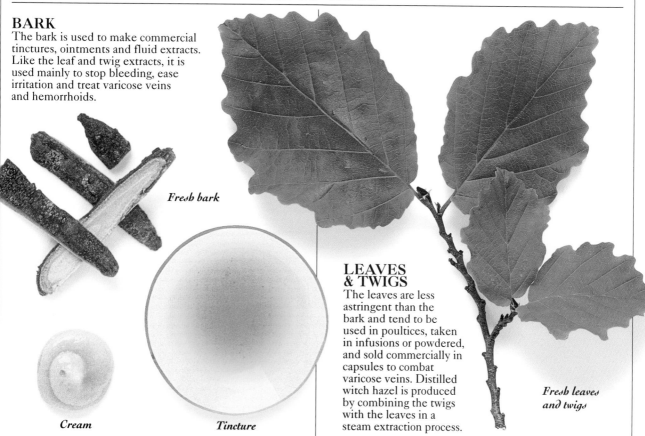

Fresh bark

LEAVES & TWIGS
The leaves are less astringent than the bark and tend to be used in poultices, taken in infusions or powdered, and sold commercially in capsules to combat varicose veins. Distilled witch hazel is produced by combining the twigs with the leaves in a steam extraction process.

Cream

Tincture

Fresh leaves and twigs

Applications

BARK

 TINCTURE Dilute and use externally instead of distilled witch hazel.

 OINTMENT/CREAM Use for cuts and scrapes or bruising, for hemorrhoids and irritated varicose veins.

LEAVES

 INFUSION Drink a standard infusion for diarrhea or bleeding hemorrhoids. A daily cup can help to combat capillary fragility.

 EYE PADS Use a cotton swab soaked in the infusion or in distilled witch hazel to relieve tired eyes.

 DISTILLATE Apply as a wash to cuts and scrapes, or soak a cotton swab as a nasal plug for nosebleeds.

 MOUTHWASH/GARGLE Use the infusion for sore throats, mouth ulcers, tonsillitis, pharyngitis, and spongy or bleeding gums.

 WASH Use the infusion to bathe irritated varicose veins, bruises, scrapes, skin rashes, and areas of capillary fragility.

TWIGS

 DECOCTION Use in the same way as an infusion of the leaves.

Harpagophytum procumbens
DEVIL'S CLAW

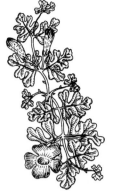

"The plant would appear to particularly benefit older patients with rheumatic complaints, obesity and hyperlipemia."
Rudolf Weiss, 1988.

NATIVE TO THE Kalahari desert in southern Africa, devil's claw was introduced to the West after a Boer farmer noticed native Bushmen gathering the roots to treat rheumatism and digestive upsets. The plant was sent to Germany for investigation and by the late 1950s its anti-inflammatory and antirheumatic properties were well established. The name devil's claw derives from the herb's characteristic claw-shaped fruits, produced in the autumn, which are reputedly used as mouse traps in Madagascar. Today the herb is used to treat arthritis and rheumatism.

Character
Bitter, astringent, cooling.
Constituents
Iridoid glycosides (inc. harpagide, harpagoside and procumbide), phenols, carbohydrates, flavonoids (inc. kempferol and luteolin), phytosterols.
Actions
Anti-inflammatory, antirheumatic, analgesic, sedative, diuretic, digestive stimulant.

Parts used

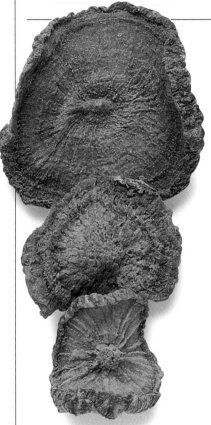

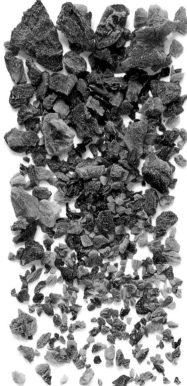

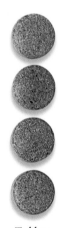

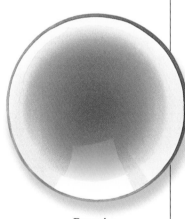

TUBER
The tubers of devil's claw, rather than the whole root structure, are used medicinally, although some commercial preparations combine the entire root mix, which dilutes the overall therapeutic effect. Researchers have found that constant use of the herb for at least six weeks significantly improves the movement of arthritic joints and reduces swelling. Devil's claw can also be used as a bitter digestive stimulant for a range of liver and gall bladder disorders.

Sliced dried tuber   *Chopped and dried tuber*   *Tablets*   *Decoction*

Applications

TUBER

 DECOCTION Drink a cup before meals to stimulate the digestion for cases of liver congestion, poor appetite, or mild gall bladder disorders.

 TINCTURE Take 20-30 drops per dose for at least six weeks for osteoarthritis or rheumatic pains.

 WASH Use the decoction as a wash for irritated and inflamed varicose veins and hemorrhoids.

 CREAM Apply to arthritic and rheumatic aches and pains three or four times a day. Add a few drops of rosemary oil to improve pain relief. Use the same mixture for sprained or strained joints and muscles.

 PILLS Take up to 600 mg three times daily for arthritic and rheumatic pains as a maintenance dose in chronic conditions. Increase to 800 mg per dose during any flare-up in symptoms.

 POWDER Use to dust open wounds to encourage healing.

CAUTIONS
• Avoid devil's claw in pregnancy, as it is believed to stimulate uterine contractions.
• Avoid the herb in cases of gastric or duodenal ulcers.

Humulus lupulus
HOPS

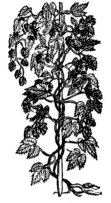

"Hops... preserves the drink, but repays the pleasure in tormenting diseases and a shorter life."
John Evelyn, 1670.

USED IN BREWING IN EUROPE since at least the 11th century, hops were never included in traditional English ale. Initially, they were thought to encourage the melancholic humor, and too many hops in German-style beer were, as Gerard records, "ill for the head". Hops were believed, however, to purge excess choleric and sanguine humors, and beer was regarded as a more "physicall drinke to keep the body in health" than English ale. Hops contain a high proportion of estrogen and, as a result, too much beer can lead to loss of libido in men.

Character
Cold, dry, bitter, slightly pungent.
Constituents
Volatile oil, valerianic acid, estrogenic substances, tannins, bitter principle, flavonoids.
Actions
Sedative, male anaphrodisiac, restoring tonic for nervous system, bitter digestive stimulant, diuretic, estrogenic effect.

Parts used

STROBILES
The flowers on the female plant, known as strobiles, are used medicinally. The character of the plant changes significantly with age as the constituents oxidize. The strobiles are best used fresh for insomnia, and the dried hops used in pillows for sleeplessness should be replaced every few months, because old, dried strobiles can be stimulating.

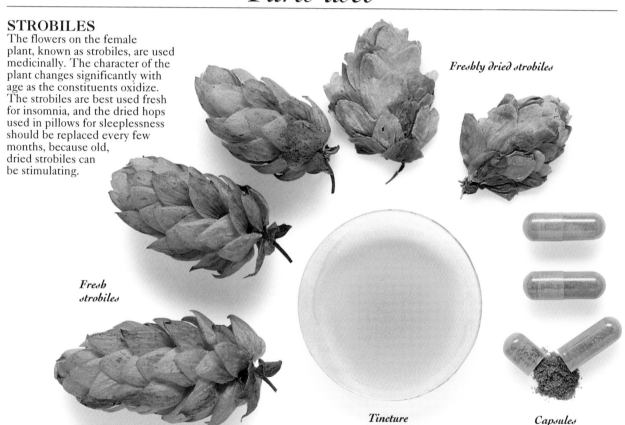

Freshly dried strobiles

Fresh strobiles

Tincture

Capsules

Applications

STROBILES

 INFUSION For insomnia, add 2 tsp fresh hops to a cup of boiling water, and infuse for five minutes. Alternatively, freshly dried or freeze-dried hops can be used.

 TINCTURE Take up to 2 ml, three times a day, as a sedative for nervous tension and anxiety. Combine with other digestive herbs, such as marshmallow, plantain, chamomile, and peppermint for irritable bowel syndrome. Take 1.5 ml on a sugar lump for a nervous stomach.

Prescribed for some sexual problems, including premature ejaculation.

 COMPRESS Use a pad soaked in the infusion or dilute tincture on varicose ulcers.

 WASH Use an infusion of fresh or freshly dried hops for chronic ulcers, skin eruptions, and wounds.

 CAPSULES Available commercially; take two before meals as an appetite stimulant. Do not use continuously for more than a few days.

CAUTIONS
• Hops act as a mild depressant on the higher nerve centers and should be avoided in depression. Do not exceed the stated doses.
• The growing plant can cause contact dermatitis.
• The estrogen-like effect may disrupt the menstrual cycles in women working in hop fields.

Hydrastis canadensis
GOLDENSEAL

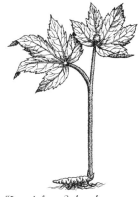

A TRADITIONAL HEALING HERB of Native Americans that has entered the European herbal repertoire, goldenseal was used by the Cherokee for indigestion, local inflammations, and to improve the appetite, while the Iroquois used it for whooping cough, liver disorders, fevers, and heart problems. The herb was introduced into Europe in 1760. During the 19th century, it became a favorite with Thomsonian and Eclectic practitioners (see pp. 20-21) and was listed in the United States *Pharmacopoeia* until 1926.

"I am informed that the Cheerake cure it [cancer] with a plant which is thought to be the Hydrastis canadensis.*"*
Benjamin Smith Barton, 1798.

Character
Bitter, astringent, dry, predominantly cold.
Constituents
Alkaloids, volatile oil, resin.
Actions
Astringent, tonic, digestive and bile stimulant, reduces phlegm, laxative, healing to gastric mucous membranes, raises blood pressure.

Parts used

RHIZOME
An excellent drying, mucus-reducing remedy for the gastric, upper respiratory tract, and vaginal mucous membranes; useful for conditions including spastic colon (mucous colitis), nasal inflammations, or ear infections. It is good for gynecological problems, can help reduce menopausal symptoms, and can ease menstrual pain or PMS symptoms linked with stagnation. Found in commercial remedies as a general tonic. Harvest in the fall.

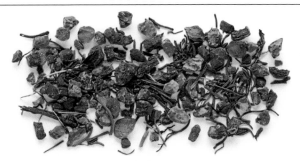

Dried rhizome

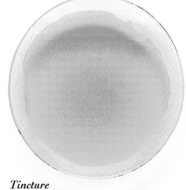

Tincture

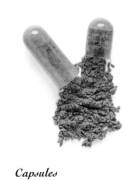

Capsules

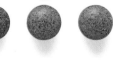

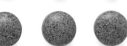

Compound tablets

Applications

RHIZOME

 TINCTURE Take 0.5-2 ml three times a day (larger doses are more laxative) for any mucous condition: nasal mucus, mucous colitis, gastro-enteritis, and vaginal discharge. Also use as a liver tonic for sluggish digestion and for digestive problems associated with food sensitivity and alcohol excess. Add to remedies for PMS or heavy menstrual bleeding.

 WASH Use 5 ml tincture in ½ cup (100 ml) water to bathe irritant skin inflammations, eczema, and measles.

 MOUTHWASH/GARGLE Use 2-3 ml tincture in a tumbler of warm water for mouth ulcers, gum disease, sore throats, and mucous conditions.

 DOUCHE Use the diluted tincture (2-3 ml in water) for vaginal discharges and yeast infections. For vaginal itching, use 5 ml tincture in ½ cup (100 ml) rosewater.

 CAPSULES Take one 200 mg capsule, three times a day, for phlegm and gastric or respiratory infections. Combine with chaste-tree berry powder to relieve menopausal flashes and sweats, and with eyebright for hay fever.

 EARDROPS Use 10 ml tincture in ½ cup (100 ml) water for serious otitis media and "blocked" ears.

 COMPOUND PILLS Some commercially available pills may be used for digestive upsets.

CAUTIONS
• Goldenseal is a uterine stimulant, so avoid in pregnancy.
• The herb is hypertensive, so avoid in cases of high blood pressure.
• Do not use eardrops if there is a risk that the ear drum is perforated.
• Eating the fresh plant can cause ulceration of the mucous membranes.
• Goldenseal is now seriously endangered in the wild; avoid buying material prepared from wild herbs and use barberry instead for digestive complaints.

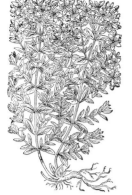

"For chilblains: boil the roots of tutsan and pour upon curds. Pound with old lard and apply as a plaster..."
Remedy of the Physicians of Myddfai, Wales, 13th century.

Hypericum perforatum
ST. JOHN'S WORT

IT IS SAID THAT ST. JOHN'S WORT takes its name from the Knights of St. John of Jerusalem, who used it to treat wounds on Crusade battlefields. It was also believed to dispel evil spirits – which is why the insane were often compelled to drink its infusions. Being yellow, the herb was associated with "choleric" humors and used for jaundice and hysteria. Old herbals often refer to tutsan (*H. androsaemum*), from the French *toutsain* or heal-all, which was also used to treat injuries and inflammations.

Character
Bitter-sweet, cool, drying.
Constituents
Glycosides, flavonoids (inc. rutin), volatile oils, tannins, resins.
Actions
Astringent, analgesic, antidepressant, antiviral, anti-inflammatory, sedative, restorative tonic for the nervous system.

Parts used

AERIAL PARTS
Now recognized as a potent antidepressant and as effective as many orthodox drugs, they also make a restorative nerve tonic, ideal for anxiety and irritability, especially during menopause. They are also good for chronic nervous exhaustion, and, as an antiviral, have been used in treating AIDS and HIV. They can relieve nerve pains such as sciatica and neuralgia. Harvest in summer.

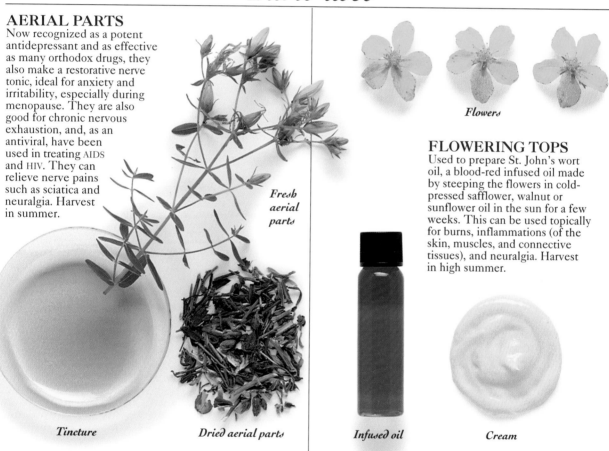

Flowers

Fresh aerial parts

FLOWERING TOPS
Used to prepare St. John's wort oil, a blood-red infused oil made by steeping the flowers in cold-pressed safflower, walnut or sunflower oil in the sun for a few weeks. This can be used topically for burns, inflammations (of the skin, muscles, and connective tissues), and neuralgia. Harvest in high summer.

Tincture

Dried aerial parts

Infused oil

Cream

Applications

AERIAL PARTS

 INFUSION Use for depression, anxiety or emotional upsets associated with menopause or premenstrual syndrome, and colds and infections combined with elderflower.

 TINCTURE Take for at least two months for long-standing nervous tension leading to exhaustion and depression. For childhood bed-wetting, give 5-10 drops at night.

 WASH Use the infusion to bathe wounds, skin sores, and bruises.

FLOWERING TOPS

 CREAM Use for localized nerve pains, such as sciatica, sprains, and cramps, or to help relieve breast engorgement during lactation. Can also be used as an antiseptic and styptic on scrapes, sores, and ulcers.

 INFUSED OIL Use on burns and muscle or joint inflammations including tennis elbow, neuralgia, and sciatica. Add a few drops of lavender oil for burns, or yarrow oil for joint inflammations.

CAUTIONS
• If on prescription drugs, seek professional advice first before taking St. John's wort.
• The herb can cause dermatitis after taking it internally, then exposing the skin to the sun.
• In very rare cases cataracts and nerve hypersensitivity have been linked to long-term or excessive use of St. John's Wort. It is also said to increase photosensitivity.

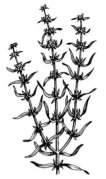

"The brethe or vapor of hisop driveth away the winde that is in the ears if they be holden over it."
William Turner, 1562.

Hyssopus officinalis
HYSSOP

PRESCRIBED BY HIPPOCRATES for pleurisy, hyssop, with rue, was recommended by Dioscorides for asthma and phlegm. Its name derives from the Greek word *azob*, or holy herb, although the "hyssop" in the Bible seems more likely to have been a local variety of marjoram. Hyssop is one of the more important of the 130 herbs flavoring the liqueur Chartreuse.

Character
Bitter, pungent, dry, slightly warming.
Constituents
Volatile oil, flavonoids, tannins, bitter substance (marrubin).
Actions
Expectorant, carminative, relaxes blood vessels, promotes sweating, reduces phlegm, topical anti-inflammatory, antiviral, antispasmodic.

Parts used

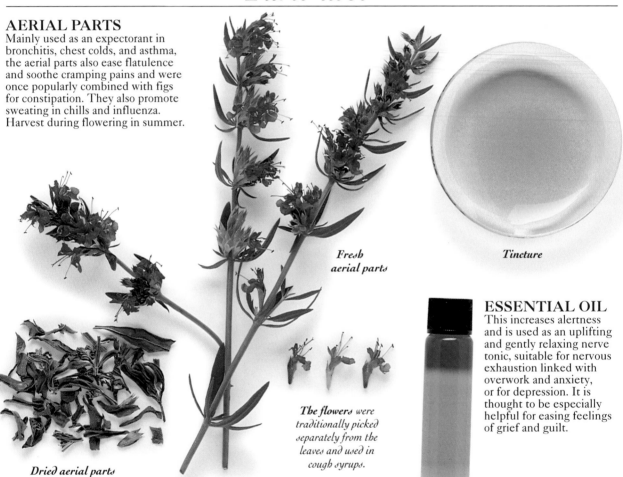

AERIAL PARTS
Mainly used as an expectorant in bronchitis, chest colds, and asthma, the aerial parts also ease flatulence and soothe cramping pains and were once popularly combined with figs for constipation. They also promote sweating in chills and influenza. Harvest during flowering in summer.

Fresh aerial parts

Tincture

ESSENTIAL OIL
This increases alertness and is used as an uplifting and gently relaxing nerve tonic, suitable for nervous exhaustion linked with overwork and anxiety, or for depression. It is thought to be especially helpful for easing feelings of grief and guilt.

The flowers were traditionally picked separately from the leaves and used in cough syrups.

Dried aerial parts

Applications

AERIAL PARTS

 INFUSION Drink hot during the early stages of colds and influenza. Also take for digestive upsets and nervous stomach.

 TINCTURE Combine with other expectorant herbs, such as licorice, elecampane, and anise, for bronchitis and stubborn coughs.

 SYRUP For coughs, use a syrup made from an infusion of either the aerial parts or the flowers. Combine with mullein flowers or licorice

for stubborn coughs and lung weakness.

ESSENTIAL OIL

 CHEST RUB Dilute 10 drops hyssop oil in 20 ml almond or sunflower oil for bronchitis and chest colds. Combines well with thyme and eucalyptus.

 OIL Add 5-10 drops to bathwater for nervous exhaustion, melancholy, or grief.

CAUTION
• The essential oil contains the ketone pino-camphone, which in high doses can cause convulsions. Do not take more than the recommended dose.

Inula spp.
ELECAMPANE

"Inula campana reddit
praecordia sana *(elecampane
will the spirits sustain)*."
Traditional Latin saying.

ONE OF THE MOST IMPORTANT herbs to the
Greeks and Romans, elecampane (*I. helenium*)
was regarded as almost a cure-all for ailments
as diverse as dropsy, digestive upsets, menstrual
disorders, and sciatica. The Anglo-Saxons used
the herb as a tonic, for skin disease, and leprosy.
By the 19th century, it was used to treat skin
disease, neuralgia, liver problems, and coughs;
today it is used almost solely for respiratory
problems. In China, *I. japonica* is used.

Character
I. HELENIUM: bitter and
slightly sweet, warm, dry.
I. JAPONICA: salty, warm.
Constituents
Mucilage, bitter principle,
volatile oil (inc. *azulenes*), inulin,
sterols, possible alkaloids.
Actions
Tonic, stimulating
expectorant, promotes sweating,
antibacterial, antifungal, antiparasitic, digestive stimulant,
immune stimulant.

Parts used

ROOT
I. HELENIUM
An excellent
tonic, especially for
weakness following
influenza or bronchitis,
the root loosens stubborn
phlegm and can help
coughs and congestion,
particularly in children.
It contains inulin, which
has been used as a sugar
substitute in diabetes.
Harvest in fall, wash, and
chop into small pieces
before drying.

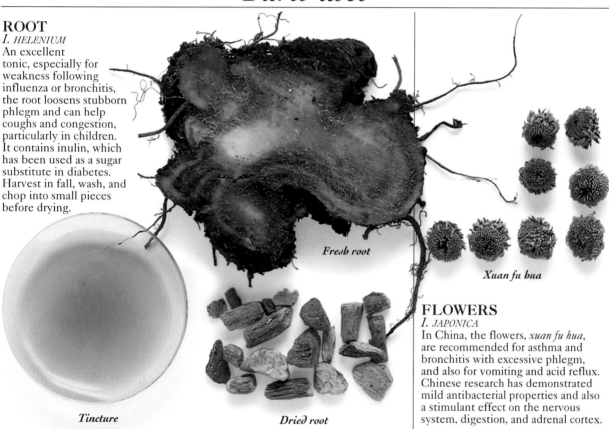

Fresh root

Xuan fu hua

Tincture

Dried root

FLOWERS
I. JAPONICA
In China, the flowers, *xuan fu hua*,
are recommended for asthma and
bronchitis with excessive phlegm,
and also for vomiting and acid reflux.
Chinese research has demonstrated
mild antibacterial properties and also
a stimulant effect on the nervous
system, digestion, and adrenal cortex.

Applications

ROOT
I. HELENIUM

DECOCTION Use for bronchitis,
asthma, upper respiratory problems,
or to ease hay fever symptoms. Take
regularly as a general tonic or for
long-standing chronic respiratory
complaints. Also acts as a digestive
tonic and liver stimulant.

TINCTURE Take as a tonic in debility
and chronic respiratory complaints.

WASH Use the decoction or diluted
tincture for eczema, rashes, and
varicose ulcers.

SYRUP Take a syrup made with
the decoction for coughs.

FLOWERS
I. JAPONICA

DECOCTION Take for nausea,
vomiting, or coughs with copious
phlegm. Alternatively, combine
10 g flowers with 10 g fresh ginger
root, 10 ml *ban xia*, and 5 ml licorice
root, and use for excess phlegm in
the stomach with nausea, abdominal
distension, flatulence, and
vomiting of mucus.

SYRUP Take a syrup made with
the infusion in 10-20 ml doses
for coughs.

CAUTION
• May cause allergic
skin reactions.

Jasminum spp.
JASMINE

"Jessamine... warms the womb and facilitates the birth... it removes diseases of the uterus and is of service in pituitous colics."
Nicholas Culpeper, 1653.

THE HIGHLY AROMATIC climbing plant, common jasmine (*J. officinale*), was brought to Europe in the 16th century and rapidly gained popularity with French perfumiers. The scented oil is extracted from the plant by layering the flowers with wax between glass sheets. A close relative, royal jasmine, or *jati* (*J. grandiflorum*), is used as an Ayurvedic tonic and cleansing remedy. Jasmine tea, popular in China, is scented using Arabian jasmine (*J. sambac*).

Character
Bitter, pungent, astringent, cooling.
Constituents
Alkaloids (inc. jasminine), essential oil (inc. linalool), salicylic acid.
Actions
Flowers: aphrodisiac, astringent, bitter, relaxing nervine, sedative, analgesic, encourages milk flow. Oil: antidepressant, antiseptic, antispasmodic, aphrodisiac, encourages milk flow, sedative, uterine tonic.

Parts used

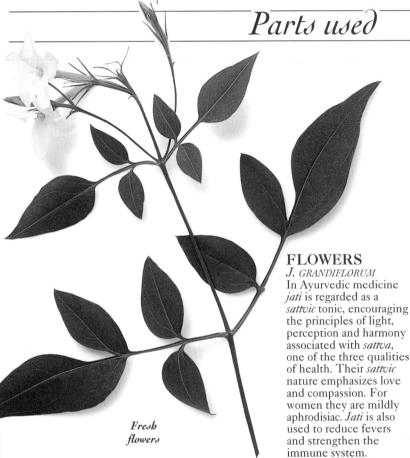

Fresh flowers

FLOWERS/ JASMINE TEA
J. SAMBAC
Arabian jasmine has been used for scenting Chinese teas since at least AD 300. The flowers, known as *mo li*, were left beside heat-dried green tea to absorb the scent. Modern commercial producers mix the petals in with the tea.

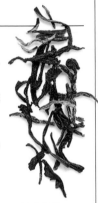

Dried flowers

FLOWERS
J. GRANDIFLORUM
In Ayurvedic medicine *jati* is regarded as a *sattvic* tonic, encouraging the principles of light, perception and harmony associated with *sattva*, one of the three qualities of health. Their *sattvic* nature emphasizes love and compassion. For women they are mildly aphrodisiac. *Jati* is also used to reduce fevers and strengthen the immune system.

ESSENTIAL OIL
J. OFFICINALE
Jasmine oil is expensive and is often adulterated with synthetic chemicals. Only the best oil should be used medicinally. In aromatherapy it is used in massage rubs for period pain, depression, impotence and frigidity, and during labor to ease pain and encourage childbirth. It is also added to chest rubs for coughs and breathing difficulties.

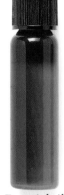

Essential oil

Applications

FLOWERS
J. GRANDIFLORUM

 INFUSION Take for infections, fevers or urinary inflammation. Combine a few flowers with lemon balm or skullcap for a calming tea at the end of a stressful day.

 WASH Apply an infusion to bathe cuts and scrapes, and stop bleeding.

COMPRESS Use a compress soaked in the cool infusion or dilute tincture and apply to the forehead for sun or heat stroke, headaches, and emotional upset.

FLOWERS/JASMINE TEA
J. SAMBAC

 INFUSION Traditionally used as a soothing and warming remedy to help relieve diarrhea.

ESSENTIAL OIL
J. OFFICINALE

 MASSAGE OIL Add 1-2 drops to massage rubs as a treatment for anxiety, insomnia or depression. Use 1-2 drops jasmine oil in 1 tsp almond oil for mutual massage before love-making to treat impotence or frigidity.

Juglans spp.
WALNUT

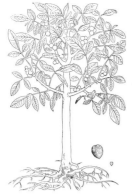

"The oyle of walnuts... maketh smooth the hands and face, and taketh away... black and blew marks that come of bruses."
John Gerard, 1597.

ACCORDING TO LEGEND, when the gods walked upon the Earth, they lived on walnuts; hence the name *Juglans* or *Jovis glans*, Jupiter's nut. The tree has been cultivated in Europe since Roman times for its nuts; these yield an important oil containing essential fatty acids, such as α-linolenic, which are vital for healthy cell function and prostaglandin development. The white walnut, or butternut (*J. cinerea*), from eastern North America is a useful laxative.

Character
Bitter, astringent, mostly warm, drying; the fresh rind is cooling.
Constituents
Quinones, oils, tannins; nuts contain essential fatty acids, including α-linolenic.
Actions
J. REGIA: astringent, expels intestinal worms, antispasmodic, digestive tonic; the nut rind is anti-inflammatory, cancer fighting, reduces cholesterol.
J. CINEREA: purgative, astringent, promotes bile flow.

Parts used

LEAVES
J. REGIA
In Europe, walnut leaves are a popular home remedy for both eczema and blepharitis (eyelid inflammation) in children. Recent research suggests antifungal properties, as well as an antiseptic action; the leaves are also used for intestinal worms and as a digestive tonic. Harvest through-out the growing season.

Fresh leaves

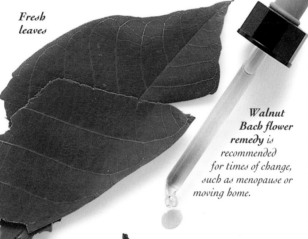

Walnut Bach flower remedy is recommended for times of change, such as menopause or moving home.

INNER BARK
J. CINEREA
The quills or inner bark are one of the few potent laxatives that are safe to use in pregnancy. Harvest in early summer.

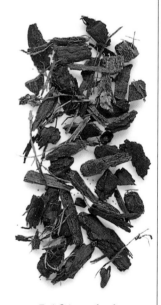

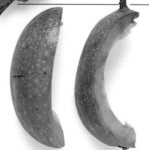

NUT & CASING
J. REGIA
The fleshy green outer casing of the nut is rich in fruit acids and minerals. Traditionally, infusions of this rind were used to darken the hair. The nuts are known to lower cholesterol levels and can help to reduce the risk of heart disease. Harvest in late summer.

Walnut and casing

Fresh outer rind

Dried inner bark

Applications

LEAVES
J. REGIA

 INFUSION Use for skin problems and eye inflammations, and as a digestive tonic for poor appetite.

 WASH Use the infusion for eczema or for wounds and scrapes.

 EYEWASH Use either a well-strained infusion or 5 drops tincture in an eyebath of water for conjunctivitis and blepharitis.

OUTER NUT RIND
J. REGIA

 INFUSION Use for chronic diarrhea or as a tonic in anemia.

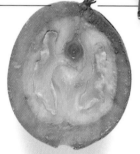 HAIR RINSE Use the infusion as a rinse for hair loss.

NUT
J. REGIA

 OIL Take 2 tsp unrefined walnut oil daily as a dietary supplement for menstrual dysfunction or for dry, flaky eczema.

INNER BARK
J. CINEREA

 DECOCTION Use for constipation, sluggish digestion, as a liver stimulant and for skin diseases.

 TINCTURE Take up to 5 ml daily for the same ailments as the decoction.

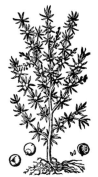

Juniperus communis
JUNIPER

LONG ASSOCIATED with ritual cleansing, juniper was burned in temples as a part of regular purification rites. Several medicinal recipes survive in Egyptian papyri dating to 1550 B.C. In central European folk medicine, the oil extracted from the berries was regarded as a cure-all for typhoid, cholera, dysentery, tapeworms, and other ills associated with poverty.

"A remedy to treat tapeworm: juniper berries 5 parts, white oil 5 parts is taken for one day."
Egyptian, c. 1550 B.C.

Character
Pungent, slightly bitter-sweet, hot, dry.
Constituents
Volatile oil, flavonoids, sugars, glycosides, tannins, podophyllotoxin (an anti-tumor agent), vitamin C.
Actions
Urinary antiseptic, diuretic, carminative, digestive tonic, uterine stimulant, antirheumatic.

Parts used

BERRIES
The ripe, blue berries are mainly used for urinary infections and prescribed to clear acid wastes from the system in arthritis and gout. They reduce colic and flatulence, stimulate the digestion, and encourage uterine contractions in labor. Pick after they have turned from green to purplish-blue; this process can take two years.

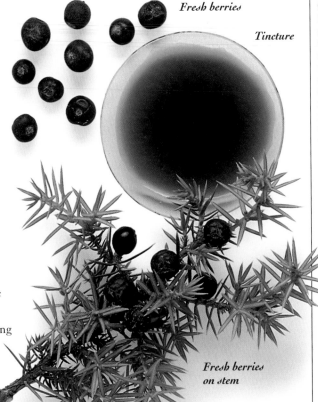

Fresh berries

Tincture

Fresh berries on stem

CADE OIL
Made by dry distillation of the heartwood of various types of juniper tree, cade oil is also known as juniper tar oil. It contains phenol and has a mild disinfectant action. Applied externally, it is a non-irritant and is mainly used for chronic skin conditions, such as scaling eczema and psoriasis.

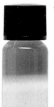

ESSENTIAL OIL
Made by steam distillation of ripe berries, the oil is a popular external remedy for arthritic and muscle pains. Internally, the oil increases the filtering of waste products by the kidneys, and is effective against many bacteria.

Cade oil

Applications

BERRIES

 INFUSION Sip a weak infusion (15 g berries to 2 cups [500 ml] water) for stomach upsets or menstrual pain.

 TINCTURE Take 2 ml, three times a day, for urinary infections, such as cystitis, or to stimulate digestion.

ESSENTIAL OIL

 LOTION Add 5 drops of oil to 50 ml equal parts rosewater and witch hazel for oily skin and acne.

 CHEST RUB Dilute 10 drops juniper oil and 10 drops thyme oil in 20 ml almond oil, and rub into the chest for stubborn coughs.

 OIL Add 5 drops to bathwater for arthritic, gout, or muscle pains.

 MASSAGE OIL Dilute 10 drops juniper oil in 5 ml almond oil, and massage into arthritic joints.

CADE OIL

OINTMENT Add 10 drops to 20 ml melted ointment base. Allow to cool, and apply to chronic, scaling eczema, or psoriasis.

 HAIR RINSE For psoriasis affecting the scalp, add 10 drops to 2 cups (500 ml) hot water and mix well. Leave on the hair for at least 15 minutes, then rinse thoroughly.

CAUTIONS
• Avoid the herb in pregnancy, because it is a uterine stimulant; may be taken during labor.
• Juniper may irritate the kidneys in long-term use, so do not take internally for more than six weeks without a break, or at all if there is already kidney damage.

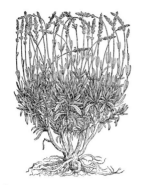

<u>*Lavandula spp.*</u>
LAVENDER

"...especiall good use for all griefes and paines of the head and brain."
John Parkinson, 1640.

ONE OF THE MOST POPULAR medicinal herbs since ancient times, lavender derives its name from the Latin *lavare*, to wash. In Arab medicine, lavender is used as an expectorant, while in European folk tradition it is regarded as a useful wound herb. Species used medicinally include *L. angustifolia* or *L. spica*, as well as French lavender (*L stoechas*) in Southern Europe.

Character
Bitter, dry, mainly cooling.
Constituents
Volatile oil, tannins, coumarins, flavonoids, triterpenoids.
Actions
Relaxant, antispasmodic, circulatory stimulant, tonic for the nervous system, anti-bacterial, analgesic, carminative, promotes bile flow, antiseptic.

Parts used

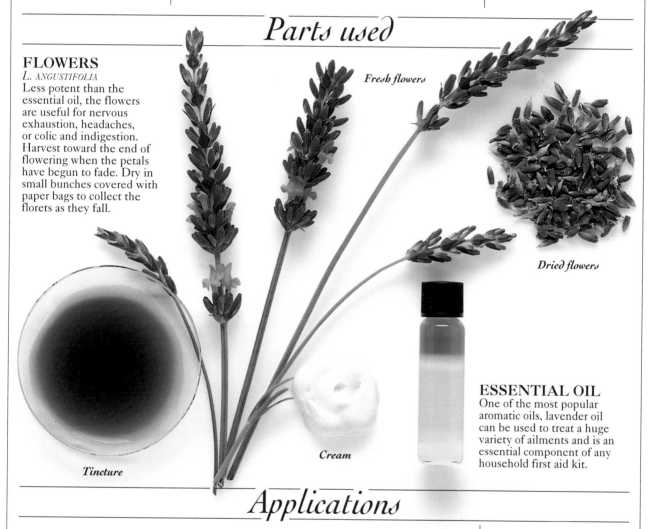

FLOWERS
L. ANGUSTIFOLIA
Less potent than the essential oil, the flowers are useful for nervous exhaustion, headaches, or colic and indigestion. Harvest toward the end of flowering when the petals have begun to fade. Dry in small bunches covered with paper bags to collect the florets as they fall.

Fresh flowers

Dried flowers

Tincture

Cream

ESSENTIAL OIL
One of the most popular aromatic oils, lavender oil can be used to treat a huge variety of ailments and is an essential component of any household first aid kit.

Applications

FLOWERS

 INFUSION Take for nervous exhaustion, tension headaches, or during labor; also for colic and indigestion. Give a weak infusion (25% normal strength) to babies for colic, irritability, and excitement.

 TINCTURE Take up to 5 ml, twice a day, for headaches and depression.

 MOUTHWASH Use for halitosis.

ESSENTIAL OIL

 CREAM Add a few drops of oil to chamomile cream for eczema.

 LOTION Add a few drops of oil to a little water for sunburn or scalds.

 CHEST RUB Add 1 ml oil and 5 drops chamomile oil to 10 ml carrier oil for asthmatic and bronchitic spasm.

 HAIR RINSE Dilute 5-10 drops of oil in water for lice, or use a few drops of neat oil on a fine comb for nits.

 MASSAGE OIL Dilute 1 ml lavender oil in 25 ml carrier oil, and massage into painful muscles. Dilute 10 drops in 25 ml carrier oil and massage into the temples and nape of the neck for tension headaches or at the first hint of a migraine.

 OIL Apply undiluted to insect bites and stings. Dilute 10 drops oil in 25 ml carrier oil for sunstroke or to help prevent sunburn. (Note: this is not an effective sunblock.)

CAUTION
• Avoid high doses of the herb during pregnancy, because it is a uterine stimulant.

Leonurus spp.
MOTHERWORT

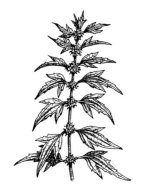

"There is no better herb to take melancholy vapours from the heart, to strengthen it, and make a merry, cheerful, blithe soul."
Nicholas Culpeper, 1653.

AN IMPORTANT HEART HERB since Roman times, motherwort, or *Leonurus cardiaca*, derives the *Leonurus* part of the botanical name from a Greek word meaning lion's tail, describing the shaggy shape of the leaves. Its common name also suggests a medicinal application for, in Gerard's words, "them that are in hard travell with childe". Early herbals also recommend the plant for "wykked sperytis". Chinese herbalists use the related species, *L. sibiricus*, mainly for menstrual disorders.

Character
Pungent, bitter, drying, cool.
Constituents
Alkaloids (inc. stachydrine), bitter glycosides, volatile oil, tannins, vitamin A.
Actions
Uterine stimulant, relaxant, cardiac tonic, carminative.

Parts used

AERIAL PARTS
L. CARDIACA/L. SIBIRICUS
Useful as a tonic and for the heart, the aerial parts are ideal for palpitations with anxiety and nervous tension. The alkaloids encourage and ease uterine contractions, so are valuable both for period pain and during labor. The herb also stimulates menstrual flow. In China, *L. sibiricus* (*yi mu cao*) is also used for eczema and sores. Harvest in summer.

SEEDS
L. SIBIRICUS
In China, the seeds, *chong wei zi*, are used mainly for menstrual irregularities and as a circulatory stimulant. The Chinese consider that they act specifically on the liver, and are therefore especially effective on the eyes to "brighten the vision".

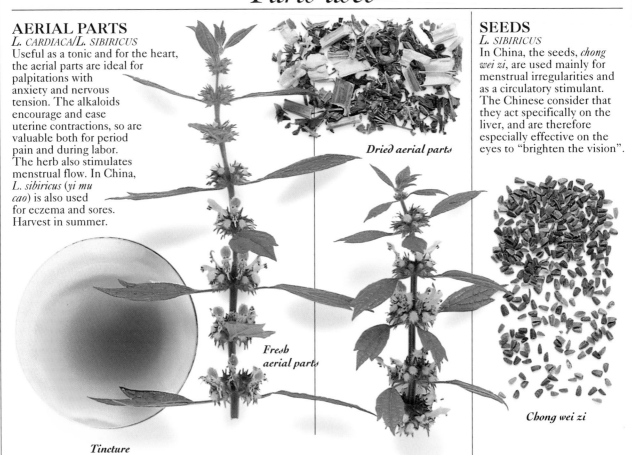

Dried aerial parts

Fresh aerial parts

Tincture

Chong wei zi

Applications

AERIAL PARTS
L. CARDIACA/L. SIBIRICUS

 INFUSION Use as a tonic for menopausal syndrome, anxiety and heart weaknesses, or for period pains. Add 2-3 cloves and drink during labor. Take after childbirth to help restore the uterus and reduce the risk of postpartum bleeding.

 SYRUP The infusion is traditionally made into a syrup to disguise the flavor. Use in similar ways.

 TINCTURE Use as the infusion. Prescribed with herbs like lily-of-the-valley and hawthorn as a heart tonic.

 DOUCHE Use the infusion or diluted tincture for vaginal infections and discharges.

SEEDS
L. SIBIRICUS

 DECOCTION Use for menstrual problems.

 EYEWASH Use a weak decoction for conjunctivitis, or sore or tired eyes.

CAUTIONS
• The herb is a uterine stimulant, so avoid in pregnancy. It may be used in labor.
• Seek professional advice for all heart conditions.

Ligusticum spp.
ALPINE LOVAGE

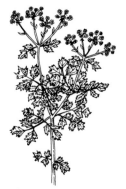

"Gao ben... promotes the growth of muscle and skin, and renders the facial complexion attractive."
Ben Cao Jing, *Shen Nong,*
c. 2500 BC.

KNOWN AS A FASHIONABLE cure-all and immune stimulant in North America, Colorado cough root, or oshá (*L. porterii*), is used for colds and coughs, as well as for digestive upsets and menstrual problems. The herb originates in the Rocky Mountains, where it was once regarded as sacred by Native Americans, who burned it to ward off evil influences. Several related species are popular in China: *gao ben* (*L. sinense*) is used for pain relief, while *chuan xiong* (*L. wallichii*) is given for menstrual and heart problems.

Character
Pungent, warm, dry.
Constituents
Essential oil, glycosides, ferulic acid, bitters.
Actions
L. PORTERII: carminative, diaphoretic, expectorant, stimulating.
L. SINENSE: antifungal, analgesic, antispasmodic.
L. WALLICHII: antibacterial, hypotensive, sedative, uterine stimulant.

Parts used

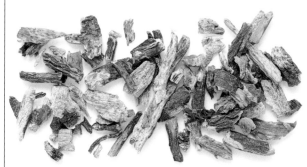

Dried root

ROOT
L. PORTERII
Colorado cough root is a warm, pungent herb that encourages sweating, and is a good remedy for the chilling winds of the Rocky Mountains. It stimulates the circulation and the kidneys, improves digestion and relieves toothache, bronchitis and spasmodic pains. It is available in over-the-counter herbal products in North America and Europe.

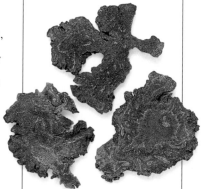

Dried rhizome

ROOT & RHIZOME
L. SINENSE
Chinese herbal folk tradition uses *gao ben* (*L. sinense*), or Chinese lovage, for menstrual problems and as a strengthening remedy after childbirth, although its main medicinal use is for chills and pain relief. It is taken for various types of headache, migraine, joint pain, toothache and arthritis, possibly associated with symptoms that develop in syndromes that the Chinese believe are caused by external wind, cold, or damp.

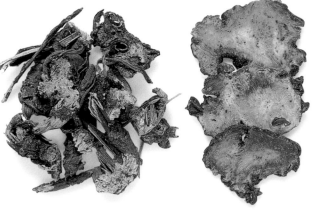

Dried root   *Dried rhizome*

RHIZOME
L. WALLICHII
Chuan xiong, Sichuan lovage, has been used in China since the 14th century as an invigorating blood remedy for menstrual and heart problems, and as a remedy for headaches. It is often combined with *dang gui, bai shao yao* and *shu di huang* for menstrual irregularities and anemia and is included in several patent remedies for coronary heart disease.

Applications

ROOT
L. PORTERII

 MACERATION Soak the root overnight to make syrups for coughs and colds. Warm a cup of maceration for period pain, digestive upsets and colds.

 TINCTURE Add 20-30 drops per dose in a little water and use in the same way as the maceration.

L. SINENSE

 DECOCTION Use for colds and chills with headaches and muscle pain.

 TINCTURE Use 10-20 drops per dose for headaches, toothache and a stiff neck. Apply a cotton swab soaked in dilute tincture to gums for toothache.

RHIZOME
L. WALLICHII

 DECOCTION Use with *shu di huang, dang gui* and *bai shao yao* for anemia and poor circulation.

 PILLS *Chuan xiong* is combined with other herbs in "*Ba Zhen Tang*" for irregular menstruation and anemia.

CAUTIONS
• Avoid Colorado cough root and *chuan xiong* during pregnancy and heavy menstrual bleeding.
• *Gao ben* and *chuan xiong* should not be used in cases of *yin* deficiency or excess heat.

Linum spp.
FLAX

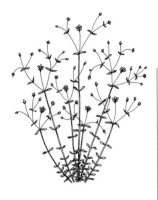

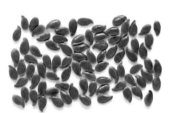

"Wherever flax seeds become a regular food item among the people, there will be better health." Mahatma Gandhi.

As THE SOURCE OF LINEN FIBER, *L. usitatissimum* has been cultivated since at least 5000 B.C.; today it is just as likely to be grown for its oil. The medicinal properties of the seeds, or linseed, were known to the Greeks: Hippocrates recommended them for inflammations of the mucous membranes. In 8th-century France, Charlemagne passed laws requiring the seeds to be consumed, to keep his subjects healthy. The related *L. catharticum* was once popular as a purgative but is little used today.

Character
Moist, warm, sweet; the oil is drying.
Constituents
Mucilage, cyanogenic glycosides, bitter principle; linseed oil contains *cis*-linoleic and α-linolenic acids, vitamins A, B, D, E, minerals, and amino acids.
Actions
L. USITATISSIMUM: demulcent, soothing antitussive, antiseptic, anti-inflammatory, laxative.
L. CATHARTICUM: laxative, antirheumatic, diuretic.

Parts used

LINSEED
L. USITATISSIMUM
The ripe seeds can be used as a relaxing expectorant, a bulking laxative, and extensively in poultices; they are also soothing for gastritis and sore throats. Linseed oil contains *cis*-linoleic and α-linolenic acids, needed for the production of hormone-like prostaglandins, vital for many bodily functions. Harvest when ripe.

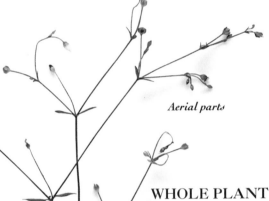

Aerial parts

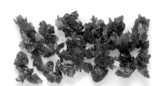

Linseed

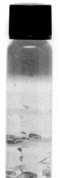

Linseed oil is an important source of essential fatty acids, which can help prevent the buildup of fatty deposits in the tissues.

Crushed seeds

WHOLE PLANT
L. CATHARTICUM
Mountain or purging flax is a potent laxative and was often used as an alternative to senna. The tea was also a traditional folk remedy for rheumatism and liver complaints, largely because its strong laxative action helps rid the body of toxins. Harvest while flowering.

Applications

LINSEED
L. USITATISSIMUM

 SEEDS For constipation, eat 1-2 tbsp of seeds, followed by 1-2 glasses of water; the seeds swell in the bowel to produce a gentle, bulking laxative. The seeds can be mixed with muesli, cereal, or honey and soft cheese, then eaten at breakfast. Simultaneous high fluid intake is important.

 INFUSION Use for coughs and sore throats; flavor with honey and lemon juice.

 POULTICE Crush the seeds, and apply to boils, abscesses, and ulcers; apply locally for pleurisy pain.

 MACERATION Soak the seeds in water to produce a thick mucilage, which can be taken for inflammations of the mucous membranes, such as gastritis and pharyngitis.

 OIL The essential fatty acids this contains can be helpful for eczema, menstrual disorders, rheumatoid arthritis, and atherosclerosis. Add 2 tsp freshly pressed oil or 1-2 tsp freshly crushed seeds to the diet every day.

WHOLE PLANT
L. CATHARTICUM

 INFUSION Take the fresh herb for constipation, liver congestion, and rheumatic pain.

CAUTIONS
• Linseed oil deteriorates rapidly, so prepare freshly as required, if possible. Do not use artists' linseed oil internally.
• The seeds contain traces of prussic acid, which is potentially toxic in large quantities. While no cases of prussic acid poisoning from linseed have ever been reported, do not exceed the stated doses.

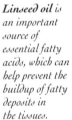

Lonicera spp.
HONEYSUCKLE

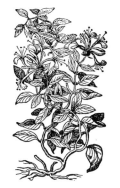

WOODBINE OR EUROPEAN honeysuckle
(*L. periclymenum*) was once widely used for
asthma, urinary complaints, and in childbirth.
Pliny recommended it to be taken in wine for
spleen disorders. Today, Chinese honeysuckle
(*L. japonica*, or *jin yin*) is more likely to be used
medicinally. This was first listed in the *Tang
Ben Cao*, written in A.D. 659, and is one of the
most important Chinese herbs for clearing
heat and poisons from the body.

*"I know of no better cure for the
asthma than this..."*
Nicholas Culpeper, 1653.

Character
Sweet, cold.
Constituents
Tannin, flavonoids, mucilage,
sugars; salicylic acid reported
in European species.
Actions
L. PERICLYMENUM: diuretic, antispasmodic, expectorant,
laxative, promotes vomiting.
L. JAPONICA: antibacterial, reduces
blood pressure, anti-inflammatory,
mild diuretic, antispasmodic.

Parts used

FLOWERS
L. PERICLYMENUM
Woodbine flowers were traditionally
made into a syrup that was taken as
an expectorant for bad coughs and
asthma and as a diuretic. The syrup
is still used for coughs today.
Harvest in summer.

FLOWER BUDS
L. JAPONICA
Known as *jin yin hua*, the
flowers are widely used in
feverish conditions, especially
those attributed to "summer
heat." They clear the toxins
or "fire poisons" that in
traditional Chinese theory
cause conditions such as
boils and dysentery. To treat
some types of diarrhea, the
Chinese warm the buds
slightly by stir-frying.
Harvest in summer.

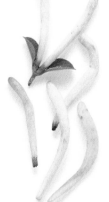

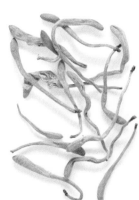

Fresh buds   *Dried buds*

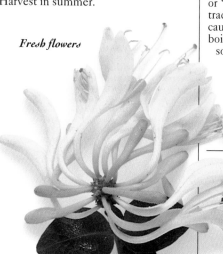

Fresh flowers

*Fresh
leaves*

STEMS
L. JAPONICA
Called *jin yin teng* and *ren dong teng*, the
stems and branches are generally used
to remove heat from the acupuncture
meridians, by stimulating the circulation
of *qi* (energy). They are also used to
treat feverish colds and dysentery, and
as a cooling remedy in combination
with other herbs for the acute stages
of rheumatoid arthritis.

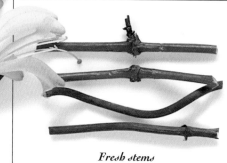

Fresh stems

Applications

FLOWERS
L. PERICLYMENUM

 INFUSION Combine with other
expectorant herbs, such as cowslip,
elecampane, or mulberry, for
coughs and mild asthma.

SYRUP Take a syrup made with
the infusion for coughs. Can
be combined with other
expectorant flowers, such
as mullein.

FLOWER BUDS
L. JAPONICA

DECOCTION Take in the early stages
of a feverish cold characterized by a
headache, thirst, and sore throat.

Use 10-15 g herb to 2½ cups
(600 ml) water. Add *huang lian* and
huang qin for high fevers.

 TINCTURE Use for diarrhea or
gastroenteritis related to
food poisoning.

STEMS
L. JAPONICA

 DECOCTION Make with 15-30 g
herb to 2½ cups (600 ml) water and
use as the flower bud decoction,
especially if there are painful joints,
as in influenza. Combine with other
cooling herbs, such as *shi hu*, for
inflammatory diseases, for example,
rheumatoid arthritis.

CAUTIONS
• Do not use honeysuckle
berries – they are toxic.
• If using the tincture for
digestive upsets, use the
hot-water method (see
p. 157) to reduce the alcohol.

Lycopersicum esculentum
TOMATO

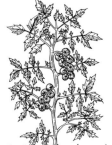

"In Spain and hose hot regions they used to eate the apples of love prepared and boiled with pepper, salt, and oile, but they yeelde very little nourishment to the bodie ..."
John Gerard, 1597.

SPANISH CONQUISTADORS introduced tomatoes into Europe from Peru in the 15th century. The first tomatoes were known by the Italian name *pomodoro*, "golden apples", because of their color. On arriving in Britain via France during the 16th century, the name became *pommes d'amours*, hence the old English name "love apples". Originally, the fruits of the tomato were thought to be poisonous because the plant's flowers are similar to those of deadly nightshade.

Character
Cold, sour, sweet.
Constituents
Vitamins: A, B₁, B₂, B₆, C, E, folic acid, malic acid, citric acid, bioflavonoids (inc. rutin), calcium, magnesium, phosphorus.
Actions
Antiscorbutic, antimicrobial, diuretic, mild laxative, digestive stimulant, reduces acidity in the blood.

Parts used

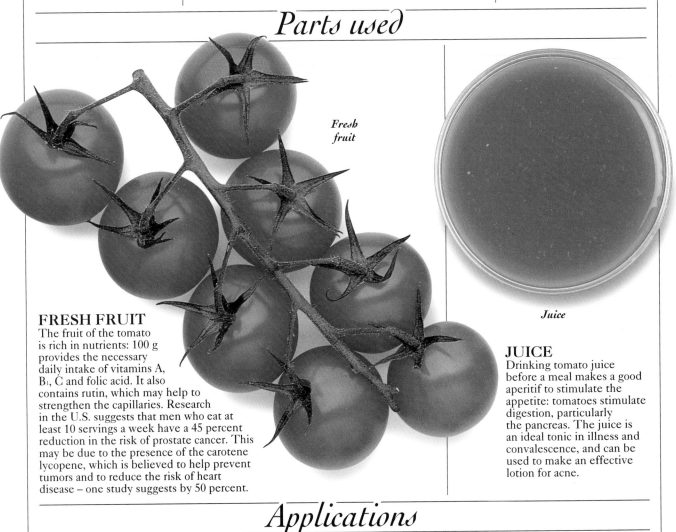

Fresh fruit

Juice

FRESH FRUIT
The fruit of the tomato is rich in nutrients: 100 g provides the necessary daily intake of vitamins A, B₁, C and folic acid. It also contains rutin, which may help to strengthen the capillaries. Research in the U.S. suggests that men who eat at least 10 servings a week have a 45 percent reduction in the risk of prostate cancer. This may be due to the presence of the carotene lycopene, which is believed to help prevent tumors and to reduce the risk of heart disease – one study suggests by 50 percent.

JUICE
Drinking tomato juice before a meal makes a good aperitif to stimulate the appetite: tomatoes stimulate digestion, particularly the pancreas. The juice is an ideal tonic in illness and convalescence, and can be used to make an effective lotion for acne.

Applications

FRESH FRUIT

 FRESH FRUIT Eat fresh tomatoes to ease arthritis, rheumatism and gout: the tomato plant is oxalate-free and will clear uric acid and toxins from the system.

 COOKED FRUIT Use tomatoes daily in sauces, casseroles and stews to help prevent prostate cancer and heart disease. Cooking the fruit makes lycopene, the main carotene in tomatoes, easier to absorb.

JUICE

 JUICE Drink three glasses of juice each day as a restorative tonic during illness and convalescence, or drink a glass before meals to stimulate digestion.

 LOTION Mix ½ cup (100 ml) tomato juice with 50 ml vodka or other strong alcohol and shake well. Use as a lotion to help prevent acne.

Malus spp.
APPLES

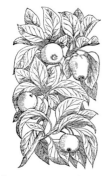

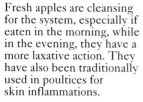

"Their syrup is a good cordial in faintings, palpitations, and melancholy."
Nicholas Culpeper, 1653.

DESPITE THE ADAGE that "an apple a day keeps the doctor away", the apple's medicinal properties are often forgotten. The fruits of *M. communis* have been cultivated since Roman times, with ripe apples used as laxatives and unripe ones to counter diarrhea. In Galenical medicine (see p.24), most apples were cool and moist; juices and infusions were prescribed for fevers and eye infections. Studies have shown that apples can reduce cholesterol levels.

Character
Ripe fruit: cool, moist, generally sweet.
Unripe fruit & some cultivated varieties: cool, moist, sour.
Constituents
Sugars, fruit acids, pectin, vitamins A, B1, C, minerals.
Actions
Tonic, digestive and liver stimulant, diuretic, anti-rheumatic, laxative, antiseptic.

Parts used

RAW FRUIT
Fresh apples are cleansing for the system, especially if eaten in the morning, while in the evening, they have a more laxative action. They have also been traditionally used in poultices for skin inflammations.

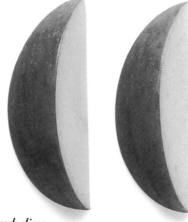

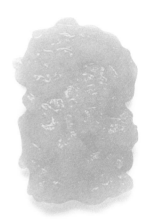

Fresh slices

Stewed apple

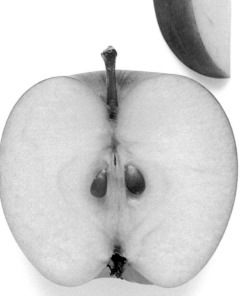

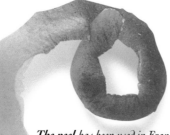

The peel has been used in France in preparations for rheumatism and gout, and as a diuretic in urinary disorders.

STEWED FRUIT
Traditionally used for diarrhea and dysentery, stewed apples can be especially helpful for babies and small children. They can also be soothing in gastric ulceration or ulcerative colitis.

Applications

RAW FRUIT

 FRESH Eat ripe apples for constipation associated with an overheated stomach. Eat sour apples as a diuretic in cystitis and other urinary infections. Apples are also a good source of minerals and vitamins in anaemia and debility.

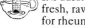 INFUSION Take an infusion of the fresh, raw fruit as a warming drink for rheumatic pains and intestinal colic, and as a cooling remedy for feverish colds.

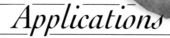 JUICE Use neat juice or juice mixed with olive oil as a household standby for cuts and scrapes.

STEWED FRUIT

 FRESH Use for diarrhea, gastro-enteritis, and intestinal infections.

 POULTICE Apply to skin infections, such as scabies.

CAUTION
• Apples are a "cold" fruit, so eating too many or eating them on a chilled stomach can lead to digestive upsets and gas.

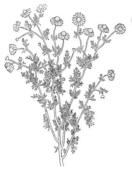

Matricaria recutita
GERMAN CHAMOMILE

CALLED "GROUND APPLE" by the Ancient Greeks because of its smell, chamomile was "maythen" to the Anglo-Saxons, one of nine sacred herbs given to the world by the god Woden. Two species are used medicinally – German chamomile and also Roman chamomile (*Chamaemelum nobile*). They have virtually identical properties and applications. German chamomile is known as "matricaria", referring to its role as a gynecological herb.

"Chamomylle …is very agreeing unto the nature of man, and … is good against weariness…"
William Turner, 1551.

Character
Bitter, mainly warm, moist.
Constituents
Volatile oil (inc. azulenes), flavonoids (inc. rutin), valerianic acid, coumarins, tannins, salicylates, cyanogenic glycosides.
Actions
Anti-inflammatory, anti-spasmodic, bitter, sedative, prevents vomiting.

Parts used

FLOWERS
One home-dried flower can give more flavor than a tea-bag of commercial offerings. Medieval herbalists developed double-flowered varieties to increase the yield of usable parts. Harvest throughout the summer; dry quickly, so that the flowers retain their rich pungent scent for months.

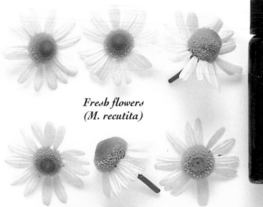

Fresh flowers (M. recutita)

ESSENTIAL OIL
Distilled from fresh flowers since medieval times, the oil is used for a wide range of complaints including eczema and asthma. True chamomile oil is extremely expensive and is a deep blue because of the azulenes it contains.

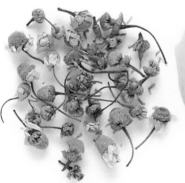

Dried flowers

Ointment

Homeopathic Chamomilla 3x pills or diluted tincture can be helpful for teething and colic in babies.

Tincture

Applications

FLOWERS

 INFUSION Take for irritable bowel syndrome, poor appetite and indigestion. Drink a cup at night for insomnia, anxiety and stress. Add ¾-1¼ cups (200-400 ml) strained infusion to a baby's bath water at night to encourage sleep.

 TINCTURE Use for irritable bowel, insomnia and tension.

 OINTMENT Use for insect bites, wounds, itching eczema, and for anal or vulval irritation.

 MOUTHWASH Use the infusion for mouth inflammations.

 EYEWASH Dissolve 5-10 drops of tincture in warm water, and use for conjunctivitis or strained eyes.

 INHALATION Add 2 tsp flowers to a basin of boiling water for catarrh, hay fever, asthma, or bronchitis.

ESSENTIAL OIL

 LOTION For eczema, use 5 drops chamomile oil to 50 ml distilled witch hazel.

 INHALATION For bad nasal catarrh, asthma or (under medical super-vision) whooping cough, put 2-3 drops in a saucer of warm water and leave in the room at night.

CAUTIONS
• Do not exceed stated doses of the herb and avoid the oil completely in pregnancy, as it is a uterine stimulant.
• This herb can cause contact dermatitis, particularly if sunbathing on damp chamomile lawns.

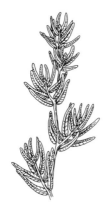

Melaleuca alternifolia
TEA TREE

TEA TREE WAS ORIGINALLY used as a remedy for colds, wounds and general illness by the Aborigines, and in World War II it was included in the field dressing kits of the Australian troops. The plant was first studied in Europe in the 1920s, when French researchers identified its antibiotic properties: the oil was found to be more antibacterial than carbolic acid. Today, the growth of a thriving tea tree industry has led to the availability of many highly adulterated oils.

"The finest antiseptic known to man".
Australian Medical Journal,
August 1930.

Character
Warm, pungent.
Constituents
Terpinen-4-ol (up to 30%), ineol, pinene, cymene, terpinenes, other monoterpenes and sesquiterpenes.
Actions
Antibacterial, antifungal, antiseptic, antiviral, diaphoretic, expectorant.

Parts used

CREAM
Tea tree cream is available commercially and is an ideal household first aid remedy for minor cuts, scrapes and skin sores.

Cream

ESSENTIAL OIL
True tea tree oil is one of the few oils that does not irritate mucous membranes and can be used undiluted on the skin. However, it is best to use diluted oil initially, as many oils are adulterated. The oil is antibacterial, antifungal, antiviral and stimulates the immune system, and is suitable as a treatment for a wide range of infectious conditions.

Essential oil

DRIED LEAVES
Leaves from the tea tree, so named by the botanist Joseph Banks because they made a pleasant tasting infusion, were used by Australian Aborigines for treating colds, fevers, and illness – the type of illnesses we now know are due to microorganisms.

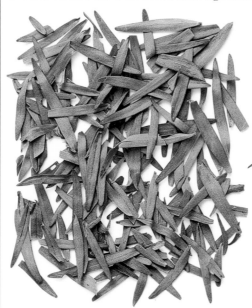

Dried leaves

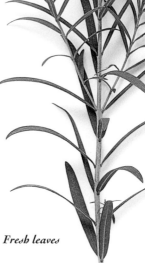

Fresh leaves

Applications

ESSENTIAL OIL
 OIL Use a drop of undiluted oil on warts 2-3 times daily. Dilute with an equal amount of almond oil for any irritation. Massage undiluted oil into the gums for tooth abscesses.

 SUPPOSITORIES Add 2-3 drops tea tree oil per 1 tsp melted cocoa butter to make suppositories (see p.157) for vaginal yeast infections.

 HAIR RINSE After shampooing use 5 ml oil in 1 cup (250 ml) warm water as a rinse for nits and headlice; or put several drops of oil on a fine-toothed comb and comb hair at night.

 LOTION Add 1 drop tea tree oil to 10 drops almond oil for cold sores. Add 5 ml of oil to 20 ml each of distilled witch hazel and rosewater and apply to acne pustules with cotton balls several times a day.

 CREAM Apply tea tree cream to athlete's foot, ringworm, cuts, scrapes, insect bites, and other skin infections.

DRIED LEAVES
 INFUSION Use 10 g leaves per 2 cups (500 ml) water or ½ tsp leaves per cup for colds, mononucleosis, cystitis, and urinary infections.

Melissa officinalis
LEMON BALM

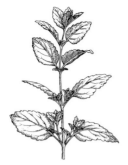

> "Balm is sovereign for the brain, strengthening the memory and powerfully chasing away melancholy."
> John Evelyn, 1679.

BALM AND BEES have been linked since ancient times. *Melissa* comes from the Greek for "honey bee," and lemon balm has the same healing and tonic properties as honey and royal jelly. Gerard said that the herb "comforteth the hart and driveth away all sadnesse," and it was a favorite in medieval "elixirs of youth;" the alchemist Paracelsus made a preparation called *primum ens melissae*, and even in the 18th century, it was still thought to "renew youth."

Character Cold, dry, sour, slightly bitter.
Constituents Volatile oil (inc. citronellal), polyphenols, tannins, bitter principle, flavonoids, rosmarinic acid.
Actions Sedative, anti-depressant, digestive stimulant, relaxes peripheral blood vessels, promotes sweating, relaxing restorative for nervous system, antiviral to *Herpes simplex* (possibly due to polyphenols and tannins), antibacterial, carminative, antispasmodic.

Parts used

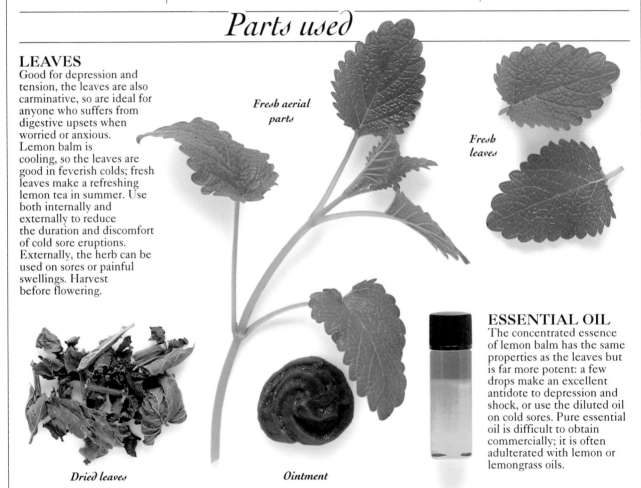

LEAVES
Good for depression and tension, the leaves are also carminative, so are ideal for anyone who suffers from digestive upsets when worried or anxious. Lemon balm is cooling, so the leaves are good in feverish colds; fresh leaves make a refreshing lemon tea in summer. Use both internally and externally to reduce the duration and discomfort of cold sore eruptions. Externally, the herb can be used on sores or painful swellings. Harvest before flowering.

Fresh aerial parts

Fresh leaves

Dried leaves

Ointment

ESSENTIAL OIL
The concentrated essence of lemon balm has the same properties as the leaves but is far more potent: a few drops make an excellent antidote to depression and shock, or use the diluted oil on cold sores. Pure essential oil is difficult to obtain commercially; it is often adulterated with lemon or lemongrass oils.

Applications

LEAVES

INFUSION Take for depression, nervous exhaustion, indigestion, nausea, and the early stages of colds and influenza. Best made with fresh leaves.

TINCTURE Has a stronger but similar action to the infusion. Best made from fresh leaves. Small doses (5-10 drops) are usually more effective.

COMPRESS Use a pad soaked in the infusion to relieve painful swellings, such as gout.

OINTMENT Use for sores, cold sores, insect bites, or to repel insects.

INFUSED OIL Use hot infused oil as the ointment or as a gentle massage oil for depression, tension, asthma, and bronchitis.

ESSENTIAL OIL

OINTMENT Combine 5 ml oil with 100 g ointment base for insect bites or to repel insects.

MASSAGE OIL Dilute 5-10 drops oil in 20 ml almond or olive oil, and use for tension or chest complaints.

Mentha spp.
MINT

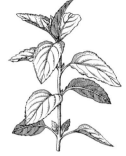

"If any man can name... all the properties of mint, he must know how many fish swim in the Indian ocean." Wilafried of Strabo, 12th century.

THERE ARE THOUGHT to be at least thirty species of mint. Until the 17th century, all mints were used in much the same way, with little attempt to differentiate between varieties. Today, peppermint (*M. x piperita*) is preferred medicinally in the West; the Chinese use field mint (*M. arvensis*), known as *bo he*. Garden mint is usually spearmint (*M. spicata*). Not as strong as peppermint, this can be used in similar ways, and is good for children.

Character Pungent, dry, generally cooling.
Constituents Volatile oil (mainly menthol), tannins, flavonoids, tocopherols, choline, bitter principle.
Actions Antispasmodic, digestive tonic, prevents vomiting, carminative, relaxes peripheral blood vessels, promotes sweating but also cooling internally, promotes bile flow, analgesic.

Parts used

AERIAL PARTS
M. X PIPERITA
These relax the muscles of the digestive tract and stimulate bile flow, so are useful for indigestion, flatulence, colic, and similar conditions. They reduce nausea and can be helpful for motion sickness; they also promote sweating in fevers and influenza. Harvest just before flowering.

AERIAL PARTS
M. ARVENSIS
The Chinese use *bo he* as a cooling remedy for head colds and influenza, and also for some types of headaches, sore throats, and eye inflammations. As a liver stimulant, it is added to remedies for digestive disorders or liver *qi* (energy) stagnation.

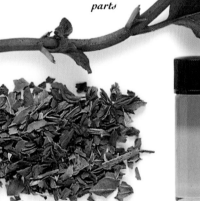

Fresh aerial parts

ESSENTIAL OIL
M. X PIPERITA
Peppermint oil contains large amounts of menthol. In fairly high doses, it is analgesic and calming. It is also cooling, so is good for skin complaints, fevers, or headaches and migraines linked to overheating. Antibacterial, it can help combat infections. Used as an inhalant, it clears nasal congestion.

Dried aerial parts

Fresh aerial parts

Applications

AERIAL PARTS
M. X PIPERITA / M. ARVENSIS

 INFUSION Take for nausea, motion sickness, indigestion, flatulence, colic, feverish conditions, and migraines.

 TINCTURE Use for the same conditions as the infusion.

 COMPRESS Soak a pad in the infusion to cool inflamed joints or for rheumatism or neuralgia.

 INHALATION Put a few fresh leaves in boiling water, and inhale to ease nasal congestion.

ESSENTIAL OIL
M. X PIPERITA

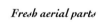 WASH Use 2-3 drops of oil in 10 ml water for skin irritations, itching, burns, inflammations, scabies and ringworm, or to repel mosquitos.

 INHALATION 2-3 drops of oil in a saucer of water left in the room at night will reduce nasal congestion.

 MASSAGE OIL Dilute 5-10 drops peppermint oil in 25 ml almond or sunflower oil for headaches, fever, or menstrual pain, or to relieve milk congestion when breast-feeding.

CAUTIONS
• Avoid prolonged use of the essential oil as an inhalant.
• Mint can irritate the mucous membranes and should not be given to children for more than a week without a break. Do not give any form of mint directly to young babies.
• Peppermint can reduce milk flow, so take internally with caution if breast-feeding, or use spearmint instead.

Morus nigra & M. alba
MULBERRY

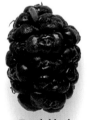

"Mulberries taken in meate... do very speedily passe thorow the belly... and make a passage for other meates, as Galen saith."
John Gerard, 1597.

IN THE 16TH CENTURY, the berries, bark, and leaves of the black mulberry (*M. nigra*) were all used medicinally: the berries for inflammations and to stop bleeding; the bark for toothache; and the leaves for "the bitings of serpents" and as an antidote to aconite poisoning. While mulberry has faded from the European *materia medica*, white mulberry (*M. alba*) is still widely used in China as a remedy for coughs, colds, and high blood pressure, and as a *yin* tonic.

Character
Mainly sweet, cold; leaves also bitter; branch bitter and neutral.
Constituents
Flavonoids, coumarin, tannins, sugars; berries also contain vitamins A, B₁, B₂, C.
Actions
Berries: tonic, laxative.
Leaves: antibacterial, promote sweating, expectorant.
Branch: antirheumatic, reduces high blood pressure, analgesic.
Root bark: sedative, diuretic, expectorant, lowers blood pressure.

Parts used

BERRIES
M. NIGRA & M. ALBA
In China, white mulberries, or *sang shen*, are used as a *yin* tonic to nourish the blood and "vital essence," and as a gentle laxative in constipation. In European tradition, black mulberries are also regarded as a tonic and taken for weakness. Harvest when ripe.

Fresh white mulberry

Dried white mulberry

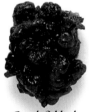

Fresh black mulberry

Crushed black mulberry

LEAVES
M. NIGRA & M. ALBA
In China, white mulberry leaves, *sang ye*, are generally used for colds with fevers, headaches, and sore throats, to cool heat in the liver channel, which can lead to sore eyes and irritability, and to cool the blood. In Europe, black mulberry leaves have recently been used to stimulate insulin production in diabetes. Harvest in summer.

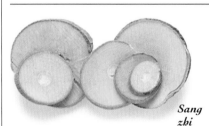

Fresh black mulberry leaves

BRANCH & TWIGS
M. ALBA
Sang zhi have been shown to be analgesic and to reduce high blood pressure, although traditionally they have been used for rheumatic disorders. The Chinese consider them more suitable for upper body pain.

Sang zhi

ROOT BARK
M. ALBA
Sang bai pi is a good expectorant for coughs associated with "hot" conditions (usually typified by thick, sticky yellow phlegm). It can help asthma and is sedative and soothing.

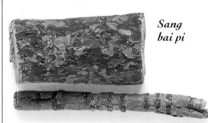

Sang bai pi

Applications

BERRIES (*M. ALBA/M. NIGRA*)

 TINCTURE Take as a tonic to nourish the blood and *yin*: combine with *wu wei zi* or *he shou wu*, or just eat the fresh fruits.

 MOUTHWASH/GARGLE Crush the fresh berries, and use the juice for mouth ulcers and sore throats.

LEAVES (*M. ALBA/M. NIGRA*)

 INFUSION Take for colds and chills: combines well with elderflower and mint.

 DECOCTION Take for colds.

 SYRUP Take a syrup made from the decoction for coughs.

TWIGS
M. ALBA

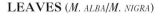 DECOCTION Use for rheumatic pains in the upper body: combine with herbs such as Siberian ginseng, *fang feng*, *gui zhi*, or *qin jiao*.

ROOT BARK
M. ALBA

 DECOCTION Use for "hot" conditions affecting the lungs, for asthma, or as a diuretic in edema (use with *fu ling*, *chen pi*, and buchu).

CAUTIONS
• Avoid excess fruits if suffering from diarrhea.
• Avoid the leaves and bark if the lungs are weak or "cold"; if in doubt, seek professional advice.

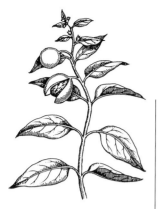

Myristica fragrans
NUTMEG

"...in large quantities it is apt to affect the head, and even to manifest an hypnotic power..."
Dr. E. Sibley, 1821.

FIRST BROUGHT TO EUROPE from the Banda Islands by Portuguese sailors in 1512, nutmeg gained the reputation of a cure-all and was widely eaten as a tonic. Its hallucinogenic properties were soon discovered, with nutmeg eaters becoming "deliriously inebriated." It was also taken, erroneously, to procure abortions and was acclaimed as a cure for the plague. Known as *rou dou kou* in China, it has been used there since the 7th century.

Character
Pungent, warm.
Constituents
Volatile oil (inc. borneol, eugenol).
Actions
Carminative, digestive stimulant, antispasmodic, prevents vomiting, appetite stimulant, anti-inflammatory.

Parts used

KERNEL
Mainly used today as a digestive remedy for nausea, vomiting, indigestion, and also for diarrhea, especially if related to food poisoning. In trials it has been used successfully to treat Crohn's disease. The Chinese take *rou dou kou* to warm the stomach and regulate *qi* (energy) flow. It is also used for the classic "cock-crow" diarrhea, which occurs on rising and can be related to *qi* weakness.

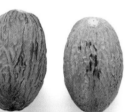

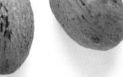
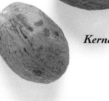

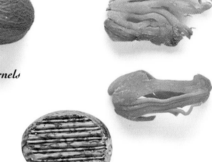
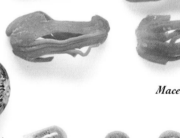

In folk medicine, the outer fleshy aril of the fruit, mace, was made into an ointment used for rheumatism.

Kernels

Mace

ESSENTIAL OIL
Externally, the oil is used for rheumatic pain and, like clove oil, can be applied as an emergency treatment to dull toothache. In France, it is given in drop doses in honey for digestive upsets and used for bad breath.

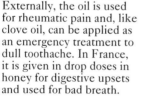
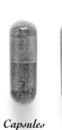

Grated nutmeg

Capsules

Applications

KERNEL

DECOCTION Decoct 5 g with 2 g ginger, 2 g licorice, 5 g *wu wei zi*, 5 g *wu zhu yu*, and 10 g *bu gu zhi* in 2½ cups (600 ml) water (three doses), and take one dose three times a day for early morning diarrhea or colitis.

CAPSULES Take 1-2 x 200 mg capsules for nausea, indigestion, gastric upsets, and chronic diarrhea.

ESSENTIAL OIL

OIL Put 1-2 drops on a cotton swab, and apply to the gums around an aching tooth until dental treatment

can be obtained. Use 3-5 drops on a sugar lump or in a teaspoon of honey for nausea, gastroenteritis, chronic diarrhea, and indigestion.

MASSAGE OIL Dilute 10 drops in 10 ml almond oil, and use for muscular pains associated with rheumatism or overexertion. Can also be combined with thyme or rosemary essential oils. To prepare for childbirth, massage the abdomen daily in the three weeks before the baby is due with a mixture of 5 drops nutmeg oil and no more than 5 drops sage oil in 25 ml almond oil.

CAUTION
• Large doses (7.5 g or more in a single dose) are dangerous, producing convulsions and palpitations.

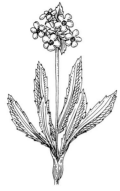

Nardostachys grandiflora
SPIKENARD

HIGHLY VALUED since Biblical times, spikenard was the substance used to anoint Jesus at the Last Supper, and was regarded as a rejuvenating tonic by the Moghul emperors. It is known as *jatamansi* in India, and shares the sedative properties of its relative, valerian (see p.133). Spikenard is listed in CITES (Convention on International Trade in Endangered Species of Wild Fauna and Flora), and trade of the wild plant is permitted only by license.

"...there came a woman having an alabaster box of ointment of spikenard very precious; and she brake the box, and poured it on his head."
Mark 14 v. 3, *The Bible.*

Character
Sweet, bitter, astringent.
Constituents
Volatile oil (inc. borneol acetates).
Actions
Antifungal, antibacterial, relaxing nervine, carminative, laxative, antispasmodic, diuretic.

Parts used

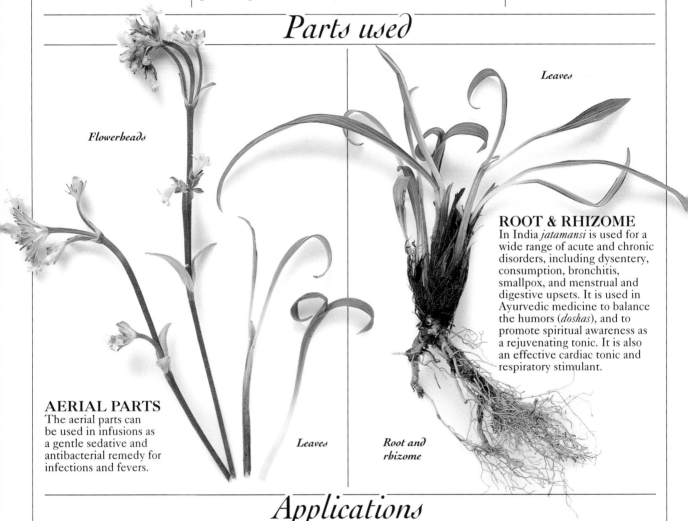

Flowerheads

Leaves

Leaves

ROOT & RHIZOME
In India *jatamansi* is used for a wide range of acute and chronic disorders, including dysentery, consumption, bronchitis, smallpox, and menstrual and digestive upsets. It is used in Ayurvedic medicine to balance the humors (*doshas*), and to promote spiritual awareness as a rejuvenating tonic. It is also an effective cardiac tonic and respiratory stimulant.

AERIAL PARTS
The aerial parts can be used in infusions as a gentle sedative and antibacterial remedy for infections and fevers.

Leaves

Root and rhizome

Applications

AERIAL PARTS

 INFUSION Drink a cup as a calming and soothing tea after a stressful day.

 WASH Use the infusion to bathe cuts, scrapes, and fungal skin infections such as athlete's foot.

ROOT & RHIZOME

 DECOCTION Simmer 1 tsp dried root in a cup of milk as a restoring tonic for tension and emotional upsets.

 SYRUP Take 1-2 tsp for coughs and bronchitis.

 MACERATION Macerate the root as for valerian (see p.133) and use as a tonic and calming sedative.

 TINCTURE Take up to 40 drops as an alternative to valerian and use as a calming sedative, or combine with *gotu kola* as a digestive and energy tonic.

 DECOCTION Use the standard decoction for constipation, poor appetite, and sluggish digestion. Add a pinch of powdered cinnamon to each cup, or combine with an equal amount of *gotu kola* infusion.

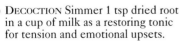

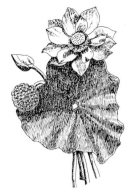

Nelumbo nucifera
LOTUS

THE LOTUS, OR *padma*, is revered as India's most sacred plant, and the unfolding petals symbolize the growth of spiritual awareness. In the East the plant holds a similar place to the rose in the West – it is a potent symbol of love and compassion. In Chinese medicine, almost all parts of the herb are used to treat a range of ailments. The nodes of the rhizome (*ou jie*) are used to stop bleeding, while in India the root and rhizome is used as a rejuvenating tonic.

"In the beginning were the waters. Matter readied itself. The sun glowed. And a lotus slowly opened, holding the universe on its golden pericarp."
Indian creation myth.

Character
Most parts are cooling or neutral, sweet and astringent.
Constituents
Rhizome nodes: asparagine, tannin, vitamin C.
Seeds: carbohydrates, calcium, phosphorus, iron, proteins.
Stamens: flavonoids, alkaloids, glucosides.
Leaves: alkaloids, flavonoids, oxalic acid, malic acid, tannin.
Actions
Aphrodisiac, astringent, stops bleeding, tonic, nervine.

Parts used

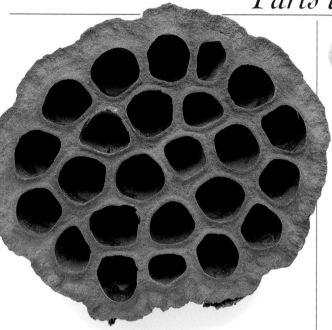

Receptacle/Flower stalk

Seeds

SEEDS
In China, the seeds (*lian zi*) are used as a tonic for the spleen and stomach to combat diarrhea and stimulate the appetite. They are also a kidney tonic and a sedative for insomnia and palpitations.

LEAVES/ LEAF STEMS
The leaves (*he ye*) and leaf stems (*lian geng*) are used in Chinese medicine mainly as a cooling remedy for fevers associated with "summer heat". They are given as a spleen tonic for weakness associated with diarrhea, and for upsets following summer fevers.

Leaf and leaf stem

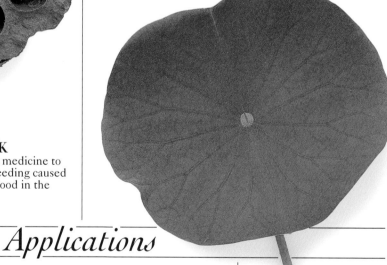

RECEPTACLE/FLOWER STALK
The flower stalk (*lian fang*) is used in Chinese medicine to disperse congealed blood and stop internal bleeding caused by gastric ulcers, abnormally heavy periods, blood in the stools, or hemorrhage following childbirth.

Applications

RECEPTACLE/ FLOWER STALK

INFUSION Combine with motherwort for heavy periods and irregularity.

LEAVES/LEAF STEMS

INFUSION Take a cup, three times daily, for summer colds and fevers.

RHIZOME NODE

DECOCTION Combine with *sheng di huang* and elecampane for bronchitis and congestive coughs with bloody phlegm; seek professional help if symptoms last for more than a day.

SEEDS

POWDER/CAPSULES Use 1-2 x 200 mg capsules or ¹/₂ tsp powder in water as a heart and kidney tonic. In India the same mix is used to strengthen the heart *chakra* and to encourage aspiration, concentration, and devotion, as well as to improve speech and reduce stammering.

DECOCTION Combine with *dang shen* and golden seal for insomnia, palpitations, irritability, and urinary dysfunction associated with kidney and heart energy weakness.

CAUTION
• Avoid lotus if suffering from constipation.

Ocimum spp.
BASIL

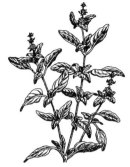

"This herb and rue will not grow together... and we know rue is as great an enemy of poison as any that grows."
Nicholas Culpeper, 1653.

FROM ITS NATIVE INDIA, sweet basil (*O. basilicum*) was introduced into Europe in ancient times. Views and traditions associated with the herb have been mixed. Some cultures associated basil with hatred and misfortune; others regarded it as a love token. Dioscorides said that it should never be taken internally, while Pliny advised smelling it in vinegar for fainting fits. In Ayurvedic medicine, holy basil (*O. sanctum*) is known as *tulsi* and the juice is an important tonic.

Character
Sweet, pungent, slightly bitter, very warm, dry.
Constituents
Volatile oil (including estragol), tannins, basil camphor.
Actions
Antidepressant, antiseptic, stimulates the adrenal cortex, prevents vomiting, tonic, carminative, febrifuge, expectorant, soothes itching, reduces blood sugar levels, lowers blood pressure.

Parts used

LEAVES
Good for rubbing on insect bites, the leaves can also be taken as a warming and uplifting tonic for nervous exhaustion or any cold condition. Harvest before flowering.

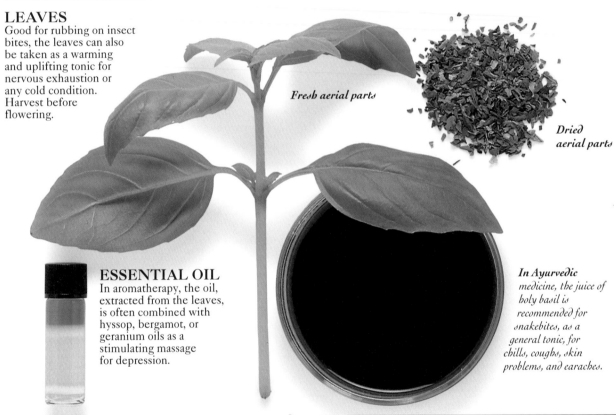

Fresh aerial parts

Dried aerial parts

ESSENTIAL OIL
In aromatherapy, the oil, extracted from the leaves, is often combined with hyssop, bergamot, or geranium oils as a stimulating massage for depression.

In Ayurvedic medicine, the juice of holy basil is recommended for snakebites, as a general tonic, for chills, coughs, skin problems, and earaches.

Applications

LEAVES

 FRESH Rub on insect bites to reduce itching and inflammation.

 INFUSION Combine with a little motherwort and drink immediately after childbirth to prevent a retained placenta.

 TINCTURE Combine with wood betony and skullcap for nervous conditions, or with elecampane and hyssop for coughs and bronchitis.

 WASH Combine the juice with an equal quantity of honey and use for ringworm and itching skin.

 JUICE Mix with a decoction of cinnamon and cloves for chills.

 SYRUP Combine the juice with an equal quantity of honey for coughs.

 INHALATION Pour boiling water onto the leaves and inhale the steam for head colds.

ESSENTIAL OIL

 OIL Add 5-10 drops to a bath for nervous exhaustion, mental fatigue, melancholy, or uneasiness.

 CHEST RUB Dilute 5 drops basil oil in 10 ml almond or sunflower oil for asthma and bronchitis.

 MASSAGE OIL Use the diluted oil for nervous weakness; can also be applied as an insect repellent.

CAUTION
• Do not use the essential oil externally (or internally) in pregnancy.

Paeonia spp.
PEONY

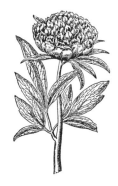

"This plant also prevents the mocking delusions that the Fauns bring on us in our sleep." Pliny, A.D. 77.

ALTHOUGH NOW REGARDED in the West as no more than a decorative garden flower, the peony has a long tradition as a medicinal herb, and was used in the past to treat nervous conditions that included epilepsy. Today, the root is still valued in Chinese medicine, where two species are used: both the red- and white-flowered *P. lactiflora*, and *P. suffruticosa*, the tree peony. The name is reputedly derived from Paeos, a physician during the Trojan Wars.

Character
P. LACTIFLORA: sour, bitter, cold.
P. SUFFRUTICOSA: more pungent.
Constituents
Alkaloids, volatile oil, benzoic acid, asparagin.
Actions
P. LACTIFLORA: antibacterial, anti-spasmodic, anti-inflammatory, analgesic, tranquilizing, lowers blood pressure.
P. SUFFRUTICOSA: antibacterial, circulatory stimulant, lowers blood pressure, analgesic, anti-inflammatory, sedative.

Parts used

ROOT
P. LACTIFLORA (RED)
Known as *chi shao yao* in China, the root of the red peony is thought to cool the blood, move stagnating blood, and relieve pain. Recent experiments in London combined red peony root with other Chinese herbs to treat childhood eczema successfully.

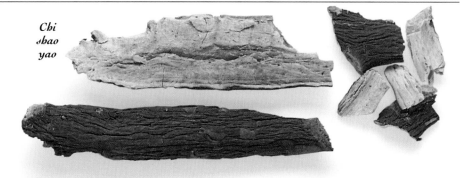

Chi shao yao

ROOT
P. LACTIFLORA (WHITE)
White peony root has a much more specific action on the liver than red peony, soothing liver energy and improving function. In Chinese medicine, *bai shao yao* is seen as nourishing the blood rather than cooling it, and is considered one of the great women's tonics, often used for menstrual disorders.

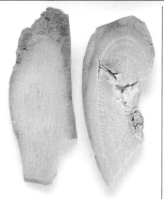

Bai shao yao

ROOT BARK
P. SUFFRUTICOSA
In China, tree peony root bark, *mu dan pi*, is considered to cool the blood, and has also been used in the childhood eczema project in London. The root bark is also a good antibacterial, used for boils and abscesses.

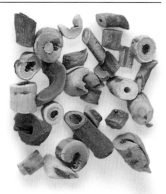

Mu dan pi

Applications

ROOT
P. LACTIFLORA (RED)

 DECOCTION Use up to 45 g herb in 2½ cups (600 ml) water (enough for three doses) for any condition involving overheated blood, including certain types of eczema, skin inflammations, nosebleeds, and pain associated with injury. Best in combination with herbs such as *mu dan pi* and *fang feng*.

ROOT
P. LACTIFLORA (WHITE)

 DECOCTION Take for liver-associated problems and some menstrual disorders. As a regular tonic, ideal for women and reputed

to beautify the skin, decoct 20 g *bai shao yao* and 5 g licorice root for 15 minutes with 2 cups (500 ml) water, and drink two half-cup doses a day.

ROOT BARK
P. SUFFRUTICOSA

 DECOCTION Use 30 g herb in 2½ cups (600 ml) water (enough for three doses) in combination with other herbs such as *sheng di huang* for feverish conditions involving nosebleeds, or add to remedies for hot, dry eczema. Combine with *shu di huang, shan zhu yu, fu ling, ze xie,* and *shan yao* for liver disharmonies.

CAUTION
• Avoid during pregnancy.

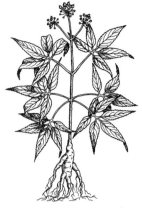

Panax spp.
GINSENG

USED IN CHINA FOR over 5,000 years, ginseng (*P. ginseng*) was known to 9th-century Arab physicians. Marco Polo wrote of this prized wonder drug and, when a delegation from the King of Siam visited Louis XIV, they presented him with a root of *gintz-aen*. From then on, ginseng was widely used by wealthy Europeans for exhaustion and debility. By the 18th century, it was also popular in America, especially when *P. quinquefolius* was found to be indigenous.

"This, with the Chinese, is the medicine par excellence, the last resort when all other drugs fail..."
G. Stuart, 1911.

Character
All species: Sweet, slightly bitter.
P. GINSENG / P. NOTOGINSENG: warm.
P. QUINQUEFOLIUS: cool.
Constituents
Steroidal glycosides, saponins, volatile oil, vitamin D, acetyleneic compounds, sterols.
Actions
Tonic, stimulant, reduces blood sugar and cholesterol levels, stimulates the immune system, helps the body to adapt to stress.

Parts used

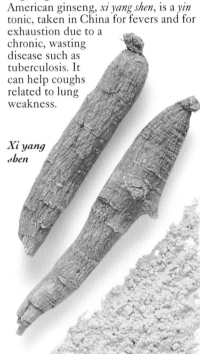

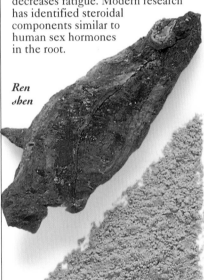

ROOT
P. GINSENG
Korean or Chinese ginseng, *ren shen*, is one of the most prized and expensive herbs. It is a *yang* tonic, replenishing *qi* (energy), especially in the spleen and lungs. It also strengthens the immune system and decreases fatigue. Modern research has identified steroidal components similar to human sex hormones in the root.

Ren shen

Powder

ROOT
P. QUINQUEFOLIUS
American ginseng, *xi yang shen*, is a *yin* tonic, taken in China for fevers and for exhaustion due to a chronic, wasting disease such as tuberculosis. It can help coughs related to lung weakness.

Xi yang shen

Powder

ROOT
P. PSEUDO-GINSENG
Known as *san qi*, or *tienchi*, in China, this is used as an analgesic and to stop internal and external bleeding. It is also added to treatments for coronary heart disease and angina. *San qi* was often used by the Vietcong during the Vietnam war to increase recovery rates from gun-shot wounds.

San qi

Sliced root

Applications

ROOT
P. GINSENG

NOTE It is often best to take P. ginseng *for one month in autumn to strengthen the body for winter. If taking* P. ginseng *regularly, have a break of at least 2-3 weeks every 2 months.*

 DECOCTION Take 3-10 g in 2 cups (500 ml) water as a *yang* tonic.

 TINCTURE Use for diarrhea related to weak digestive function. For asthma and chronic coughs, combine with walnut and ginger.

 POWDER Use in capsules or pills in 500 mg to 4 g doses as a tonic.

ROOT
P. QUINQUEFOLIUS

 TINCTURE Take as a tonic or combine with herbs such as elecampane and mulberry bark for chronic coughs and weak lungs.

 POWDER Use in capsules or pills in 1-2 g doses for *yin* deficiency.

ROOT
P. PSEUDO-GINSENG

 POWDER Use in capsules or pills in 1-2 g doses for wounds, bleeding or pain. Combine with slippery elm for the pain of gastric ulceration.

CAUTIONS
• Avoid *P. pseudo-ginseng* in pregnancy; it may adversely affect the fetus.
• Although *P. ginseng* is generally safe, side effects have been reported: avoid high doses or prolonged use in pregnancy and if affected by hypertension.
• Avoid other stimulants such as tea, coffee and cola drinks when taking *P. ginseng*.

Passiflora incarnata
PASSION FLOWER

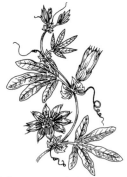

"The Mayas used the crushed plant as a poultice for swellings and in internal decoctions for ringworm…the juice was applied with cotton to sore eyes."
Virgil Vogel, *American Indian Medicine*, 1970.

THE NAME PASSION FLOWER derives from the Christian symbolism of its flowers: three stigmas for the nails of the Crucifixion, five anthers for Christ's five wounds, a finely cut corona for the Crown of Thorns, and ten sepals representing the Apostles present at the Cross. The herb originates in North America, where it is known as maypop, and was first sent to Europe as a gift for Pope Paul V in 1605. By the 19th century, it was given for epilepsy and later for insomnia.

Character
Cooling, bitter.
Constituents
Flavonoids (inc. rutin), cyanogenic glycosides, alkaloids, sapanarin.
Actions
Analgesic, antispasmodic, bitter, cooling, hypotensive, sedative, heart tonic, relaxes blood vessels.

Parts used

AERIAL PARTS

The Houmas tribe of Louisiana traditionally used passion flower as a blood tonic, and the Maya Indians used the crushed plant for swellings and ringworm. Today, it is primarily used as a sedative and painkiller, to reduce blood pressure, and as a homeopathic remedy for nervous insomnia. Although a potent remedy, it is gentle enough for children and can be used for hyperactivity and restlessness. It can ease tremors in the elderly, including those associated with Parkinson's disease, and can help to relieve the vertigo and dizziness of Ménière's disease.

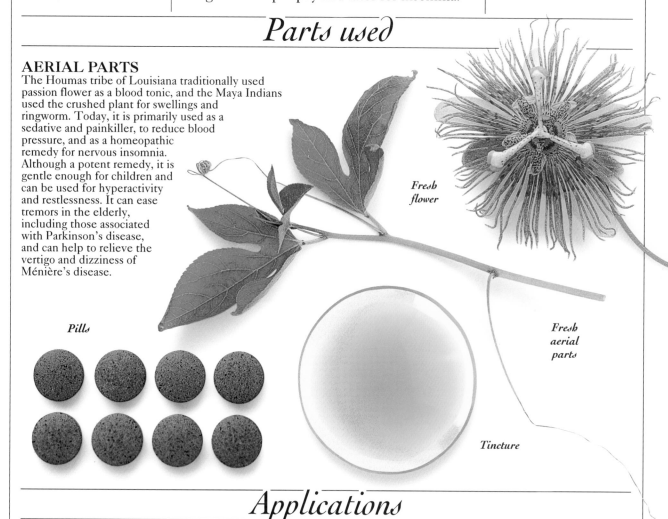

Fresh flower

Fresh aerial parts

Pills

Tincture

Applications

AERIAL PARTS

 PILLS Take 1-2 pills at night (or as directed on the pack) for insomnia. Use for nervous tension during the day, although excess can cause drowsiness.

 TINCTURE Combine with equal amounts of valerian and hops for insomnia and nervous tension or for high blood pressure. Take 50 drops three times daily in a little water.

 TINCTURE Use up to 4 ml, three times daily, for tremors and vertigo, or to ease the pain associated with shingles and toothache.

 POWDER/PILLS Use 1-2 x 200 mg capsules or ½ tsp powder night and morning for anxiety, tension and stress headaches.

 INFUSION Take a cup for period pain, tension headaches, and to calm underlying tension in irritable bowel syndrome or for irregular heart beats. Dilute a standard infusion with an equal amount of water and give half a cup for hyperactivity in children.

 INFUSION Combine the infusion with an equal amount of raspberry leaf for period pain.

CAUTIONS
• Use only low doses of passion flower in pregnancy.
• The herb may cause drowsiness.

Phyllostachys nigra
BAMBOO

BAMBOO IS AN important Asian cash crop, used to make objects ranging from drainpipes and scaffolding to musical instruments. Extracts of bamboo are used in Chinese and Ayurvedic medicine, primarily as a cooling lung remedy for coughs and congestion and as a rejuvenating tonic after chronic illness. Bamboo extracts can be rich in silica, leading some Western suppliers to promote it for bone and joint disorders, and for the prevention of bone loss after menopause.

"The palace has arisen firm as the roots of a clump of bamboo."
Chinese proverb.

Character
Sweet, cold.
Constituents
Cellulose, sugars, triterpenes.
Actions
Antispasmodic, antimicrobial, demulcent, expectorant, tonic, stops bleeding.

Parts used

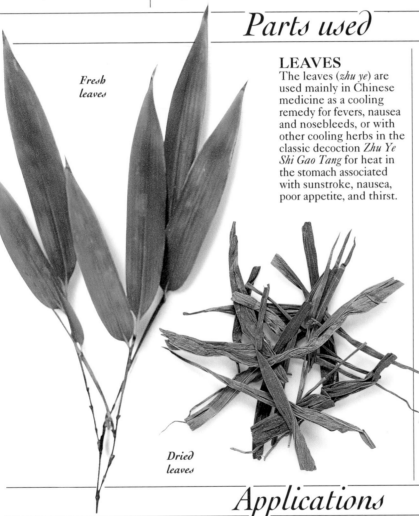

Fresh leaves

Dried leaves

Shavings

LEAVES
The leaves (*zhu ye*) are used mainly in Chinese medicine as a cooling remedy for fevers, nausea and nosebleeds, or with other cooling herbs in the classic decoction *Zhu Ye Shi Gao Tang* for heat in the stomach associated with sunstroke, nausea, poor appetite, and thirst.

SHAVINGS
Bamboo shavings (*zhu ru*) are usually supplied by Chinese herbalists in balls, and are similar to raffia in appearance. They are used as a cooling remedy for the blood, to clear dampness and phlegm, and to clear heat from the stomach, which in Chinese terms may include symptoms such as bad breath and nausea. In Ayurvedic medicine they can be used as *vamsha rochana*, or bamboo manna, and are regarded as anti-*pitta* to stop bleeding and reduce fevers.

Applications

LEAVES

INFUSION Take a cup for feverish colds and nausea. Soak a swab in the infusion and use to plug nosebleeds. The infusion can be taken internally.

SHAVINGS

DECOCTION Combine the decoction with an equal amount of elecampane as a tonic following influenza, or use with a pinch of ginger for congestive coughs. The decoction is often made with milk in Ayurvedic medicine.

TINCTURE Take 20-40 drops to soothe the nervous system.

POWDER Use 250 mg to 1 g (up to 1 tsp) powder per dose as a lung tonic following influenza or other debilitating disorder.

CAUTIONS
• Avoid taking bamboo if suffering from diarrhea or coughs associated with colds.

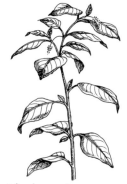

Phytolacca americana
POKEROOT

CALLED POCON BY NATIVE AMERICANS, pokeroot was used mainly in two ways: as an emetic, and externally for skin diseases. The Delaware Indians took it as a heart stimulant and in Virginia it was regarded as a strong purgative. Even today Appalachian backwoodsmen chew the seeds and berries for arthritis – all the more remarkable because the fresh plant is very toxic. It arrived in Europe in the 19th century and is used as an important lymphatic cleanser.

"...it has been used as an alterative in syphilis, rheumatism and chronic eruptions. The berries have also been praised in the same complaints."
R. Eglesfield Griffiths, 1859.

Character
Pungent, drying, slightly cold.
Constituents
Saponins, tannins, alkaloids, bitter principle, sugars.
Actions
Antirheumatic, stimulant, anticatarrhal, purgative, causes vomiting, antiparasitic, anti-inflammatory, immune stimulant, lymphatic stimulant, mild analgesic.

Parts used

DRIED ROOT
Used today as a lymphatic cleanser, particularly for mononucleosis and tonsillitis, the dried root can also be helpful for mastitis, and is added to rheumatic remedies. Externally, it is used occasionally for skin infections such as scabies and ringworm; it can also be applied in poultices to soothe ulcers, hemorrhoids and inflamed joints.

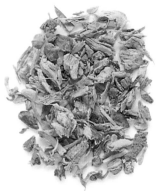
Dried root

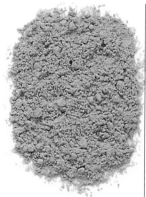
Powdered root

BERRIES
Generally described as "milder" in action than the root, the fresh and dried berries are toxic, so the Appalachian practice of chewing them is not recommended. In the past, they were used externally for skin complaints and in poultices for rheumatism. The juice was applied for ulcers and tumors, but is not particularly effective.

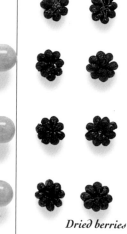

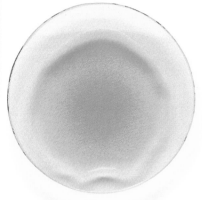
Tincture

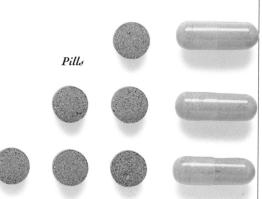
Pills

Dried berries

Applications

DRIED ROOT

 TINCTURE Use a maximum dose of 1 ml (20 drops) for acute lymphatic congestion and infection, including mastitis, tonsillitis, scrofula and mononucleosis. Combine with wild indigo, purple coneflower or cleavers. Add to herbal remedies for rheumatism and rheumatoid arthritis. Can also be added to remedies used to stimulate the liver, or in prescriptions for gastric ulceration.

 POULTICE Apply to inflamed joints, varicose ulcers, hemorrhoids, or for mastitis.

 LOTION Use the diluted tincture or powder dispersed in water for lymphatic swellings.

 POWDER Take internally in small doses (50-250 mg) for lymphatic disorders including mastitis and tonsillitis, or for rheumatism. Use a little powder as a dust for skin fungal infections, dry eczema, psoriasis and scabies.

 CREAM Use with a little ginger in a cream for mastitis and other glandular inflammations.

CAUTIONS
• All parts of the fresh plant are toxic and can cause vomiting. Avoid growing pokeroot in the garden if you have young children, as fatalities have been reported.
• The dried berries are toxic.
• In large doses, the dried root is an extremely violent emetic (causes vomiting) and purgative. Do not exceed stated doses.
• Avoid pokeroot in pregnancy, as it can cause fetal abnormalities.

Piper spp.
PEPPER

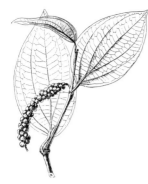

"A sparing diet did her health assure;
Or sick, a pepper posset was her cure."
John Dryden.

MANY FORMS OF PEPPER are used medicinally – notably black pepper (*P. nigrum*), which is a common seasoning, and long pepper (*P. longum*), which is known in India as *pippali* and in China as *bi ba*. These peppers originated in the East Indies, but have been imported into Europe since ancient times. Pliny cites pepper for many ailments, for example coughs, and the mystic Hildegard of Bingen used it in a remedy for strengthening the liver and cleansing the lungs.

Character
Pungent, hot.
Constituents
Alkaloids (inc. piperine), camphene, ß-bisabolene and other terpenes, proteins, minerals.
Actions
Antiseptic, antibacterial, carminative, digestive, and circulatory stimulant. Topical: increases blood flow to an area.

Parts used

FRUIT
P. NIGRUM
Black pepper is an effective warming stimulant for the digestive tract. It is traditionally known to balance out gas caused by eating cold, damp vegetables such as beans. In China, the herb is known as *hu jiao* and is used as a warming remedy for stomach chills.

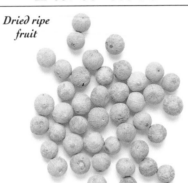
Dried ripe fruit

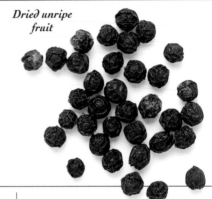
Dried unripe fruit

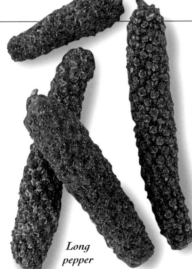
Long pepper

FRUIT
P. LONGUM
Pippali is regarded as an aphrodisiac, and is used in Ayurvedic medicine to strengthen *pitta* and control the *vata* and *kapha* humors. It is also given for digestive and respiratory problems associated with bronchitis, laryngitis, coughs, and colds, indigestion, and abdominal bloating. In China, the fruits (known as *bi ba*) are used for abdominal chills and discomfort, and are believed to reverse the upward flow of *qi* to combat nausea and acid reflux, as well as being a useful painkiller for headaches, toothache, and sinus pain.

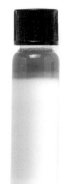

ESSENTIAL OIL
P. NIGRUM
Black pepper oil is used in aromatherapy massage for aches and pains, coughs, chills, and digestive upsets, but should be used in moderation. It can be combined with rosemary oil for treating muscular aches and pains, or with sandalwood for respiratory problems.

Essential oil

Applications

FRUIT
P. NIGRUM

 DECOCTION Simmer 10 peppercorns with a slice of galangal for nausea, vomiting, diarrhea and bloating.

FRUIT
P. LONGUM

 INFUSION Use as a tonic for chronic respiratory problems. In Ayurvedic medicine, three pods are simmered in a cup of milk.

 DECOCTION Simmer three pods with a slice of galangal and take a cup for stomach chills and diarrhea.

 POWDER Combine crushed black pepper, long pepper and powdered ginger and use a pinch in cooking to stimulate the digestion. Rub a pinch of powder on the affected area for toothache.

ESSENTIAL OIL
P. NIGRUM

 MASSAGE RUB Use 10 drops oil in 20 ml infused cayenne oil (see p. 50) for rheumatic aches and pains associated with cold.

 CREAM Add 10 drops oil to 20 g arnica cream for inflammation of the hands and feet caused by exposure.

Piper methysticum
KAVA KAVA

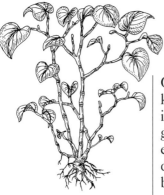

"Feed with kava so that the spirit may gain strength."
Hawaiian proverb.

GREAT RITUAL SIGNIFICANCE is attributed to kava kava in the South Sea Islands – it is used in religious ceremonies, offered to honored guests and recommended as a remedy for an extensive range of ailments. Traditional ritual drinks made from the macerated root are believed to act as a calming potion to increase mental awareness. In recent years, kava kava has become highly commercialized, and in North America its usage is widespread.

Character
Pungent, bitter, warm.
Constituents
Resin containing kava lactones, glycosides, piperidine alkaloids (inc. pipermethysticine).
Actions
Analgesic, antispasmodic, antiseptic, sedative, diuretic, tonic, urinary antiseptic, encourages sleep.

Parts used

STUMP
In many parts of Polynesia, the underground stump of the plant is prepared by chewing and soaking. It is an effective remedy for rheumatic pains, digestive upsets, obesity, asthma and chest infections, and is applied as a poultice in the treatment of skin diseases. The stump is up to 2 feet (60 cm) long and the roots up to 10 feet (3 meters).

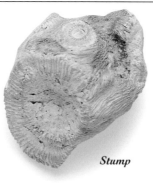

Stump

LEAVES
On some South Sea islands, the leaves are burned as a general fumigant for infectious diseases, and in the past they were inserted into the vagina to cause abortion.

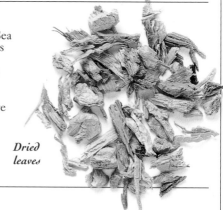

Dried leaves

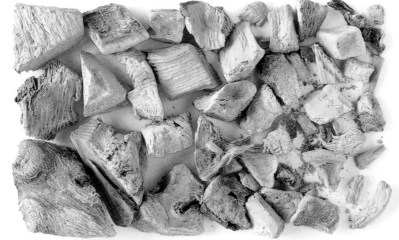

Dried root

ROOT
The root of kava kava is the most commonly used part of the herb. Traditionally, it was chewed to a pulp by young girls to ferment it with saliva, then infused in cold water, strained, and served in coconut shells. Today, as a more hygienic alternative, the root is mechanically ground. An extract of the root is given for urogenital infections, menstrual problems, headaches, general debility, colds, chills, chest pains, or as a general tonic. The root is usually harvested after three or four years.

Applications

ROOT
 TINCTURE Apply drops to the tongue to relieve pain.

 INFUSION Drink a cup as a calming sedative, to relieve tension or insomnia, or for the pain of rheumatic complaints and urinary tract infection. Regular cups will help in debility and convalescence. High doses of the infusion can induce euphoria, although excess will lead to stupor and drowsiness.

 CAPSULES Use for pains, stress, and tension headaches or to increase resistance to infection.

 MOUTHWASH Use the infusion as a mouthwash and gargle for toothache and gum disorders.

 WASH Use the infusion as an antiseptic to bathe cuts and scrapes.

STUMP
 POULTICE Apply the crushed and soaked root or stump on skin infections and pus secreting sores.

 JUICE Take 5-10 ml per dose for chronic respiratory disorders.

CAUTION
• Kava kava should not be taken in pregnancy or for longer than one month without a break.

Plantago spp.
PLANTAIN

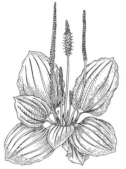

"And thou, waybread, Mother of worts, Open from Eastward, Mighty within."
The Lacnunga, 9th century.

CALLED WAYBREAD by the Anglo-Saxons, common plantain (*P. major*) was considered an important healing herb: Pliny even suggests that if several pieces of flesh are put in a pot with plantain it will join them back together again. Common plantain is still used as a healing astringent to stop both external and internal bleeding, while ribwort plantain (*P. lanceolata*) is more often used as a treatment for catarrhal conditions.

Character
Slightly sweet, salty, and bitter; cool, mainly drying.
Constituents
Leaves: mucilage, glycosides, tannins, minerals.
Seeds: mucilage, oils, protein, starch.
Actions
Leaves: relaxing expectorant, tonify mucous membranes, reduce phlegm, antispasmodic, topically healing.
Seeds: demulcent, laxative.

Parts used

LEAVES
P. MAJOR & P. LANCEOLATA
The leaves soothe urinary tract infections and irritations and ease dry coughs. Applied externally, both are healing for sores and wounds. Ribwort leaves reduce phlegm (useful in allergic rhinitis) while those from common plantain tend to be more suitable for gastric inflammations. Harvest year-round.

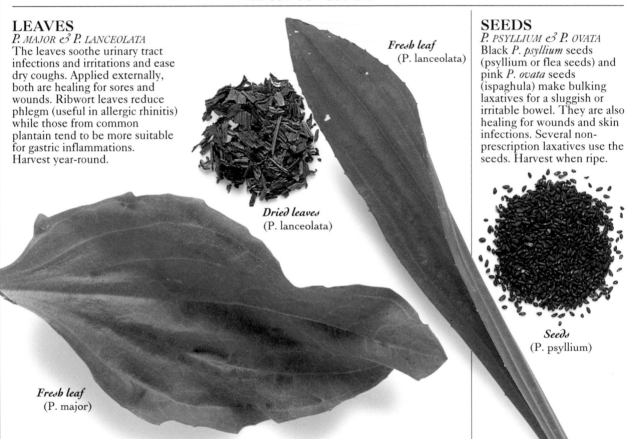

Fresh leaf
(P. lanceolata)

Dried leaves
(P. lanceolata)

Fresh leaf
(P. major)

SEEDS
P. PSYLLIUM & P. OVATA
Black *P. psyllium* seeds (psyllium or flea seeds) and pink *P. ovata* seeds (ispaghula) make bulking laxatives for a sluggish or irritable bowel. They are also healing for wounds and skin infections. Several non-prescription laxatives use the seeds. Harvest when ripe.

Seeds
(P. psyllium)

Applications

LEAVES
P. MAJOR/P. LANCEOLATA

 JUICE Press from fresh leaves. Take 10 ml, three times a day, for inflamed mucous membranes in cystitis, diarrhea, and lung infections.

 TINCTURE (*P. lanceolata*) Make from fresh leaves if possible. Good for heavy mucus, as in allergic rhinitis, or if astringency is needed.

 POULTICE Apply fresh leaves to bee stings and slow-healing wounds.

 OINTMENT (*P. major*) Apply to wounds, burns, and hemorrhoids.

 WASH Use the juice for inflammations, sores, and wounds.

 GARGLE Use the diluted juice for sore throats and mouth or gum inflammations.

 SYRUP Take a syrup made from the juice for coughs, particularly if the throat is sore or inflamed.

SEEDS
P. PSYLLIUM/P. OVATA

 INFUSION For constipation, pour a cup of boiling water over 1 tsp of either seed. Cool, then drink the mucilage and the seeds at night.

Primula spp.
COWSLIP & PRIMROSE

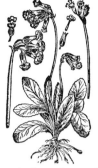

"...our city dames know well enough the ointment or distilled water of it aids beauty."
Nicholas Culpeper, 1653.

COWSLIPS (*P. VERIS*) TAKE THEIR NAME from the Anglo-Saxon *cu-sloppe*, a reminder of the days when they bloomed in meadows among dairy herds. Given their current rarity, primroses (*P. vulgaris*) are now regarded as a good second best, and the two plants are used almost interchangeably. The roots are high in saponins, irritating chemicals with expectorant properties. They are also a rich source of salicylates, which have similar actions to aspirin.

Character
Sweet, dry, slightly warm.
Constituents
Flowers: Volatile oil, glycosides, bitters.
Root: Saponins, glycosides, salicylates, volatile oil, tannin, flavonoids, sugars, silicic acid.
Actions
Flowers: sedating nervine, calming, astringent, promote sweating.
Root: stimulating expectorant, antispasmodic, anti-inflammatory, astringent.

Parts used

FLOWERS
Containing neither salicylates nor saponins, the flowers have markedly different properties from the root. The petals are very sedating, ideal for overexcited states or what Gerard described as "the frensies." They are also astringent and promote sweating, and can be used for feverish colds with headaches and nasal congestion. Harvest in spring.

ROOT
Once a popular European standby for arthritis, the root is mainly used today for chest coughs, as in chronic bronchitis. It helps to stimulate and warm the lungs and can be very effective where there is a lot of sticky, white phlegm suggesting a "cold" condition. Harvest roots of established plants in the fall.

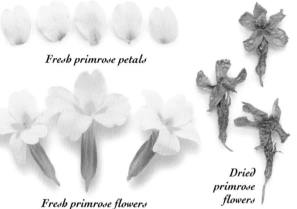

Fresh primrose petals

Fresh primrose flowers

Dried primrose flowers

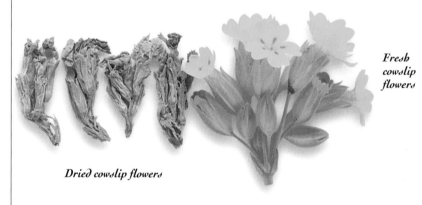

Fresh cowslip flowers

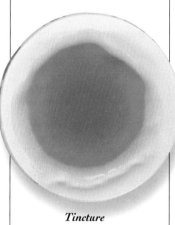

Dried cowslip flowers

Tincture

Applications

FLOWERS

 INFUSION Sip for headaches, feverish chills, or head colds and mucus.

 TINCTURE Take 5-10 drops for insomnia, anxiety, or over-excitement.

 COMPRESS Soak a pad in the hot infusion and apply to facial or trigeminal neuralgia.

 OINTMENT Use for sunburn and skin blemishes.

 ESSENTIAL OIL For insomnia, use 5-10 drops in bathwater at night.

MASSAGE OIL Dilute 5-10 drops oil in 25 ml almond or sunflower oil. Use for nerve pains, or apply to the temples for migraine.

ROOT

 DECOCTION Take to clear the phlegm of stubborn coughs, especially chronic bronchitis. Can also relieve arthritis and rheumatism.

 TINCTURE Take a standard dose for the same ailments as the decoction.

 COMPRESS Soak a pad in the decoction for painful arthritic joints.

CAUTIONS
• Avoid the root if sensitive to aspirin.
• Do not take high doses of either herb during pregnancy, because they are uterine stimulants.
• Neither herb should be used by patients taking blood-thinning drugs.

Prunella vulgaris
SELF-HEAL

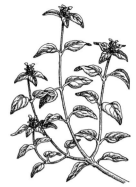

A HIGHLY REGARDED EUROPEAN wound herb, self-heal is widely used to stop bleeding. In the past, the flower spikes were considered to resemble the throat, and under the Doctrine of Signatures theory, whereby plants cured those parts of the body that they most resembled, self-heal was also used for inflammations of the mouth and throat. In Chinese medicine, the flower spikes are used, and are known as *xia ku cao*, literally meaning "summer dry herb".

"...it serveth for the same that Bugle doth, and in the world, there are not two better wound herbes, as hath been often prooved."
John Gerard, 1597.

Character
Slightly bitter, pungent, cold, drying.
Constituents
Flavonoids (inc. rutin), vitamins A, B, C, K, fatty acids, volatile oil, bitter principle.
Actions
Aerial parts: antibacterial, reduce blood pressure, diuretic, astringent, heal wounds.
Flower spikes: liver stimulant, reduce blood pressure, antibacterial, cooling.

Parts used

AERIAL PARTS
The leaves and young shoots are used by Western herbalists to stop bleeding and applied fresh in poultices as emergency first aid on clean cuts. Culpeper recommended them for "green" (fresh) wounds, suggesting that they would be ideal to "close the lips of them" in the days before stitches. Harvest before flowering.

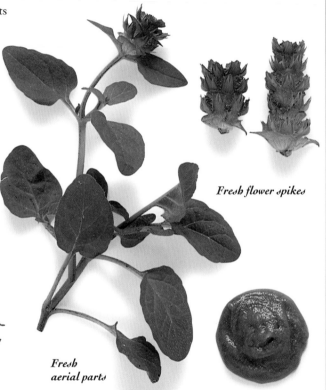

Fresh flower spikes

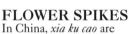

Dried flower spikes

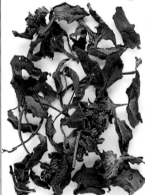

Dried aerial parts

Fresh aerial parts

Ointment

FLOWER SPIKES
In China, *xia ku cao* are regarded as being very specific for the liver and gall bladder: cooling in over-heated conditions and soothing to the eyes, which the Chinese associate with the liver in traditional theory. The slang phrase, "gung-ho", is derived from the Chinese for "liver fire", *gan hao*; self-heal is ideal for cooling this over-exuberance.

Applications

AERIAL PARTS

 TINCTURE Use for all sorts of bleeding, including heavy periods and blood in the urine.

 INFUSION Use cool for the same ailments as the tincture. Can be helpful as an astringent, bitter herb in diarrhea, and as a spring tonic.

 POULTICE Apply the fresh leaves to clean wounds.

 OINTMENT Apply to bleeding hemorrhoids.

 EYEWASH Use a very weak, well-strained infusion for hot, tired eyes.

 MOUTHWASH/GARGLE Use a weak infusion or dilute tincture for bleeding gums, mouth inflammations and sore throats.

FLOWER SPIKES

 DECOCTION In China, used to clear "liver fire" associated with irritability and anger, over-excitability, high blood pressure, headaches, hyperactivity in children, or eye problems. Often combined with *ju hua* (Chinese chrysanthemum flowers).

CAUTION
• Always seek professional advice for abnormal uterine bleeding or blood in the urine.

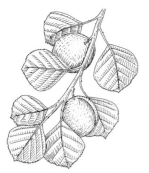

Prunus spp.
PLUM FAMILY

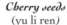

VARIOUS MEMBERS of the plum family are used in herbal medicine, including Chinese plums and cherries (*P. mume* and *P. japonica*), wild apricots (*P. armeniaca*), peaches (*P. persica*) and wild cherries (*P. serotina*). Chemicals in these herbs break down in the body to form small amounts of a compound similar to cyanide that stimulates the digestive, respiratory and nervous systems. Seeds, stalks, fruits, bark and flowers have all been used medicinally.

"Tao hua [peach flowers] kills malign demonic influx and gives one a good facial complexion. Tao xiao [ripe peach fruits] kills hundreds of ghosts and spiritual matters."
Ben Cao Jing, *Shen Nong*, *c*. 2500 BC.

Character
P. ARMENIACA: bitter, warm, toxic.
P. JAPONICA: pungent, sweet, bitter, neutral.
P. MUME: sour, warm.
P PERSICA: sweet, bitter, neutral.
P. SEROTINA: pungent, astringent, warm, toxic.
Constituents
Amygdalin, amygdalase, prunase, salicylates, plant sterols, vitamin C, fruit acids, sugars.
Actions
Antitussive, analgesic, diuretic, antibacterial, anti-inflammatory.

Parts used

SEEDS
In Chinese medicine, cherry seeds (*yu li ren*) are a laxative and diuretic. Peach seeds (*tao ren*) are used to invigorate the blood and circulation, as a laxative, and for coughs. They are included in remedies for menstrual problems and constipation due to old age or debility. Wild apricot seeds (*xing ren*) are a cough remedy for asthma and bronchitis.

Cherry seeds (yu li ren)

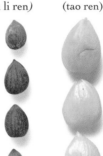

Peach seeds (tao ren)

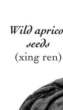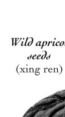

Wild apricot seeds (xing ren)

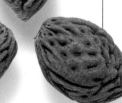

Fresh leaves

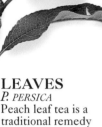

BARK
P. SEROTINA
The bark of the North American wild cherry is one of the most widely used cough remedies in Anglo-American herbalism.

Fresh fruit

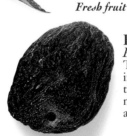

LEAVES
P. PERSICA
Peach leaf tea is a traditional remedy for morning sickness.

FRUIT
P. ARMENIACA
The fruit is rich in iron and is used in the West in tonic mixtures for anemia and debility.

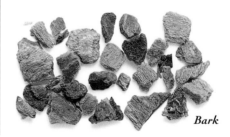

Bark

Applications

SEEDS
P. ARMENIACA

 TINCTURE Use 10 drops in 1 tsp mulberry leaf tincture for dry coughs associated with feverish colds.

P. PERSICA

 DECOCTION Use with rhubarb root, liquorice, cinnamon twigs (*gui zhi*) and *dang gui* for menstrual problems.

P. JAPONICA

 DECOCTION Use as a gentle laxative for mild constipation.

FRUIT
P. ARMENIACA

 TONIC Add 9 oz (250 g) apricots to 2 cups (500 ml) water and simmer for 8-12 hours. Remove the pits and blend. Add 2 cups (500 ml) red wine and $\frac{1}{2}$ cup (100 ml) *dang gui* tincture and mix well. Take 10 ml twice a day for iron deficiency anemia.

BARK
P. SEROTINA

 DECOCTION Use $\frac{1}{2}$ tsp dried bark per cup and take in half cup doses, up to three cups daily.

CAUTIONS
• Use in moderation, as all *Prunus spp.*, especially the seeds, are potentially toxic in high doses due to the cyanogenic glycosides.
• High doses may also cause drowsiness.
• Avoid wild cherry bark for productive coughs, because it acts as a cough suppressant rather than an expectorant.

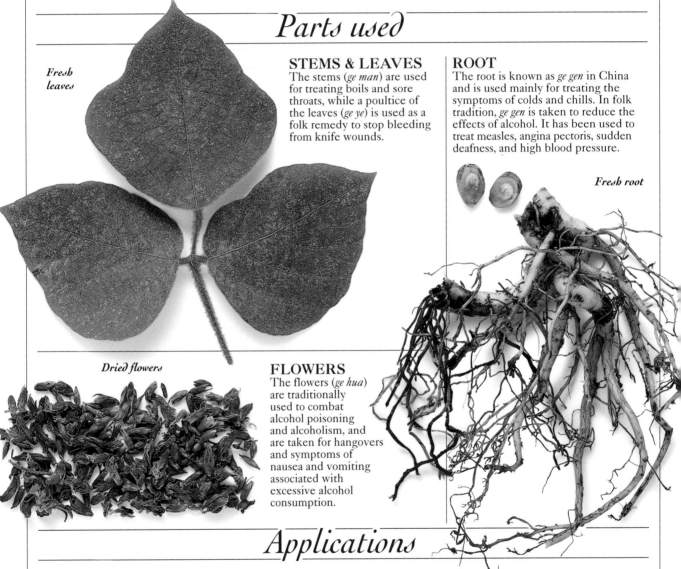

Pueraria lobata
KUDZU

"It mainly treats wasting, thirst, generalized great fever, retching, vomiting and various impediments. It lifts yin qi *and resolves various toxins."*
Ben Cao Jing, *Shen Nong,*
c. 2500 BC.

INTRODUCED INTO THE United States from Japan in the 1870s as a food, fodder, and fiber crop, kudzu vine was found growing in some 500,000 acres of the southeastern states by 1945. Today, the plant is described as a "vegetative plague" throughout many of the southern states, and is the subject of an eradication program. Kudzu is an important Chinese remedy for headaches, fevers and heart disease, and is used effectively to combat alcohol addiction.

Character
Sweet, pungent, cool.
Constituents
Isoflavonoids, ß-sitosterol, arachidinic acid, daidzein (estrogenic), genistein, starch.
Actions
Circulatory stimulant, diaphoretic, mild hypotensive, febrifuge, reduces blood sugar.

Parts used

Fresh leaves

STEMS & LEAVES
The stems (*ge man*) are used for treating boils and sore throats, while a poultice of the leaves (*ge ye*) is used as a folk remedy to stop bleeding from knife wounds.

ROOT
The root is known as *ge gen* in China and is used mainly for treating the symptoms of colds and chills. In folk tradition, *ge gen* is taken to reduce the effects of alcohol. It has been used to treat measles, angina pectoris, sudden deafness, and high blood pressure.

Fresh root

Dried flowers

FLOWERS
The flowers (*ge hua*) are traditionally used to combat alcohol poisoning and alcoholism, and are taken for hangovers and symptoms of nausea and vomiting associated with excessive alcohol consumption.

Applications

ROOT

 TINCTURE Use with half as much each of *huang qin*, licorice, and golden seal for diarrhea associated with food poisoning. Take 5 ml of the mix per dose. Use 10-20 drops in hot water for alcohol poisoning.

 DECOCTION Combine with ginger, cinnamon twigs and licorice for treating colds, chills and headaches.

 JUICE Drink 12 shot-sized glasses to reduce severe drunkenness.

PILLS/CAPSULES Used to stimulate blood flow through the coronary artery in angina pectoris (30-120 mg daily, in two doses). Pills containing the equivalent of 5 g of crude root (two, three times daily) can help for headaches and sudden deafness associated with spasms of the internal auditory artery.

FLOWERS

 INFUSION Drink a cup for nausea associated with hangovers.

Rheum palmatum
RHUBARB

ORIGINATING FROM NORTHWEST China and Tibet, rhubarb has been used in medicine for more than 2,000 years. Its use gradually spread through India, reaching Europe during the Renaissance overland via Asia Minor – hence the common name, Turkey rhubarb. The plant was a favorite remedy with early Persian and Arabian physicians. The rhubarb grown for cooking and eating is usually *R. rhabarbarum*, an 18th-century cultivar.

"...so effective for the liver that it is called the life, soul and treacle of the liver, purging... choler, phlegme and water humours."
William Cole, 1656.

Character
Bitter, cold, dry.
Constituents
Anthraquinones, tannins, calcium oxalate, resins, minerals.
Actions
Laxative, digestive remedy, astringent, antibacterial.

Parts used

ROOT
This is known as *da huang* in China, which translates as "big yellow" – the color of rhubarb tinctures and decoctions. It is used very similarly in both East and West, as a purgative and liver cleanser. It is intrinsically "cold", and the Chinese use it to clear "heat" from the liver, stomach and blood; they also believe that it moves stagnant blood. Harvest in fall.

Fresh sliced root

Tincture

Powdered root

Fresh root

Dried root

Applications

ROOT

 TINCTURE The action of the root varies considerably depending on dose. Low doses (5-10 drops) are astringent and can be used for diarrhea. A slightly higher dose (1 ml) acts as a good liver stimulant and gentle laxative. Very high doses (up to 2.5 ml) have a strong cooling and purgative effect. Use increasing doses (0.5-2 ml) of carminatives such as fennel or mint with higher doses of rhubarb to prevent cramping.

 DECOCTION A weak decoction (up to 0.5 g root per dose) can be used for diarrhea, while a strong decoction (3 g root per dose) is effective for chronic constipation or period cramps with delayed menstruation.

 WASH The root is also antibacterial and astringent, and a strong decoction can be used on boils and suppurating skin diseases.

CAUTIONS
• Avoid the herb in pregnancy as it is a strong purgative.
• Rhubarb contains oxalates, and is best avoided in arthritic conditions and gout.
• Do not use the leaves, as they are potentially toxic and fatalities have been reported.

Rosa spp.
ROSE

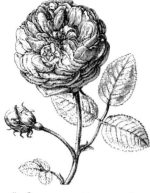

THERE IS A SAYING that roses are good for "the skin and the soul," and they have a long tradition of medicinal use. In Roman times, the wild rose, *R. canina*, was recommended for the bites of rabid dogs. Roses continued as an official medicine well into the 1930s, when tincture of apothecary's rose, *R. gallica* var. *officinalis*, was prescribed for sore throats. Today, roses are still highly prized: the oil is expensive, and is one of the most important oils in aromatherapy. In Ayurvedic medicine, roses are considered cooling and a tonic for the mind.

"...drye roses put to ye nose to smell do comforte the braine and the harte and quencheth sprite."
Askham's Herbal, 1550.

Character Sweet, astringent, generally either neutral or slightly cooling.
Constituents Volatile oil, vitamins C, B, E, K, tannins. Rose oil contains some 300 chemical constituents, of which only around 100 have been identified so far.
Actions Antidepressant, antispasmodic, aphrodisiac, astringent, sedative, digestive stimulant, increases bile production, cleansing, expectorant, antibacterial, antiviral, antiseptic, kidney tonic, blood tonic, menstrual regulator, anti-inflammatory.

Parts used

ROSEHIPS
R. CANINA
Valued as an important source of vitamin C, rosehips from the dog rose are still used in commercial teas, syrups, and fruit drinks. The leaves were once used as a substitute for tea. Harvest in the fall.

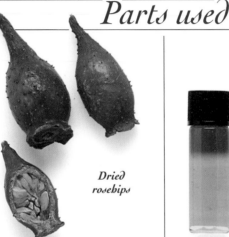

Dried rosehips

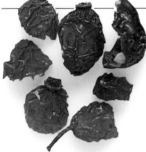

ROSEHIPS
R. LAEVIGATA
In China, the hips from this rose are known as *jin ying zi* and are mainly used as a kidney *qi* (energy) tonic, prescribed for urinary dysfunction. Like other rose remedies, they are astringent and taken for chronic diarrhea. Harvest in the fall.

Jin ying zi

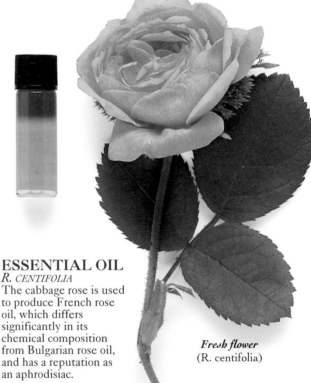

ESSENTIAL OIL
R. CENTIFOLIA
The cabbage rose is used to produce French rose oil, which differs significantly in its chemical composition from Bulgarian rose oil, and has a reputation as an aphrodisiac.

Fresh flower
(R. centifolia)

Applications

ROSEHIPS
R. CANINA

 TINCTURE Take as an astringent for diarrhea, to relieve colic, or as a component in cough remedies.

 SYRUP Use to flavor other medicines, add to cough mixtures, or take as a source of vitamin C.

ROSEHIPS
R. LAEVIGATA

 DECOCTION Take with *dang shen*, *bai zhu*, and *shan yao* for chronic diarrhea with stomach weakness.

ESSENTIAL OIL
R. CENTIFOLIA/R. DAMASCENA

 CREAM Add a few drops of oil to creams for dry or inflamed skin.

 LOTION Apply 1 ml lady's mantle tincture in 10 ml rosewater for vaginal itching. The same combination can be made into a cream using a standard base. Combine rosewater with an equal amount of distilled witch hazel, and use as a cooling, moisturizing lotion for skin prone to pimples or acne.

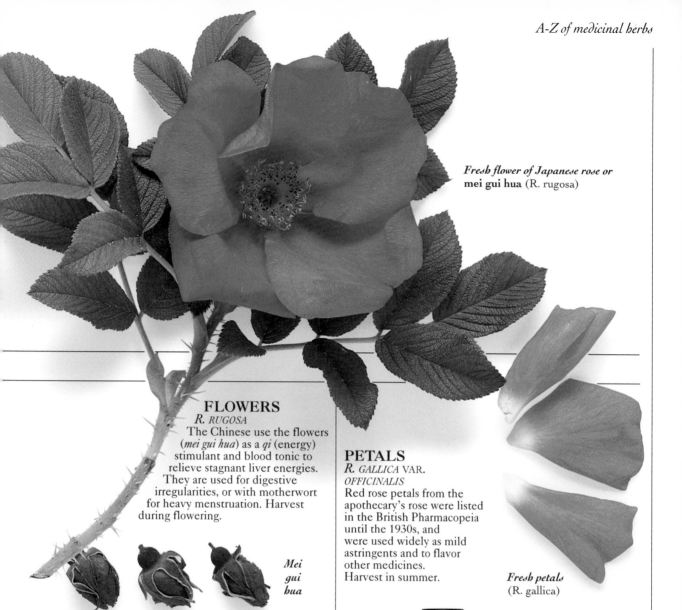

Fresh flower of Japanese rose or **mei gui hua** (R. rugosa)

FLOWERS
R. RUGOSA
The Chinese use the flowers (*mei gui hua*) as a *qi* (energy) stimulant and blood tonic to relieve stagnant liver energies. They are used for digestive irregularities, or with motherwort for heavy menstruation. Harvest during flowering.

Mei gui hua

PETALS
R. GALLICA VAR. *OFFICINALIS*
Red rose petals from the apothecary's rose were listed in the British Pharmacopeia until the 1930s, and were used widely as mild astringents and to flavor other medicines. Harvest in summer.

Fresh petals (R. gallica)

ESSENTIAL OIL
R. DAMASCENA
Damask rose petals are steam-distilled to produce Bulgarian rose oil, used in about 96% of all women's perfumes. Medicinally, it is an important nervine, used for depression and anxiety, and is thought to help those who lack love in their lives. It can also be added to skin remedies or taken for digestive problems. Recent research also suggests that the oil has anti-HIV activity.

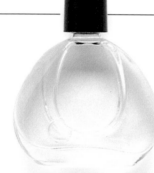

Rosewater is a by-product of the steam distillation of Bulgarian rose oil, and makes a good skin remedy.

Applications

 OIL Add 2 drops of oil to bathwater for depression, grief, or insomnia.

 MASSAGE OIL Add up to 2 ml rose oil to 20 ml almond or wheatgerm oil, and use to relieve stress and exhaustion, or for a sluggish digestion.

FLOWERS
R. RUGOSA

 DECOCTION Take with motherwort for heavy menstruation. Combine with *bai shao yao* and *xiang fu* for liver *qi* dysfunction.

PETALS
R. GALLICA

 TINCTURE Take up to 3 ml three times a day for diarrhea or sluggish digestion. Combine with lady's mantle, white deadnettle, or shepherd's purse for irregular or heavy menstruation.

 GARGLE Use the infusion as a gargle for sore throats. Can also be combined with sage.

CAUTIONS
• Because of the high price of rose oil, adulteration is commonplace. Only use the best quality, genuine oil medicinally.
• Rose oil is nontoxic and can be taken internally, but seek professional advice first if you are unfamiliar with dosages.
• Use only the rose species listed here, and not garden hybrids.

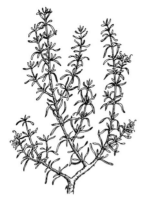

Rosmarinus officinalis
ROSEMARY

A FAVORITE HERB both medicinally and as a symbol for remembrance, rosemary is a Mediterranean shrub that gradually spread north and was reputedly first grown in England by Philippa of Hainault, wife of Edward III, in the 14th century. The plant is an excellent tonic and all-around stimulant, and has always been regarded as uplifting and energizing: Gerard said that it "comforteth the harte and maketh it merie."

"If thou be feeble boyle the leaves in cleane water and washe thyself and thou shalt be shiny... smell it oft and it shall keep thee youngly."
Banckes' Herbal, 1525.

Character
Warming, dry, pungent, bitter.
Constituents
Volatile oil, bitter, tannin.
Actions
Aerial parts: astringent, digestive remedy, nervine, carminative, antiseptic, diuretic, promote sweating and bile flow, antidepressant, circulatory stimulant, antispasmodic, nervous tonic, cardiac tonic, analgesic.
Essential oil: Topical: increases blood flow to an area, analgesic, antirheumatic, stimulant.

Parts used

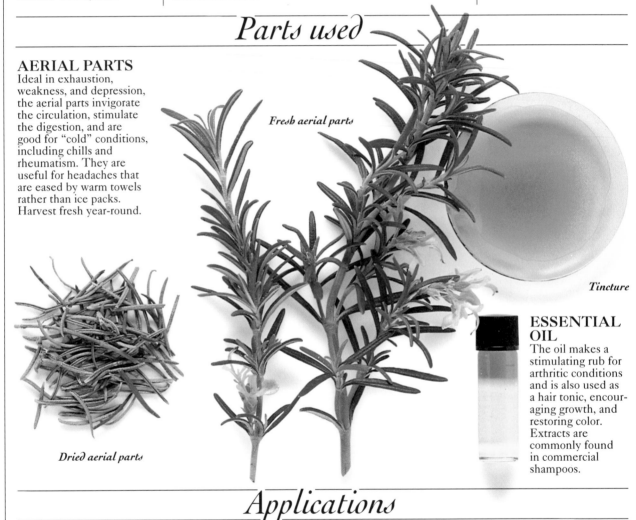

AERIAL PARTS
Ideal in exhaustion, weakness, and depression, the aerial parts invigorate the circulation, stimulate the digestion, and are good for "cold" conditions, including chills and rheumatism. They are useful for headaches that are eased by warm towels rather than ice packs. Harvest fresh year-round.

Fresh aerial parts

Tincture

Dried aerial parts

ESSENTIAL OIL
The oil makes a stimulating rub for arthritic conditions and is also used as a hair tonic, encouraging growth, and restoring color. Extracts are commonly found in commercial shampoos.

Applications

AERIAL PARTS

 INFUSION Take the hot infusion for colds, influenza, rheumatic pains, and indigestion; also as a stimulating drink for fatigue or headaches.

 TINCTURE Take as a stimulant tonic. Combine with oats, skullcap, or vervain for depression.

 COMPRESS Soak a pad in the hot infusion and use for sprains. Alternate two to three minutes of the hot compress with two to three minutes of applying an ice pack to the injury.

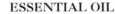

 HAIR RINSE Use the infusion as the final rinse for dandruff.

ESSENTIAL OIL

 OIL Add 10 drops to the bath to soothe aching limbs or to act as a stimulant in nervous exhaustion.

 MASSAGE OIL Dilute 1 ml rosemary oil in 25 ml sunflower or almond oil and massage into aching joints and muscles, into the scalp to stimulate hair growth, or use on the temples for headaches.

CAUTION
• Avoid essential oil use during pregnancy.

Rubus idaeus
RASPBERRY

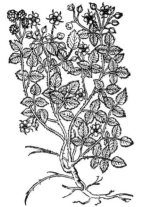

> "The fruit is good to be given to those that have weake and queasie stomackes."
> John Gerard, 1597.

THE RASPBERRY PLANT was a favorite household remedy. Raspberry vinegars were used for sore throats and coughs; the leaves in infusions for diarrhea or as poultices for hemorrhoids; and raspberry syrup to prevent a buildup of tartar on teeth. Gerard considered the fruit "of a temperate heat," so it was easier on the stomach than strawberries, which could cause excess phlegm and chilling. Today, raspberry leaf tea is still taken to prepare for childbirth.

Character
Dry, astringent, generally cooling.
Constituents
Leaves: fragarine (uterine tonic), tannins, polypeptides.
Fruit: vitamins A, B, C, E, sugars, minerals, volatile oil.
Actions
Leaves: astringent, preparative for childbirth, stimulant, digestive remedy, tonic.
Fruit: diuretic, laxative, diaphoretic, cleansing.

Parts used

LEAVES
Used for period cramps and discomfort, the leaves taken during late pregnancy also help to prepare the womb for childbirth. They are also astringent, so are useful for diarrhea, wounds, sore throats, and mouth ulcers. They have been included in rheumatic remedies as a cleansing diuretic, and in France they are regarded as a tonic for the prostate gland. Harvest in summer before the fruit ripens.

BERRIES
Traditionally taken for indigestion and rheumatism, the berries are rich in vitamins and minerals, and highly nutritious. Harvest when ripe in late summer.

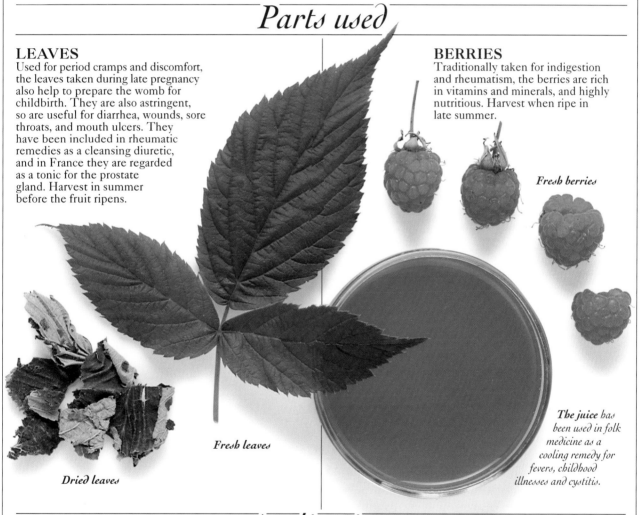

Fresh berries

The juice has been used in folk medicine as a cooling remedy for fevers, childhood illnesses and cystitis.

Fresh leaves

Dried leaves

Applications

LEAVES

 INFUSION To ease childbirth, take one cup daily in the last six to eight weeks of pregnancy, and drink plenty of the warm tea during labor. Can also be used for mild diarrhea, menstrual problems, or as a gargle for mouth ulcers and sore throats.

 TINCTURE More astringent than the infusion, the diluted tincture is used on wounds and inflammations, or as a mouthwash for ulcers and gum inflammations.

 WASH Use the infusion for bathing wounds, and apply regularly to varicose ulcers and sores. It also makes a soothing eyewash.

BERRIES

 VINEGAR Steep 500 g fruit in 4 cups (1 liter) wine vinegar for two weeks, then strain. This thick red liquid can be added to cough mixtures or used in gargles for sore throats. Its pleasant taste can help disguise the flavor of other herbal expectorants.

CAUTION
• Avoid high doses of the leaves during early pregnancy, because they can stimulate the uterus.

Salix alba
WILLOW

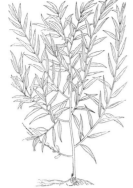

"The leaves... stay the heat of lust in man or woman, and quite extinguishes it, if it be long used; the seed also has the same effect."
Nicholas Culpeper, 1653.

IN TRADITIONAL HERBAL MEDICINE, white willow was widely used for fevers and other "hot" conditions. It was one of the first herbs to be scientifically investigated, and in the 19th century, a French chemist, Leroux, extracted the active constituent and named it "salicine." By 1852 this chemical was being produced synthetically, and by 1899 a less irritant and unpleasant-tasting variant of the substance (acetylsalicylic acid) was manufactured and marketed as aspirin, the first of the modern generation of plant-derived drugs.

Character
Cool, dry, slightly bitter.
Constituents
Salicin, tannins, flavonoids, glycosides.
Actions
Antirheumatic, anti-inflammatory, reduces heat, antihydrotic, analgesic, antiseptic, astringent, bitter digestive tonic.

Parts used

BARK
In modern herbalism only the bark is generally used. It is prescribed for many inflammatory conditions, including rheumatism and arthritis; it helps control fevers, and relieves neuralgia, headaches, and pain in general. As a gentle bitter, it also acts as a mild digestive stimulant and is used for gastroenteritis, and diarrhea related to heat and inflammation. Harvest in summer.

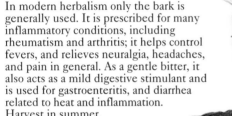

Dried bark

LEAVES
In the past, the leaves were a popular home remedy, used much as the bark today. Willow leaf tea was taken for fevers or colicky pains, and the infusion was recommended for dandruff.

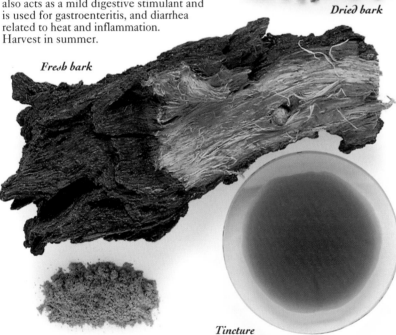

Fresh bark

Tincture

Powdered bark

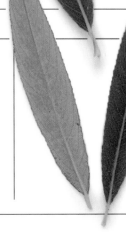

Fresh leaves

Applications

BARK

 FLUID EXTRACT Stronger than the tincture; take for rheumatic conditions, headaches, and neuralgia.

 TINCTURE Take up to 15 ml per dose for fever, or combine with boneset, elder, and bitter remedies like gentian. Use with soothing herbs such as plantain for infections and gastric inflammations (take nonalcoholic tincture, see p. 157).

 POWDER Take in doses of up to 10 g for fevers and headaches; mix with a teaspoon of honey.

 DECOCTION Take for feverish chills and headaches, or as part of arthritic treatments.

LEAVES

 INFUSION Drink after meals for digestive problems.

Salvia spp.
SAGE

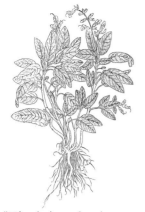

"Why of seknesse deyeth man Whill sawge in gardeyn he may han?"
Macer's herbal, 10th century.

TRADITIONALLY ASSOCIATED with longevity, sage has a reputation for restoring failing memory in the elderly. Like other memory-enhancing herbs, it was also planted on graves. It is said that when the British started importing tea from China, the Chinese so valued the herb they would trade two cases of tea for one of dried English sage. Green sage (*S. officinalis*) is often adulterated with Greek sage (*S. fruticosa*), although the two have very similar properties. Purple sage (*S. officinalis* "Purpurescens Group") is often preferred by herbalists instead.

Character
Pungent, bitter, cool, drying.
Constituents
S. OFFICINALIS: volatile oil, diterpene bitters, tannins, triterpenoids, resin, flavonoids, estrogenic substances, saponins.
S. MILTIORRHIZA: vitamin E.
Actions
S. OFFICINALIS: carminative, anti-spasmodic, astringent, antiseptic, relaxes peripheral blood vessels, reduces perspiration, salivation, and lactation, uterine stimulant, antibiotic, reduces blood sugar levels, promotes bile flow.
S. MILTIORRHIZA: circulatory stimulant, sedative, clears heat.

Parts used

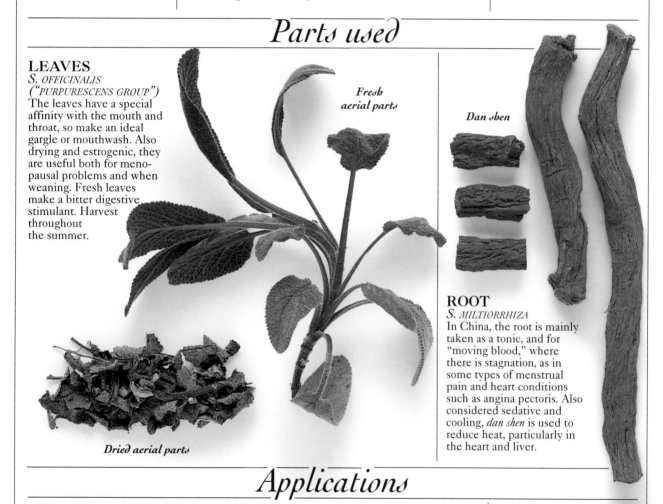

LEAVES
S. OFFICINALIS ("PURPURESCENS GROUP") The leaves have a special affinity with the mouth and throat, so make an ideal gargle or mouthwash. Also drying and estrogenic, they are useful both for meno-pausal problems and when weaning. Fresh leaves make a bitter digestive stimulant. Harvest throughout the summer.

Fresh aerial parts

Dan shen

Dried aerial parts

ROOT
S. MILTIORRHIZA
In China, the root is mainly taken as a tonic, and for "moving blood," where there is stagnation, as in some types of menstrual pain and heart conditions such as angina pectoris. Also considered sedative and cooling, *dan shen* is used to reduce heat, particularly in the heart and liver.

Applications

LEAVES
S. OFFICINALIS/S. FRUTICOSA

 INFUSION Use 20 g leaves to ¼ cup (50 ml) water as a tonic and liver stimulant, or to improve digestive function and circulation in debility. Can reduce lactation when weaning, and relieve menopausal night sweats.

 TINCTURE Use for menopausal problems. Prescribed to reduce salivation in Parkinson's disease.

 CREAM Popular in France to treat minor skin sores, scrapes, and insect bites.

 GARGLE/MOUTHWASH Use a weak infusion for sore throats, tonsillitis, mouth ulcers, or gum disease.

 HAIR RINSE Use the infusion as a rinse for dandruff, or to restore color to graying hair.

ROOT
S. MILTIORRHIZA

 DECOCTION Prescribed for menstrual pain caused by blood stagnation; also prescribed in Chinese medicine for angina pectoris and coronary heart disease.

CAUTIONS
• Avoid therapeutic doses in pregnancy. Small amounts of sage used in cooking are quite safe.
• Only take *dan shen* where the condition is caused by blood stagnation. Seek professional help for all heart disorders.
• Sage contains thujone, which can trigger fits in epileptics, who should avoid the herb.

Sambucus nigra
ELDER

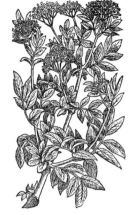

*"The decoction of the root...
cureth the biting of an adder."*
Nicholas Culpeper, 1653.

A WEALTH OF FOLKLORE attaches to this plant, often described as a "complete medical chest," because of its countless therapeutic and prophylactic qualities. Classed as "hot and dry" by Galen, the herb was used for cold, damp conditions, such as phlegm, or excessive mucus. In the 17th century, it was a favorite remedy for "clearing phlegm," both as an expectorant for coughs, and as a diuretic and violent purgative. Elderflower water was much praised in the 18th century for whitening the skin and removing freckles.

Character
Flowers/Berries: bitter, drying, cool, slightly sweet.
Bark: hot, bitter, drying.
Constituents
Volatile oil, flavonoids, mucilage, tannins, vitamins A, C, cyanogenic glycoside, viburnic acid, alkaloid.
Actions
Flowers: expectorant, diuretic, circulatory stimulant, promote sweating, anti-inflammatory.
Berries: promote sweating, diuretic, laxative.
Bark: purgative, promotes vomiting (in large doses), diuretic. Topical: emollient.

Parts used

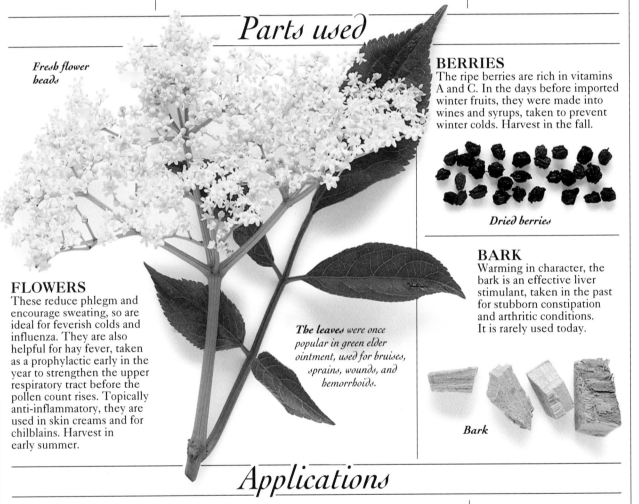

Fresh flower heads

FLOWERS
These reduce phlegm and encourage sweating, so are ideal for feverish colds and influenza. They are also helpful for hay fever, taken as a prophylactic early in the year to strengthen the upper respiratory tract before the pollen count rises. Topically anti-inflammatory, they are used in skin creams and for chilblains. Harvest in early summer.

The leaves were once popular in green elder ointment, used for bruises, sprains, wounds, and hemorrhoids.

BERRIES
The ripe berries are rich in vitamins A and C. In the days before imported winter fruits, they were made into wines and syrups, taken to prevent winter colds. Harvest in the fall.

Dried berries

BARK
Warming in character, the bark is an effective liver stimulant, taken in the past for stubborn constipation and arthritic conditions. It is rarely used today.

Bark

Applications

FLOWERS

INFUSION Drink hot for feverish and mucous conditions of the lungs or upper respiratory tract, including hay fever. Can be combined with yarrow, boneset, and peppermint.

TINCTURE Take for colds and influenza, or in early spring to help reduce later hay fever symptoms.

CREAM Apply to chapped skin and sores on the hands or to chilblains.

EYEWASH Use the cold, strained infusion for inflamed or sore eyes.

MOUTHWASH/GARGLE Use the infusion for mouth ulcers, sore throats, and tonsillitis.

BERRIES

SYRUP Make from the decoction and take as a prophylactic for winter colds or in combination with other expectorant herbs, such as thyme, for coughs.

TINCTURE Use in combination with other herbs, such as bogbean or willow, for rheumatic conditions.

CAUTIONS
• Do not take any parts of elder if the condition would be worsened by further drying or fluid depletion.
• Do not use the bark in pregnancy as it is very strongly purgative.

Scrophularia spp.
FIGWORT

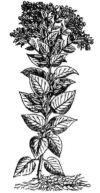

"...it taketh away all redness, spots and freckles in the face, as also the scurf, and any foul deformity therein..."
Nicholas Culpeper, 1653.

IN BOTH EASTERN AND WESTERN traditions, figwort (*S. nodosa*) is a very cleansing herb. In the past, it was known as the scrofula plant (hence the botanical name), and used to treat abscesses, purulent wounds, and the "King's Evil" or scrofula (tuberculosis of the lymph glands in the neck). Culpeper calls the herb throatwort because of its use in treating this disease. The Chinese use *xuan shen*, the root of a related species, *S. ningpoensis*, as a prime remedy for "fire poisons," the kind of purulent conditions associated with the herb in the West.

Character
Bitter, cold, drying; salty (*S. ningpoensis*).
Constituents
S. NODOSA: saponins, cardioactive glycosides, alkaloids, flavonoids, iridoids.
S. NINGPOENSIS: saponins, phytosterol, essential fatty acids, asparagine.
Actions
S. NODOSA: diuretic, laxative, heart stimulant, circulatory stimulant, anti-inflammatory.
S. NINGPOENSIS: tonic, cooling, anti-inflammatory, antibacterial, heart tonic, lowers high blood pressure, sedative.

Parts used

AERIAL PARTS
S. NODOSA
Best known for treating skin problems, the aerial parts are suitable for any sort of cleansing – for example, in rheumatic disorders and gout, when there is stagnation in the lymphatic system, or for a sluggish digestion with constipation. Harvest after flowering in summer.

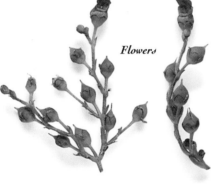

Flowers

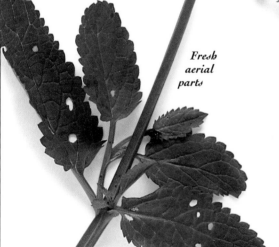

Fresh aerial parts

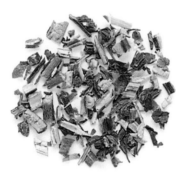

Dried aerial parts

ROOT
S. NINGPOENSIS
Unlike *S. nodosa*, the Chinese variety relaxes the heart, lowering blood pressure, and sedating slightly. It also replenishes *jing* (vital essence).

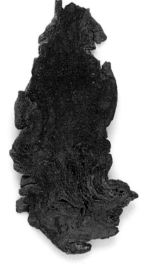

Xuan shen

Applications

AERIAL PARTS
S. NODOSA

 INFUSION Use whenever there is a buildup of toxins to cleanse: for rheumatic conditions, lymphatic disorders, or skin conditions such as eczema and psoriasis.

 TINCTURE Take in combination with other digestive herbs such as dandelion, barberry, or rhubarb root for constipation and sluggishness, or with herbs such as yellow dock or burdock for skin conditions.

 COMPRESS Soak a pad in the infusion and apply to painful swellings, wounds, and ulcers.

 WASH Use the infusion for eczema, skin inflammations, and fungal infections.

ROOT
S. NINGPOENSIS

 DECOCTION Use for throat problems, including swollen glands and tonsillitis. Prescribed for deep-seated abscesses and lymphatic swellings. As a *yin* tonic, it is taken with salt in China.

CAUTION
• *S. nodosa* stimulates the heart, so avoid in cases of abnormally rapid heartbeat.

Scutellaria spp.
SKULLCAP

"Skullcap is perhaps the most widely relevant nervine available to us in the materia medica."
David Hoffman, *The Holistic Herbal*, 1983.

A COMPARATIVE NEWCOMER to the European herbal repertoire, Virginian skullcap was used by Native Americans for rabies and to promote menstruation. It is characterized by dish-shaped seed pods and flowers that grow on only one side of the stem; hence its botanical name, *S. lateriflora*. Today, it is one of the best herbs for treating nervous disorders. The Chinese use a related plant, *S. baicalensis*, or *huang qin*.

Character
Bitter, cold, drying.
Constituents
S. LATERIFLORA: flavonoids, tannins, bitter, volatile oil, minerals.
S. BAICALENSIS: flavonoids, sitosterols.
Actions
S. LATERIFLORA: relaxing nervine, antispasmodic.
S. BAICALENSIS: antibacterial, cooling, diuretic, anti-spasmodic, promotes bile flow.

Parts used

Fresh aerial parts

Dried aerial parts

AERIAL PARTS
S. LATERIFLORA
Calming for many nervous conditions, the aerial parts also have a tonic effect on the central nervous system, so are ideal for nervous exhaustion. They can be helpful in premenstrual tension and have been used for epilepsy. Harvest late in the flowering period, when the characteristic, skullcap-shaped seed pods have appeared on the plant.

Tincture

ROOT
S. BAICALENSIS
In China, *huang qin* is mainly used to clear heat from the respiratory and digestive systems. It is thought to contain melatonin to help ease headaches and insomnia. Korean research suggests the herb can combat gum and tooth disease.

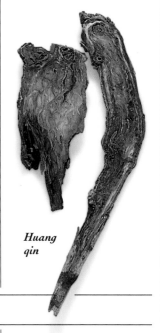

Huang qin

Applications

AERIAL PARTS
S. LATERIFLORA

 INFUSION Use the herb fresh, if possible, to make a soothing tea for nervous exhaustion, excitability, overanxiety, and premenstrual tension. For insomnia, combine skullcap with wild lettuce or passion flower and take at night.

TINCTURE Best made from the fresh herb, this is a potent remedy for calming the nerves. Take 5 ml or combine with 10 drops lemon balm for nervous stress or depression.

ROOT
S. BAICALENSIS

 DECOCTION Use in combination with other cold, bitter herbs, such as *huang lian* or goldenseal, to purge heat from the system in gastric, chest and urinary infections, including diarrhea, jaundice, gastroenteritis, bronchitis, and cystitis. Combine with herbs such as *ju hua* to reduce high blood pressure.

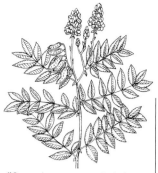

Senna alexandrina
SENNA

FOR CENTURIES, senna leaves and pods have been used as a potent laxative. In China, the leaves are known as *fan xie ye*, and in sanskrit the whole plant is known as *rajavriksha* – "king of trees". When using senna in herbal remedies, it is best initially to take small doses of the pods, which are milder than the strongly purgative leaves. The herb is commonly found today in many conventional over-the-counter remedies.

"Senna is ... very certain in its operation; it is admissable in most diseases and is only objectionable from its nauseous taste."
George Graves, *Hortus Medicus*, 1834.

Character
Bitter, sweet, cold.
Constituents
Sennosides (rhein-dianthrone diglucosides), aglycones, monoanthraquinone glycosides, dianthrone diglucosides, flavonoids.
Actions
Stimulating laxative, cooling, antibacterial, expels worms.

Parts used

LEAVES
Generally the leaves are used in infusions, powders and pills. They irritate the digestive tract and encourage peristalsis. Long-term, habitual use can weaken the digestive system, and senna should be avoided if there is inflammation in the gut, as in Crohn's disease or ulcerative colitis. Senna can produce soft stools, and is therefore used for problems with bleeding hemorrhoids or anal fissures.

PODS
Western practitioners often prefer the pods to the leaves because they are milder. Adulteration of commercial senna was often a problem in the past.

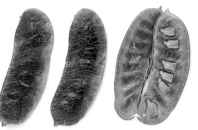
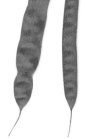

Dried pods   *Fresh pods*

DRIED LEAVES
The Chinese use dried senna leaf (*fan xie ye*) as a purgative to help habitual constipation, and as a cooling remedy to clear heat that can lead to abdominal bloating and discomfort in the digestive system.

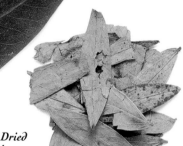

Fresh leaves

Dried leaves

Applications

LEAVES

TINCTURE 10-30 drops per dose, taken in the morning with water.

INFUSION Use ¹/₂ tsp dried leaves with 1 tsp fennel seeds per cup of boiling water for severe constipation. Do not continue for more than seven days and ensure a break of at least two weeks before repeating the treatment.

PODS

INFUSION Always start with a low dose. Use 15-30 mg per dose, or 3-6 pods. Leave the pods in a cup of warm water overnight and drink first thing in the morning. Add a slice of fresh ginger root, or 1 tsp of fennel seeds to combat cramps.

PILLS/POWDERS 1-2 tsps granules or 2-4 pills, taken in the morning.

CAUTION
• Do not take senna in pregnancy, while breast-feeding, or in cases of inflammatory bowel disease.

Silybum marianus
MILK THISTLE

DUBBED MILK THISTLE, or Mary thistle, because of its traditional use in stimulating milk flow in nursing mothers, this plant is a good example of the medieval Doctrine of Signatures (see p. 19): its white-streaked leaves were said to symbolize splashes of milk. Milk thistle was once cultivated as a highly versatile vegetable. Today, it is regarded as one of the most important herbal liver tonics and restoratives.

"It staieth bleedings, wasteth away colde swellings, easeth the paine of the teeth…and that it is thought to drive away serpents …"
John Gerard, 1597.

Character
Bitter, astringent, warm.
Constituents
Flavolignans (inc. silymarin), bitters.
Actions
Bitter tonic, promotes bile flow, antidepressant, antioxidant, antiviral, promotes milk flow.

Parts used

SEEDS
The seeds are rich in silymarin, which has been shown to help combat liver damage. Extracts have been used to treat hepatitis and cirrhosis of the liver. The seeds can also help to reduce high cholesterol levels and soothe inflammation of the gall bladder. Studies have shown that milk thistle is a more powerful antioxidant than vitamin E, and can help to prevent damage to tissues caused by free radicals.

FLOWERS/ LEAVES
Eaten before the flowers open, the heads are prepared in the same way as artichokes, and are used to help stimulate the liver and digestive system. The leaves are eaten like spinach, and are used to stimulate milk flow in mothers and to ease menstrual problems. They can also be used in infusions to stimulate digestion.

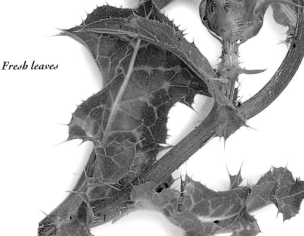

Flower head

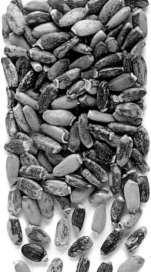
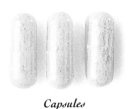

Seeds

Fresh leaves

Tincture

Capsules

Applications

SEEDS

 TINCTURE Take 20-50 drops with water for liver and gall bladder problems, or as a digestive stimulant. Take up to 5 ml daily in water as a preventative if there is a history of gallstones or liver disease, or combine with an equal amount of dandelion root tincture. Adding milk thistle tincture to a cup of peppermint infusion also makes a good digestive tonic.

CAPSULES Use 1-2 x 200 mg capsules to combat hangovers, or before drinking alcohol.

POWDER Use topically to dust swollen skin ulcers.

INFUSION Drink a cup for liver and gall bladder weakness: combines well with vervain. Use with lady's mantle and St. John's wort for premenstrual syndrome.

FLOWERS/LEAVES

INFUSION Drink a cup to stimulate milk production when breast-feeding. Also helps to stimulate digestion.

FRESH LEAVES Use as a vegetable in the traditional way.

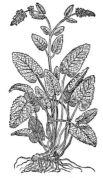

Stachys officinalis
WOOD BETONY

"...it is good whether for a man's soul or his body; it shields him against visions and dreams."
Herbarium Apuleii, Saxon translation, c. 9th century.

THE MOST IMPORTANT Anglo-Saxon herb, wood betony had no fewer than 29 uses in treating physical diseases, and was also possibly the most popular amulet herb, used well into the Middle Ages to ward off evil or ill humors. Gerard, in 1597, gives a long list of applications, adding that "it maketh a man to pisse well". Today, wood betony is neglected by many herbalists: it is, however, worth rediscovering.

Character
Cool, drying, bitter-sweet.
Constituents
Alkaloids (inc. stachydrine and trigonelline), tannins, saponins.
Actions
Sedative, bitter digestive remedy, nervine, mild diuretic, circulatory tonic particularly for the cerebral circulation, astringent.

Parts used

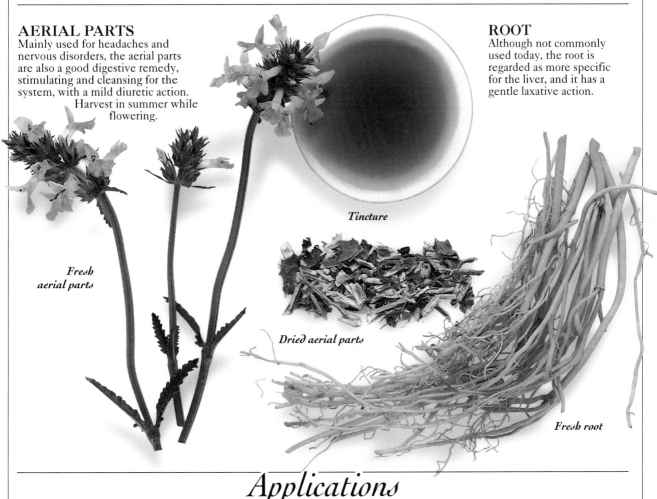

AERIAL PARTS
Mainly used for headaches and nervous disorders, the aerial parts are also a good digestive remedy, stimulating and cleansing for the system, with a mild diuretic action. Harvest in summer while flowering.

Fresh aerial parts

Tincture

Dried aerial parts

ROOT
Although not commonly used today, the root is regarded as more specific for the liver, and it has a gentle laxative action.

Fresh root

Applications

AERIAL PARTS

 INFUSION Take low doses (1 tsp per cup) as a relaxing and tonic herb for general use. Take in therapeutic doses for period pain, migraines, and other headaches, nervous tension, or as a digestive stimulant and cleanser. During difficult or painful labor, drink a hot infusion.

 TINCTURE Use as the infusion. It is especially helpful for nervous headaches; combines well with lavender. Also useful as a cleansing herb in toxic and arthritic conditions.

 POULTICE Apply pounded fresh herb to wounds and bruises.

 WASH Bathe leg ulcers and infected wounds in the infusion.

 MOUTHWASH/GARGLE Use the infusion for mouth ulcers, gum inflammations, and sore throats.

 TONIC WINE Macerate 50 g betony with 25 g each of vervain and hyssop in 75 cl white wine for two weeks. Take shot-glass doses for nervous headaches and tension.

CAUTION
• The herb is a uterine stimulant, so avoid high doses in pregnancy; may be taken during labor.

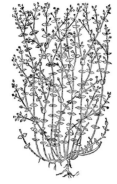

"...in a word, it comforteth, digesteth, defendeth and suppurateth very notably."
John Gerard, 1597.

Stellaria spp.
CHICKWEED

IN GERARD'S DAY, chickweed (*S. media*) was given as a tonic to caged birds. It is probably the most common of weeds, growing in virtually all corners of the world. Instead of rooting it out, it is worth remembering that chickweed was traditionally harvested as a vegetable. It was also used to heal wounds, and in poultices for drawing boils. In China, the root of *S. dichotoma*, or *yin chai hu*, is used.

Character
Sweet, moist, cool.
Constituents
Mucilage, saponins, silica, minerals, vitamins A, B, C, fatty acids.
Actions
Astringent, antirheumatic, heals wounds, demulcent.

Parts used

AERIAL PARTS
S. MEDIA
Made into creams, the aerial parts are still used today for eczema and skin irritations. In mainland Europe, they are a traditional folk remedy, mainly taken internally as a cleansing diuretic and tonic for rheumatic pains and weak conditions. Harvest throughout the growing period.

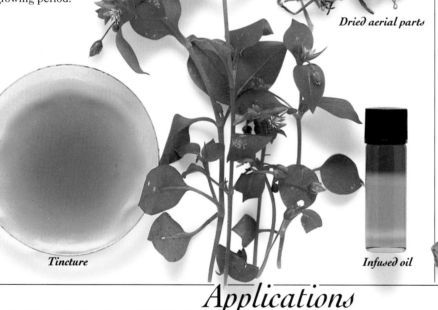

Fresh aerial parts

Dried aerial parts

Tincture

Infused oil

ROOT
S. DICHOTOMA
In China, *yin chai hu* is used as a cooling herb in fevers and to stop nosebleeds and heavy menstrual bleeding. It is also given as a tonic for malnourished children, reflecting its use, in poor European rural areas, as a "free food" in hard times.

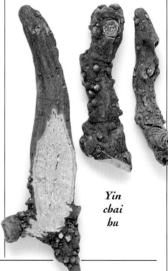

Yin chai hu

Applications

AERIAL PARTS
S. MEDIA

 DECOCTION Use the herb fresh, if possible, for a cleansing, tonic mixture to relieve fatigue and debility. Also helpful for urinary tract inflammations, such as cystitis.

 TINCTURE Add to remedies for rheumatism.

 POULTICE Apply the fresh plant to boils and abscesses; also to painful rheumatic joints.

 COMPRESS Soak a pad in the hot decoction, or tincture diluted in hot water, and apply to painful joints.

 CREAM Apply to eczema, especially if it is itching. Use to draw insect stings or splinters, and on burns and scalds.

 INFUSED OIL Follow the hot infusion method (see p. 122), and apply the oil as an alternative to creams for skin rashes, or add 1 tbsp to bathwater for eczema.

ROOT
S. DICHOTOMA

 DECOCTION Use for hot fevers related to weakness in chronic illness.

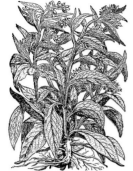

"... given to drinke against the paine of the backe, gotten by violent motion as wrastling or overmuch use of women…"
John Gerard, 1597.

Symphytum officinale
COMFREY

A COUNTRY NAME for comfrey was knitbone, a reminder of its traditional use in healing fractures. The herb contains allantoin, which encourages bone, cartilage, and muscle cells to grow. When the crushed herb is applied to an injured limb, the allantoin is absorbed through the skin and speeds up healing. In the past, comfrey baths were popular before marriage to repair the hymen and thus "restore virginity."

Character
Cool, moist, sweet.
Constituents
Mucilage, steroidal saponins, allantoin (mainly flowering tops), tannins, pyrrolizidine alkaloids (mainly root), inulin, vitamin B12, protein.
Actions
Cell proliferator, astringent, demulcent, heals wounds, expectorant.

Parts used

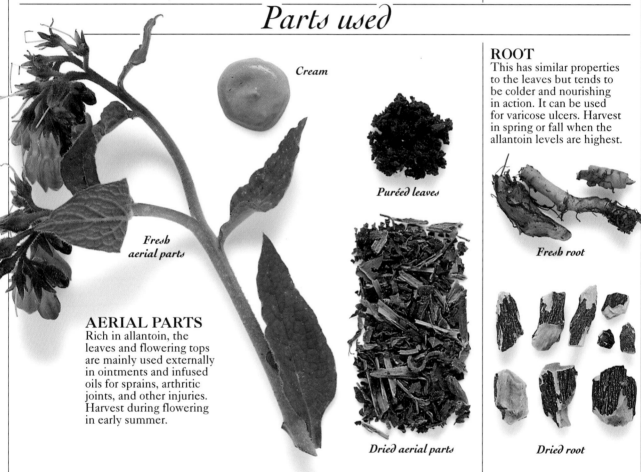

Cream

Puréed leaves

ROOT
This has similar properties to the leaves but tends to be colder and nourishing in action. It can be used for varicose ulcers. Harvest in spring or fall when the allantoin levels are highest.

Fresh aerial parts

Fresh root

AERIAL PARTS
Rich in allantoin, the leaves and flowering tops are mainly used externally in ointments and infused oils for sprains, arthritic joints, and other injuries. Harvest during flowering in early summer.

Dried aerial parts

Dried root

Applications

AERIAL PARTS

 POULTICE Purée the leaves only, and apply to minor fractures that would not normally be set in plaster, such as broken toes, ribs, or hairline cracks in larger bones.

 CREAM Use for bone or muscle damage, including osteoarthritis.

 INFUSED OIL Make by the hot infusion method (see p. 122), and use on arthritic joints, bruises, sprains, and other traumatic injuries; also for inflamed bunions.

 INFUSION Used for inflammations and ulcerations of the digestive tract.

 SYRUP Take a syrup made from the infusion for dry coughs or stubborn, thick phlegm.

ROOT

 POULTICE Make a paste of powdered root with a little water and use on varicose ulcers and other stubborn wounds; also for bleeding hemorrhoids.

CAUTIONS
• Use only under professional supervision because of pyrrolizidine akaloids, which in isolation have been linked by some research to liver cancer in rats. Concentration is highest in the root, which is best avoided for internal use.
• Avoid using on dirty wounds, because rapid healing can trap dirt or pus.
• Use is restricted in Australia, New Zealand, Canada, and Germany.

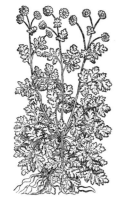

Tanacetum parthenium
FEVERFEW

RECENTLY, FEVERFEW has been hailed as a "cure" and prophylactic for migraines. In the past, the herb was also used for headaches, but it was largely applied externally; feverfew was thought too bitter and potentially damaging to be taken internally. Nevertheless, it was popularly taken by women, to expel the placenta after birth and for various uterine disorders. The name feverfew is a corruption of featherfew, referring to the plant's fine petals.

"...the herb bruised... and applied to the wrists before the coming of the ague-fits, does take them away."
Nicholas Culpeper, 1653.

Character
Bitter, warm, drying.
Constituents
Sesquiterpene lactones, volatile oil, pyrethrin, tannins.
Actions
Anti-inflammatory, relaxes blood vessels, relaxant, digestive stimulant, promotes menstruation, expels worms.

Parts used

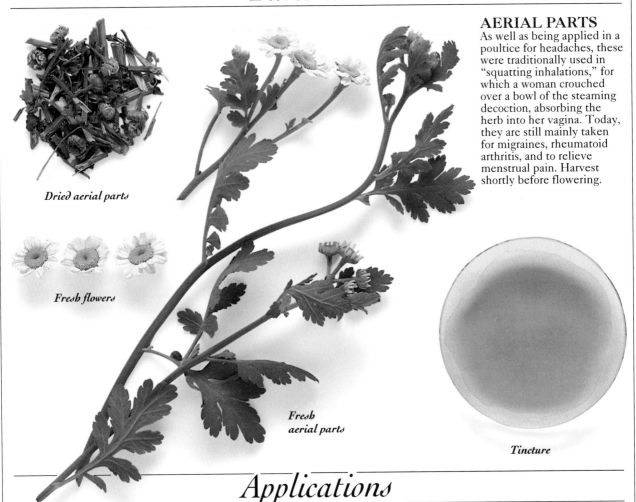

Dried aerial parts

Fresh flowers

Fresh aerial parts

Tincture

AERIAL PARTS
As well as being applied in a poultice for headaches, these were traditionally used in "squatting inhalations," for which a woman crouched over a bowl of the steaming decoction, absorbing the herb into her vagina. Today, they are still mainly taken for migraines, rheumatoid arthritis, and to relieve menstrual pain. Harvest shortly before flowering.

Applications

AERIAL PARTS

 FRESH Eat one large leaf daily as a prophylactic against migraines.

 INFUSION Drink a weak infusion (15 g herb to 2 cups [500 ml] water) after childbirth to encourage cleansing and tonifying of the uterus; also for menstrual pain associated with sluggish flow and congestion.

 TINCTURE Take 5-10 drops every 30 minutes at the onset of a migraine; it is best for "cold"-type migraines, involving tightening of the cerebral blood vessels and eased by applying a hot towel to the head. For the acute stages of rheumatoid arthritis, add up to 2 ml tincture, three times a day, to other herbal remedies.

 POULTICE Sauté the fresh herb in a little oil, and apply hot to the abdomen for colicky pains.

CAUTIONS
• Mouth ulcers are a common side effect of eating fresh leaves: if this is a problem, try sautéing the leaves first.
• The herb should be avoided by patients taking blood-thinning drugs because it can affect clotting rates.

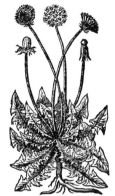

Taraxacum officinale
DANDELION

A RELATIVELY RECENT ADDITION to the medicinal repertoire, dandelion was not mentioned in Chinese herbals until the 7th century, and in Europe it first appears in the *Ortus Sanitatis* of 1485. The name dandelion was apparently invented by a 15th-century surgeon, who compared the shape of the leaves to a lion's tooth, or *dens leonis*. In the West, we separate the leaves and root; the Chinese use the whole plant, which they call *pu gong ying*.

"It is colde, but drieth more and doth withall clense and open by reason of the bitternes which it hath joined with it…"
John Gerard, 1597.

Character
Cold, bitter, sweet.
Constituents
Leaves: bitter glycosides, carotenoids, terpenoids, choline, potassium salts, iron, and other minerals, vitamins A, B, C, D.
Root: bitter glycosides, tannins, triterpenes, sterols, volatile oil, choline, asparagin, inulin.
Actions
Leaves: diuretic, liver and digestive tonic.
Root: liver tonic, promotes bile flow, diuretic, antirheumatic.

Parts used

WHOLE HERB
In China, the flowers, leaves, root, and seed heads of either the common dandelion or an Oriental species, *T. mongolicum*, are used as a diuretic and liver stimulant. They are also considered to clear heat and toxins from the blood, so are used for boils and abscesses.

LEAVES
An effective diuretic, the leaves are rich in potassium, which is generally lost with frequent urination. They are used for fluid retention, especially with heart problems, and for other urinary disorders. The leaves are also an effective liver and digestive tonic. Harvest throughout the growing season.

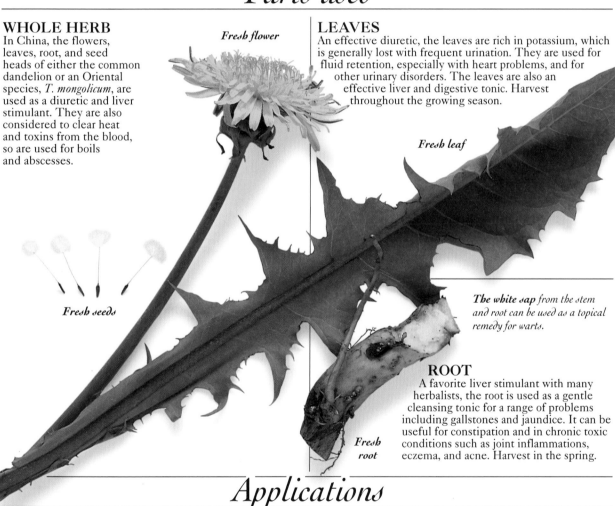

Fresh flower

Fresh leaf

Fresh seeds

The white sap from the stem and root can be used as a topical remedy for warts.

ROOT
A favorite liver stimulant with many herbalists, the root is used as a gentle cleansing tonic for a range of problems including gallstones and jaundice. It can be useful for constipation and in chronic toxic conditions such as joint inflammations, eczema, and acne. Harvest in the spring.

Fresh root

Applications

LEAVES

 FRESH Add to spring salads as a cleansing remedy.

 JUICE Purée the leaves when a diuretic action is needed. Take up to 20 ml juice, three times a day.

 INFUSION A less effective diuretic than the juice, the infusion makes a cleansing remedy for toxic conditions including gout and eczema. Also use as a gentle liver and digestive stimulant. Make with freshly dried leaves.

 TINCTURE Often added to remedies for a failing heart to ensure adequate potassium intake.

ROOT

 TINCTURE Use the fresh root for toxic conditions such as gout, eczema, or acne. Also prescribed as a liver stimulant in liver disorders and related constipation.

 DECOCTION Use for the same conditions as the tincture.

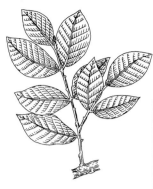

Terminalia spp.
MYROBALAN

"... haritaki should be taken with salt during the rainy season, with sugar in the autumn ... with honey in the spring and with treacle in the hot months."
Ayurvedic prescription.

SEVERAL SPECIES of the *Terminalia* genus of trees are used in Ayurvedic medicine, among them *T. belerica* (*bibhitaki*, or *beleric myrobalan*), *T. arjuna* (*arjuna*, or *indradrum*) and *T. chebula* (*haritaki*, or *chebulic myrobalan*). They are all important rejuvenating and tonic herbs that are only now being thoroughly researched. *Haritaki* is known as *he ti* in Chinese medicine, and is used for persistent coughs and dysentery; in Tibet, it is regarded as "the king of medicines".

Character
Astringent, sour, sweet, bitter, warm.
Constituents
Tannins, triterpenoid saponins, flavonoids, phytosterols.
Actions
T. BELERICA/T. CHEBULA: astringent, restorative tonic, expectorant, laxative, antiseptic, expels worms.
T. ARJUNA: cardioprotective, liver-protective, mild diuretic.

Parts used

BARK
T. ARJUNA
Arjuna has been used for treating heart problems for at least 3,000 years. Modern studies have had mixed results, but most have confirmed a degree of efficacy and the plant is known to reduce cholesterol levels, improve the supply of nutrients to heart muscles, and reduce the risk of heart attacks among people with angina pectoris.

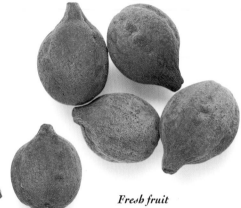
Fresh fruit

FRUIT
T. BELERICA
Bibhitaki is mainly used in Ayurveda as a *kapha* tonic, helping to strengthen the lungs, voice, and eyesight. The unripe fruit is an effective laxative for cleansing the digestive system and is used to expel intestinal parasites. The ripe fruit is preferred for indigestion and diarrhea. *Bibhitaki* is often combined with *haritaki* in the classic "three fruits", or *triphala*, remedy.

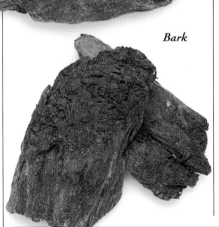
Bark

FRUIT
T. CHEBULA
Haritaki is an important Ayurvedic tonic herb. It is the main ingredient in the "three fruits", or *triphala*, remedy – with *amalaki* (*Emblica officinalis*) and *bibhitaki* – a widely used laxative and antiseptic tonic for the digestive system. *Haritaki* is believed to strengthen the brain and nerves, and to increase spiritual awareness. Like *bibhitaki*, it is used for both diarrhea and constipation and is said to promote vision, voice, and longevity. As an astringent, it is also used for vaginal discharges and excessive menstrual bleeding.

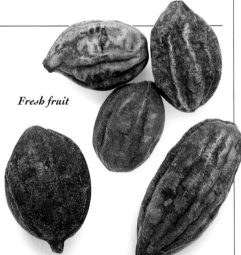
Fresh fruit

Applications

BARK
T. ARJUNA

 TINCTURE Take 3 doses of 40 drops to 5 ml daily for heart disorders.

 DECOCTION To boost the heart's energy, take ½ cup three times daily.

FRUIT
T. BELERICA

 POULTICE Use crushed fruits spread on gauze as a poultice for sore eyes.

 POWDER Mix 1 tsp powder with 1 tsp honey for sore throats.

FRUIT
T. CHEBULA

 DECOCTION Use 1 tsp dried fruit per cup of decoction to strengthen the respiratory and digestive systems.

 WASH Use the infusion or decoction as a wash for ulcerated skin sores and infections. The same wash can also be used as a douche for vaginal discharges and infections.

 EYEWASH Use a well-strained, weak decoction as an eyewash for inflammations such as conjunctivitis.

CAUTION
• Avoid all *Terminalia spp.* in pregnancy, and in cases of severe exhaustion, or excess heat exhaustion.

Thymus spp.
THYME

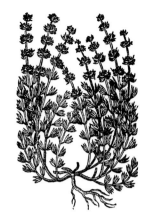

"For headaches a decoction in vinegar is applied to the temples..."
Pliny, AD 77.

GARDEN THYME (*T. vulgaris*) is the cultivated form of wild thyme (*T. serpyllum*). Known as "mother of thyme", probably because of its traditional use for menstrual disorders, wild thyme derives its Latin name from the plant's serpent-like growth. Pliny recommends it as an antidote for snake bites, "poison of marine creatures", and headaches. The Romans also burned the plant in the belief that the fumes would repel scorpions.

Character
Pungent, slightly bitter, warm, drying.
Constituents
Volatile oil, bitter principle, saponins, triterpenes, flavonoids, tannins.
Actions
Antiseptic expectorant, antispasmodic, antiseptic, astringent, antibacterial, antifungal, diuretic, soothes coughs, antibiotic, heals wounds. Topical: increases blood flow to an area.

Parts used

AERIAL PARTS
T. VULGARIS
An antiseptic expectorant, the aerial parts are ideal for deep-seated chest infections marked by thick yellow phlegm. They are also a useful digestive remedy, warming for stomach chills and associated diarrhoea, and have been shown to inhibit *Heliobactor pylorii*, associated with gastric ulcers. Discard the woody stems.

Fresh aerial parts

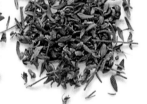

Dried aerial parts

AERIAL PARTS
T. SERPYLLUM
The leaves and flowers have similar actions to the cultivated garden variety, but are slightly more stimulating and effective at preventing spasms. They can also be taken for period pain. Harvest before and during flowering.

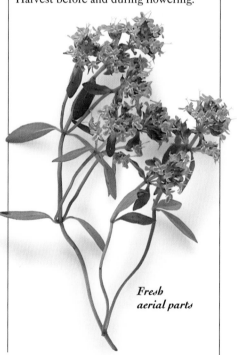

Fresh aerial parts

ESSENTIAL OIL
T. VULGARIS
Extremely antimicrobial, thyme oil also stimulates the immune system, and is good for respiratory and digestive problems. Used with evening primrose and fish oils, it can help to improve concentration skills in hyperactive and dyslexic children. Several qualities of thyme oil are available commercially: all have similar actions.

Applications

AERIAL PARTS
T. VULGARIS/T. SERPYLLUM

 INFUSION Use for chest infections, stomach chills, or irritable bowel.

 TINCTURE Use for diarrhea associated with stomach chills, or as an expectorant in chest infections.

 GARGLE Use the infusion or diluted tincture for sore throats.

 SYRUP Take a syrup made from the infusion for coughs and lung infections.

ESSENTIAL OIL

 CHEST RUB Dissolve 10 drops thyme oil in 20 ml almond or sunflower oil for chest infections.

 OIL Dissolve 10 drops in 20 ml water, and apply to insect bites and infected wounds. Add 5 drops to bath water for weakness and arthritic conditions.

 MASSAGE OIL Dissolve 10 drops each of thyme and lavender oil in 25 ml almond or sunflower oil for rheumatic pains or strained muscles.

CAUTIONS
• Recommendations to avoid thyme and thyme oil in pregnancy are often not based on secure clinical evidence, and some argue that the herb is actually quite safe to use then.
• Thyme oil can irritate the mucous membranes, so always dilute it well.

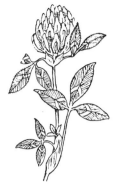

Trifolium pratense
RED CLOVER

THE RED CLOVER we now use medicinally was mainly used in the past as a fodder crop for cattle. Gerard knew it as meadow trefoil or "three-leaved grasse," and its familiar three-lobed leaves were associated by medieval Christians with the Trinity. The Romans used strawberry-leaved clover (*T. fragiferum*), a Mediterranean plant, which Pliny suggested taking in wine for urinary stones, and recommended the root for dropsy.

"Plinie writeth and setteth it downe for certaine, that the leaves hereof do tremble and stande right up against the comming of a storme or tempest."
John Gerard, 1597.

Character
Slightly sweet, cool.
Constituents
Phenolic glycosides, flavonoids, salicylates, coumarins, cyanogenic glycosides, mineral acids.
Actions
Alterative, antispasmodic, diuretic, anti-inflammatory, possible estrogenic activity.

Parts used

FLOWERS
Mainly used as a cleansing herb for skin complaints, the flowers are also useful for coughs and have been widely used for bronchitis and whooping cough. In the 1930s, they became popular as a cancer fighting remedy and may still be prescribed to breast, ovarian, and lymphatic cancer sufferers. Harvest during flowering.

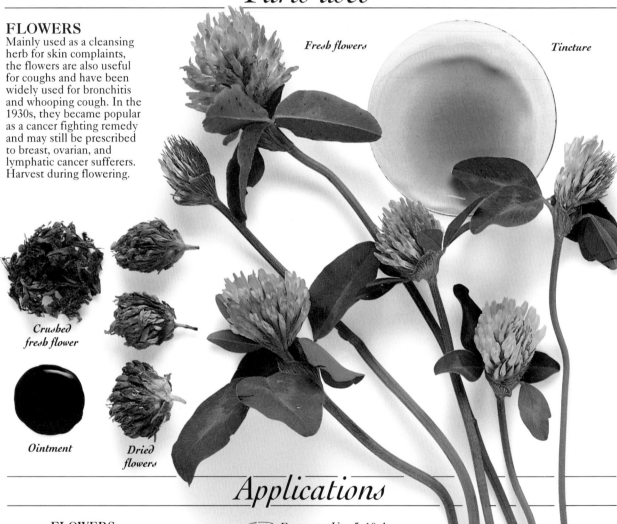

Fresh flowers

Tincture

Crushed fresh flower

Ointment

Dried flowers

Applications

FLOWERS

 FRESH Crush the flowers, and apply to insect bites and stings.

 TINCTURE Take internally for eczema and psoriasis.

 COMPRESS Use for arthritic pains and gout.

 OINTMENT For lymphatic swellings, cover fresh flowers with water and simmer in a slow cooker for 48 hours. Strain, evaporate the residue to semi-dryness, and combine with an equal amount of ointment base.

 EYEWASH Use 5-10 drops tincture in 20 ml water (a full eyecup) or a well-strained infusion for conjunctivitis.

 DOUCHE Use the infusion for vaginal itching.

 SYRUP Take a syrup made from the infusion for stubborn, dry coughs.

Trigonella foenum-graecum
FENUGREEK

"When the body is rubbed with it, the skin is left beautiful without any blemishes."
Ancient Egyptian recipe for fenugreek ointment, c. 1500 B.C.

HIGHLY REGARDED BY HIPPOCRATES, fenugreek is one of the oldest medicinal herbs. In ancient Egypt, it was used to ease childbirth and to increase milk flow; today, it is still taken by Egyptian women for menstrual pain, and as *hilba* tea it is a popular standby to ease stomach cramps for tourists afflicted by gastric upsets. In China, fenugreek or *hu lu ba* is also used for abdominal pain. Western research has recently highlighted hypoglycemic properties.

Character
Very warming, pungent, bitter.
Constituents
Steroidal saponins, alkaloids (inc. trigonelline and gentianine), mucilage, protein, vitamins A, B, C, minerals.
Actions
Seeds: anti-inflammatory, digestive tonic, promote milk flow, locally demulcent, uterine stimulant, lowers blood sugar levels, aphrodisiac, lowers cholesterol levels.
Aerial parts: antispasmodic.

Parts used

SEEDS
Traditionally used as an aphrodisiac, the seeds are warming for the kidneys and reproductive organs and are used in China to treat male impotence. They can be taken for menstrual pain and menopausal problems related to kidney *qi* (energy) weakness. They are also a bitter digestive remedy, and can be used in diabetes and, externally, for skin inflammations. Harvest when ripe.

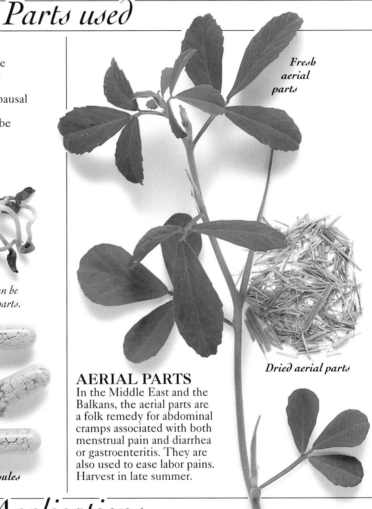

Fresh aerial parts

Dried aerial parts

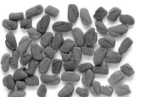

Seeds

Sprouted seeds can be used as the aerial parts.

Tincture

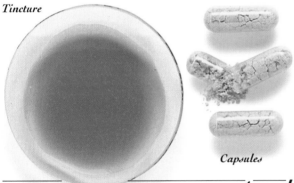

Capsules

AERIAL PARTS
In the Middle East and the Balkans, the aerial parts are a folk remedy for abdominal cramps associated with both menstrual pain and diarrhea or gastroenteritis. They are also used to ease labor pains. Harvest in late summer.

Applications

SEEDS

 DECOCTION Take as a warming drink for menstrual pain, stomach upsets, and, if a nursing mother, to increase milk flow. Disguise the bitter taste with a little fennel.

 TINCTURE Take for reproductive disorders and conditions involving kidney *qi* (energy) weakness. Prescribed with other hypo-glycemic herbs in diabetes.

 CAPSULES Prescribed to help control glucose metabolism in late-onset diabetes, and to lower cholesterol levels in those at risk from heart disease.

 POULTICE Make the powdered herb into a paste and apply to boils and cellulitis.

AERIAL PARTS

 INFUSION Take for abdominal cramps, labor and menstrual pain. May be made from sprouted seeds.

CAUTIONS
• Fenugreek is a uterine stimulant, so avoid in pregnancy. The aerial parts may be used in labor.
• Insulin-dependent diabetics should seek professional advice before using fenugreek as a hypoglycemic.

Tussilago farfara
COLTSFOOT

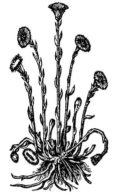

"The smoke of this plant, dried with the root and burnt, is said to cure, if inhaled deeply through a reed, an inveterate cough."
Pliny, A.D. 77.

SMOKING COLTSFOOT for coughs and asthma was recommended by the Greek physician Dioscorides. The plant's Latin name means "cough dispeller" and even now, herbal cigarettes often contain coltsfoot. The plant flowers in early spring. and the leaves only appear when the flowers have died down; hence the plant's old name, *filius ante patrem* ("the son before the father"). In China, only the flowers, known as *kuan dong hua*, are used.

Character
Warm, pungent, slightly sweet.
Constituents
Mucilage, tannins, pyrrolizidine alkaloids, inulin, zinc, bitter principle, sterols, flavonoids (inc. rutin), potassium, calcium.
Actions
Relaxing expectorant, reduces phlegm, antispasmodic, demulcent. Topically: tissue healer, emollient.

Parts used

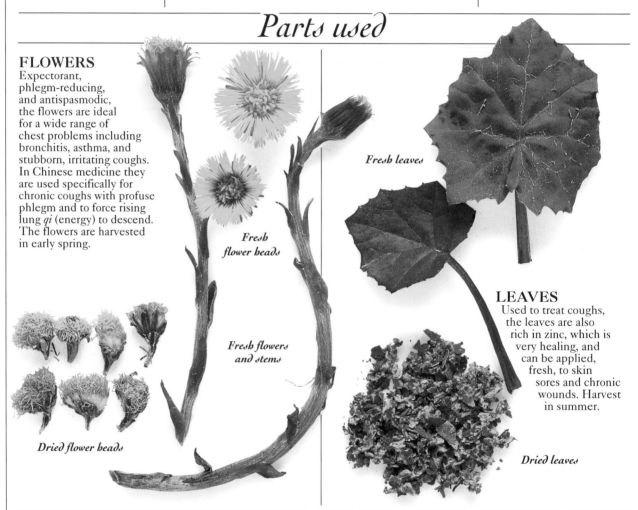

FLOWERS
Expectorant, phlegm-reducing, and antispasmodic, the flowers are ideal for a wide range of chest problems including bronchitis, asthma, and stubborn, irritating coughs. In Chinese medicine they are used specifically for chronic coughs with profuse phlegm and to force rising lung *qi* (energy) to descend. The flowers are harvested in early spring.

Fresh leaves

Fresh flower heads

Fresh flowers and stems

LEAVES
Used to treat coughs, the leaves are also rich in zinc, which is very healing, and can be applied, fresh, to skin sores and chronic wounds. Harvest in summer.

Dried flower heads

Dried leaves

Applications

FLOWERS

 DECOCTION Prescribed for irritable coughs and phlegm; also for coughs associated with colds or influenza.

 TINCTURE Prescribed for chronic or persistent coughs; combines well with thyme and elecampane.

 SYRUP Prescribed for coughs; a syrup made from the decoction is more moistening for dry, stubborn, coughs than the infusion.

LEAVES

 DECOCTION Prescribed for coughs and phlegm.

 TINCTURE Prescribed for chronic or persistent coughs.

 POULTICE Apply the fresh leaf externally to ulcers, sores, and other slow-to-heal wounds.

CAUTION
• Use internally only under professional guidance. Some herbalists and medical texts recommend avoiding it altogether. The herb contains pyrrolizidine alkaloids, which, in isolation, have caused liver damage in rats. (The quantities in the plant are, however, minute, and Swedish research also suggests that in coltsfoot they are destroyed when making a decoction.)

Urtica dioica
STINGING NETTLE

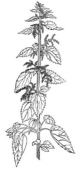

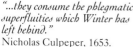

"...they consume the phlegmatic superfluities which Winter has left behind."
Nicholas Culpeper, 1653.

ACCORDING TO TRADITION, Caesar's troops introduced the Roman nettle (*U. pilulifera*) into Britain because they thought that they would need to flail themselves with nettles to keep warm, and until recently "urtication," or beating with nettles, was a standard folk remedy for arthritis and rheumatism. Nettles are still used medicinally and make a cleansing spring tonic and a nourishing vegetable if gathered when the leaves are young.

Character
Cool, dry; astringent, slightly bitter taste.
Constituents
Histamine, formic acid, acetylcholine, serotonin, glucoquinones, many minerals (inc. silica), vitamins A, B, C, tannins.
Actions
Astringent, diuretic, tonic, nutritive, stops bleeding, circulatory stimulant, promotes milk flow, lowers blood sugar levels, prevents scurvy.

Parts used

AERIAL PARTS
Nettles take minerals, including iron, from the soil and the aerial parts are a good tonic for anemia; the high vitamin C content in the plant helps ensure that the iron is properly absorbed by the body. They clear uric acid from the system to relieve gout and arthritis, and their astringency stops bleeding. Nettles "sting" because of histamine and formic acid in the hairs that trigger the familiar allergic response. Harvest while flowering.

ROOT
Traditionally used as a hair conditioner, recent research has confirmed that it is also effective in controlling benign prostate enlargement.

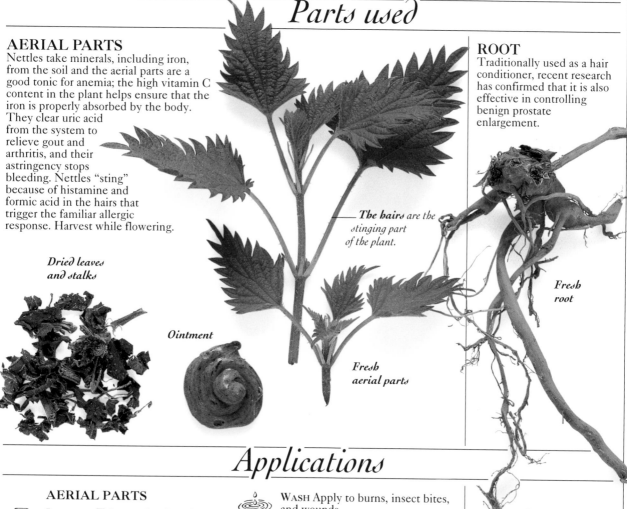

The hairs are the stinging part of the plant.

Dried leaves and stalks

Ointment

Fresh aerial parts

Fresh root

Applications

AERIAL PARTS

 INFUSION Take to stimulate the circulation and to cleanse the system in arthritis, rheumatism, gout, and eczema. Also increases milk flow in nursing mothers. The fresh shoots make a revitalizing spring tonic.

 TINCTURE Used in combinations for arthritic disorders, skin problems, and heavy uterine bleeding.

COMPRESS Soak a pad in the tincture, and apply to painful arthritic joints, gout, neuralgia, sprains, tendinitis, and sciatica.

 OINTMENT Apply to hemorrhoids.

 WASH Apply to burns, insect bites, and wounds.

 JUICE Liquidize the whole fresh plant to make a good tonic for debilitated conditions and anemia, and to soothe nettle stings.

 POWDER The powdered leaves are inhaled as snuff for nosebleeds.

ROOT

 POULTICE Use the decoction as a rinse for dandruff, hair loss and as a general conditioner.

 DECOCTION Use with saw palmetto for benign prostate enlargement.

131

Vaccinium spp.
BILBERRY & COWBERRY

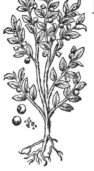

"...they cure the bloody flixe proceeding of choler..."
John Gerard, 1597.

ONCE HIGHLY REGARDED medicinal herbs, the bilberry and cowberry plants are near relatives of bearberry (*Arctostaphylos uva-ursi*), an important urinary antiseptic, and their leaves have been used in very similar ways in folk medicine. Elizabethan apothecaries made a syrup of the berries with honey, called *rob*, as a remedy for diarrhea. In recent trials, the juice of another relative, cranberry (*V. oxycoccus*), has proved to be very effective in treating cystitis.

Character
Sour, astringent, cold, drying.
Constituents
Tannins, sugars, fruit acids, glucoquinone, glycosides. Cowberry leaves contain arbutin.
Actions
Astringent, lowers blood sugar levels, tonic, antiseptic, prevent vomiting, urinary antiseptic.

Parts used

FRUIT
V. MYRTILLUS
Bilberries contain a pigment believed to kill or inhibit the growth of bacteria, so they are especially useful for diarrhea caused by microorganisms, such as dysentery. Large quantities of fresh fruit, how-ever, have a laxative effect. Children find bilberries a palatable remedy. Harvest in late summer and early fall.

Fresh berries

Powdered berries

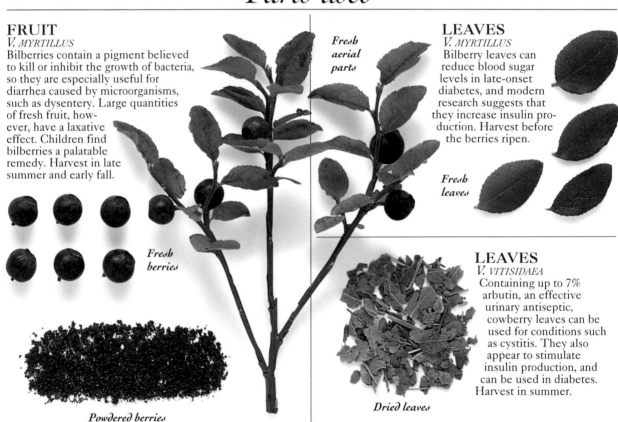

Fresh aerial parts

Fresh leaves

LEAVES
V. MYRTILLUS
Bilberry leaves can reduce blood sugar levels in late-onset diabetes, and modern research suggests that they increase insulin pro-duction. Harvest before the berries ripen.

LEAVES
V. VITISIDAEA
Containing up to 7% arbutin, an effective urinary antiseptic, cowberry leaves can be used for conditions such as cystitis. They also appear to stimulate insulin production, and can be used in diabetes. Harvest in summer.

Dried leaves

Applications

FRUIT
V. MYRTILLUS

 FRESH Eat a large bowl of the whole fresh berries (with sugar and milk or cream, if preferred) for constipation.

 JUICE The unsweetened juice is most effective for diarrhea: take in 10 ml doses.

 DECOCTION Take one glass daily for chronic diarrhea.

 MOUTHWASH Use the diluted juice for ulcers and gum inflammations.

 LOTION Dilute the juice with an equal amount of witch hazel to make a cooling lotion for sunburn and skin inflammations.

 POWDER For babies and infants with diarrhea: mix 75 mg per 1 lb body weight into the baby's bottle.

LEAVES
V. MYRTILLUS

 INFUSION Take as an adjunct to dietary controls in late-onset, non-insulin-dependent diabetes.

 MOUTHWASH/GARGLE Use for ulcers and throat inflammations.

LEAVES
V. VITISIDAEA

 INFUSION Use a strong infusion (40 g herb to 2 cups [500 ml] water) for urinary infections or diarrhea.

CAUTION
• The leaves lower blood sugar levels, so insulin-dependent diabetics should not take them in infusions without professional guidance.

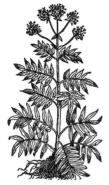

Valeriana officinalis
VALERIAN

NATURE'S TRANQUILIZER, valerian calms the nerves without the side effects of comparable orthodox drugs. It has a distinctive, rather unpleasant smell, and was aptly called *phu* by the Greek physician Galen. In recent years, it has been well researched, with chemicals called valepotriates developing in valerian extracts. These seem to depress the nervous system, and the fresh plant is more sedating.

"...for such as be troubled with the crampe and other convulsions, and for all those that are brused with falles."
John Gerard, 1597.

Character
Pungent, slightly bitter, cool, dry.
Constituents
Volatile oil (inc. isovalerianic acid, borneol), valepotriates, alkaloids, iridoids.
Actions
Tranquilizer, antispasmodic, expectorant, diuretic, lowers blood pressure, carminative, mild anodyne.

Parts used

ROOT
Good for nervous tension, especially anxiety and insomnia, the root also strengthens the heart and can sometimes reduce high blood pressure. It encourages healing in wounds and ulcers and is effective, topically, for muscle cramps. It may also be used as an expectorant and can help tickling, nervous coughs. Harvest in the fall.

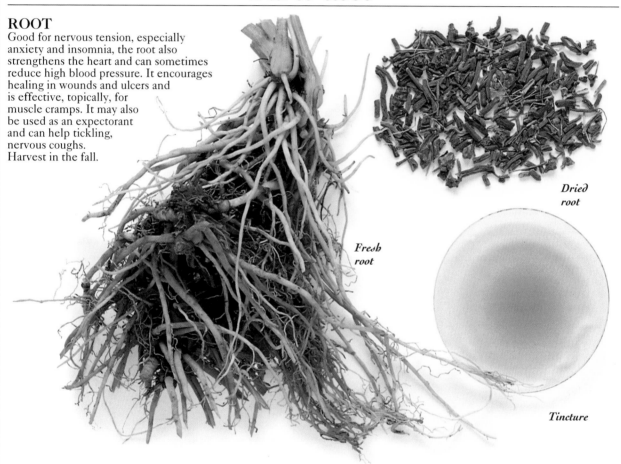

Dried root

Fresh root

Tincture

Applications

ROOT

 MACERATION Soak 2 tsp of the chopped, preferably fresh root for 8-10 hours in a cup of cold water. Use as a sedating brew for anxiety and insomnia. Add 2-3 drops of peppermint water (available from pharmacies) to disguise the flavor.

 INFUSION Use for anxiety and insomnia.

 TINCTURE Use as a sedative or for insomnia. The dosage can vary considerably with individuals: up to 5 ml may be required, but in some

people this can cause headaches, so start with low doses of 1-2 ml. Combine with licorice and other expectorants such as hyssop for coughs. Can be added to mixtures for high blood pressure where tension or anxiety is a contributory factor.

 COMPRESS Soak a pad in the tincture to ease muscle cramps.

 WASH Use the infusion or maceration for chronic ulcers and wounds, and for drawing splinters.

CAUTIONS
• Do not take for more than 2-3 weeks without a break, as continual use or high doses may lead to headaches and palpitations.
• Valerian enhances the action of sleep-inducing drugs, so avoid if taking this type of medication.
• Do not confuse with the garden plant, red "American" valerian (*Centranthus ruber*), which has no medicinal properties.

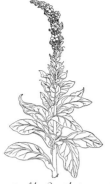

Verbascum thapsus
MULLEIN

THE TALL STEMS OF MULLEIN, covered in fine down, were once burned as tapers in funeral processions. Dioscorides used the herb for scorpion stings, eye complaints, toothache, tonsillitis, and coughs. It was also traditionally taken for wasting diseases such as tuberculosis. An infused oil made from the flowers was a standby in many parts of Europe for ailments as diverse as hemorrhoids and ear infections.

"...beasts of burden that are not only suffering from cough but also broken-winded, are relieved by a draft."
Pliny, A.D. 77.

Character
Slightly sweet, cool, moist.
Constituents
Mucilage, saponins, volatile oil, flavonoids, bitter glycosides (inc. aucubin).
Actions
Expectorant, demulcent, mild diuretic, sedative, heals wounds, astringent, anti-inflammatory.

Parts used

FLOWERS
A relaxing expectorant for dry, chronic, hard coughs such as in whooping cough, tuberculosis, asthma, and bronchitis. The flowers are also effective for throat inflammations. Still made today, the infused oil is used to soothe inflammations, wounds, and earache. Harvest flowers individually.

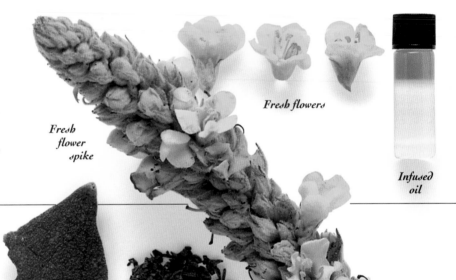

Fresh flower spike

Fresh flowers

Infused oil

LEAVES
Used mainly for respiratory disorders, the leaves were at one time made into herbal "tobacco" and smoked for asthma and tuberculosis. Traditionally, the plant was regarded as antiseptic and the large leaves produced in the second season were wrapped around fruits to preserve them. Harvest before flowering in the second year.

Fresh leaf

Flowers and leaves are not often separated in commercially dried mullein; leaves generally predominate.

Applications

FLOWERS

 TINCTURE Take up to 20 ml a day for chronic, dry coughs, and throat inflammations.

 GARGLE Use an infusion for throat inflammations.

 SYRUP Take a syrup made from the infusion for chronic, hard coughs.

 INFUSED OIL Make by the cold infusion method and use drops for earache (only if certain that the eardrum is not perforated). Use as a salve on wounds, hemorrhoids, eczema, or inflamed eyelids.

LEAVES

 INFUSION Use a strong infusion of dried herb (50 g to 2 cups [500 ml] water) for chronic coughs and throat inflammations. Promotes sweating, so can be useful for feverish chills with hard coughs.

 TINCTURE Use for chronic respiratory disorders; combine with stimulating expectorants if required, such as mulberry bark, cowslip root, elecampane, sweet violet, or thyme.

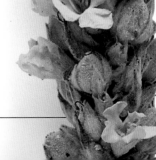

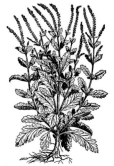

Verbena officinalis
VERVAIN

ONE OF THE DRUIDS' most sacred herbs, vervain was called *hiera botane* (sacred plant) by the Romans, who used it to purify homes and temples. Its association with magic and ritual was still popular in the 17th century, and Gerard warns against using it for "witchcraft and sorceries." The herb was traditionally used for dropsy; cardioactive glycosides have been identified in the plant to support this use.

"...the Magi make the maddest statements about the plant: that people who have been rubbed with it will obtain their wishes, banish fever... and cure all diseases..."
Pliny, A.D. 77.

Character
Pungent, bitter, cool.
Constituents
Volatile oil (inc. citral), bitter glycosides (inc. iridoids), tannins.
Actions
Relaxant tonic, promotes milk flow, promotes sweating, nervine, sedative, antispasmodic, liver restorative, laxative, uterine stimulant, bile stimulant.

Parts used

AERIAL PARTS
An effective nerve tonic, liver stimulant, urinary cleanser and fever remedy, the aerial parts also encourage milk flow and can be taken during labor to stimulate contractions. They have a number of topical uses for sores, wounds, and gum disorders. In China, the plant is known as *ma bian cao*, and the aerial parts are used mainly as a fever remedy for malaria and influenza. Gather while flowering in summer.

Fresh aerial parts

Vervain is one of Dr. Bach's original 12 flower remedies, used for mental stress and overexertion, with related insomnia and inability to relax.

Dried aerial parts

Ointment

Applications

AERIAL PARTS

 INFUSION Take for insomnia and nervous tension or to encourage sweating and stimulate the immune system in feverish conditions. Can also be used as a liver stimulant to improve poor appetite and digestive function. Sip during labor to encourage contractions and during lactation to stimulate milk flow.

 TINCTURE Take for nervous exhaustion and depression (combines well with oats); as a liver stimulant for sluggish digestion, toxic conditions, or jaundice; and with other urinary herbs for stones and conditions related to excess uric acid, such as gout.

 POULTICE Apply to insect bites, sprains, and bruises.

 OINTMENT Use on eczema, wounds, and weeping sores. Also for painful neuralgia.

 MOUTHWASH Use the infusion for mouth ulcers and soft, spongy gums.

CAUTIONS
• Avoid the herb in pregnancy, as it is a uterine stimulant; may be taken during labor.
• May cause vomiting in excessive doses.

Viburnum spp.
GUELDER ROSE & BLACK HAW

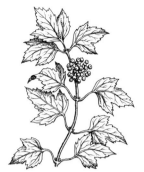

"...for sympathetic disturbances of the heart, stomach and nervous system, common to ladies..."
Finley Ellingwood, 1910.

AN ALTERNATIVE NAME for the guelder rose (*V. opulus*) is cramp bark, which neatly sums up its main medicinal action as a muscle relaxant. The plant was known in the 14th century, since Chaucer suggests eating the berries. It was also used by Native Americans for mumps and other swellings. A close relative, black haw (*V. prunifolium*), is an even more important American variety, known for its significant relaxing action on the uterus. Black haw was a favorite with the Eclectics of 19th-century America (see pp. 20-21).

Character
Astringent, bitter, cool, dry.
Constituents
Bitter substance (viburnin), valerianic acid, tannins, saponins. *V. prunifolium* also contains scopoletin (a coumarin).
Actions
Antispasmodic, sedative, astringent, muscle relaxant, cardiac tonic, uterine relaxant, anti-inflammatory.

Parts used

BARK
V. OPULUS

Guelder rose bark is a muscle relaxant. It also sedates the nervous system, and is useful when physical and emotional tensions combine: typical symptoms include tense, raised shoulders and tight breathing. It relaxes the cardiovascular system in high blood pressure and eases constipation associated with tension. Applied externally, it relieves muscle cramps. Strip from stems in spring before flowering.

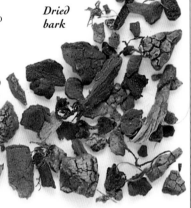

Dried bark

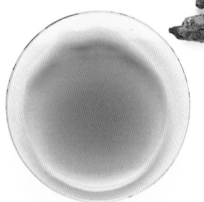

Tincture

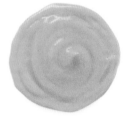

Cream

ROOT BARK
V. PRUNIFOLIUM

A potent muscle relaxant, black haw root bark has a very specific action on the uterus and is one of the best remedies for menstrual pain. It can be helpful for pain and bleeding after childbirth and for heavy menstrual bleeding linked to menopausal syndrome. It can also help to reduce high blood pressure and relieve cramp. Dig up the root in fall and strip off the bark.

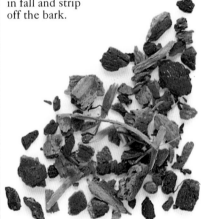

Dried root bark

Applications

BARK
V. OPULUS

 TINCTURE Take as a relaxant for nervous or muscular tension. Use for colicky conditions of the intestines, gallbladder, or urinary system. Add to digestive remedies for an irritable bowel, or combine with butternut or rhubarb root for constipation caused by tension.

 CREAM Mix the tincture with a standard base (such as emulsifying ointment) to make a cream, and apply for muscle cramps or shoulder tension.

ROOT BARK
V. PRUNIFOLIUM

 TINCTURE Use for menstrual pain or pain after childbirth, either in 1-1.5 ml doses every 15-20 minutes, or as a single 20 ml dose taken at the first hint of muscle cramps. Use in standard doses for other menstrual irregularities and menopausal syndrome. Can be added to remedies for high blood pressure.

 DECOCTION Less effective than the tincture. Drink a cup of strong decoction for menstrual pain.

Viola spp.
SWEET VIOLET & HEARTSEASE

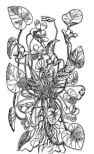

"The lytylnes... in substaunce is nobly rewarded in gretnesse of sauour and of vertue."
Bartholomaeus Anglicus, c. 1250.

SWEET VIOLET AND HEARTSEASE (*V. odorata* and *V. tricolor*) have been used medicinally since ancient times. Homer relates how the Athenians used violets to "moderate anger," while Pliny recommends wearing a garland of violets to prevent headaches and dizziness. Heartsease was once used in love potions, hence the name. The Chinese use a related species, *V. yedoensis*, in similar ways. This has also been used successfully, with other herbs, to treat severe childhood eczema.

Character
Moist, pungent, cold, slightly bitter.
Constituents
Saponins, salicylates, alkaloids, flavonoids, volatile oil.
Actions
V. ODORATA: anti-inflammatory, stimulating expectorant, diuretic, antitumor remedy.
V. TRICOLOR: expectorant, anti-inflammatory, diuretic, anti-rheumatic, laxative, stabilizes capillary membranes.
V. YEDOENSIS: antimicrobial, anti-inflammatory.

Parts used

AERIAL PARTS
V. TRICOLOR
Used for a wide range of skin disorders, from diaper rash to varicose ulcers. A good cough expectorant because of the high saponin content, the aerial parts also tonify and strengthen the blood vessels.
Harvest while flowering.

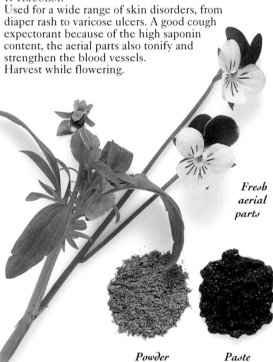

Fresh aerial parts

Powder   *Paste*

AERIAL PARTS
V. ODORATA
Mainly used for coughs, bronchitis, and phlegm. In the 1930s, widely used for breast and lung cancer and may still feature in alternative cancer therapies, especially after surgery to prevent the development of secondary tumors.
Harvest in spring.

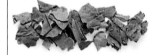

Fresh leaves

Dried leaves

The flowers were once popularly made into a syrup, which was used for an enormous array of disorders.

WHOLE PLANT
V. YEDOENSIS
Called *zi hua di ding* in China, the plant is mainly used for infectious skin conditions, including boils, and for snakebite. It is also taken for lymphatic inflammations and breast abscesses.

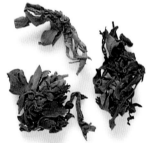

Zi hua di ding

Applications

AERIAL PARTS
V. ODORATA

 SYRUP Take a syrup made from the infusion for coughs.

 MOUTHWASH Use the infusion for mouth and throat infections.

AERIAL PARTS
V. TRICOLOR

 INFUSION Take for chronic skin disorders and as a gentle circulatory and immune system stimulant.

 TINCTURE Use for lung and digestive disorders, capillary fragility, and urinary problems.

 POULTICE Make a paste of the powdered herb with water, and apply to skin sores and ulcers.

 CREAM Use for skin rashes and irritant eczema.

 WASH Use the infusion for diaper rash, cradle cap, weeping sores, or insect bites, or varicose ulcers.

WHOLE PLANT
V. YEDOENSIS

 DECOCTION Use in combination with other cooling, cleansing herbs such as *chi shao yao* and *fang feng* for skin diseases and abscesses.

CAUTION
• Avoid very high doses of the plants, as they contain saponins, which can induce nausea and vomiting.

Withania somnifera
ASHWAGANDHA

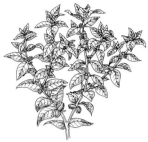

"It nurtures and clarifies the mind, calms and strengthens the nerves, and promotes sound, restful sleep."
Robert Svoboda, 1992.

ASHWAGANDHA, the sanskrit name for winter cherry, translates as "that which has the smell of a horse" – the plant was thought to endow people with the strength, vitality, and sexual energy of a horse. Also called "Indian ginseng", it is one of the most important Ayurvedic tonic herbs. It is currently less expensive than Korean ginseng, can be just as effective, and is becoming readily available in the West. Extensive recent studies have shown it to be an invigorating tonic for the elderly and to have antitumor properties.

Character
Bitter, astringent, sweet, hot.
Constituents
Alkaloids (inc. anaferine and isopelietierine), steroidal lactones (inc. withanolides and withaferins), saponins, iron.
Actions
Tonic, nervine, sedative, anti-inflammatory, antitumor.

Parts used

ROOT
The root is used as a tonic to encourage healthy growth in children. In the elderly it improves vigour and sexual performance. Studies have also shown that it can help increase body weight, slow the development of lung cancer in laboratory animals, and encourage tumor regression. Some studies suggest that winter cherry can nourish the blood, improving hemoglobin levels in anemia.

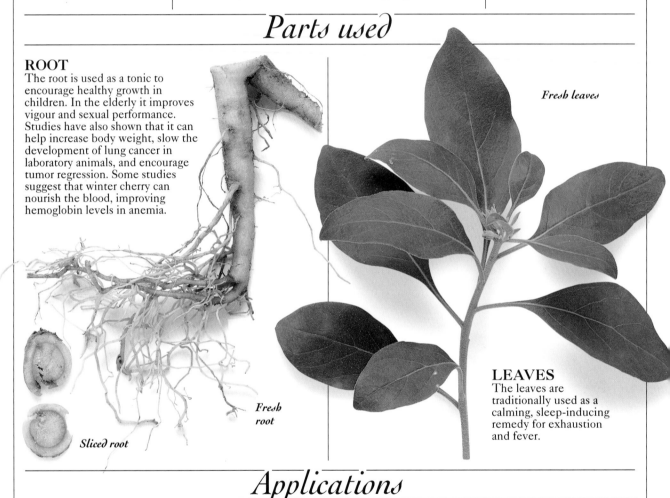

Fresh leaves

Fresh root

Sliced root

LEAVES
The leaves are traditionally used as a calming, sleep-inducing remedy for exhaustion and fever.

Applications

ROOT

POWDER/CAPSULES Use 250 mg to 1 g per dose for exhaustion, sleep problems, stress and debility caused by chronic disease. Up to 5 g per day can be taken in warm milk sweetened with sugar. Regular use can help ease degenerative disorders.

DECOCTION Drink a cup for weakness in pregnancy. Use ½ cup to encourage healthy growth in children, or to help strengthen weak or emaciated children. The root is also decocted in milk to enhance its tonic effects, or it can be combined with half as much long pepper.

WASH Use the decoction externally as a wash for wounds, sores, and skin inflammations.

TONIC WINE Use the tonic wine or tincture as the basis for an iron tonic in anemia and to encourage hemoglobin production.

LEAVES

INFUSION Use as a calming sedative for treating debilitating fevers and stress. Drink a cup at night.

POWDER Studies suggest the leaves may help to reduce the risk of cancer: take ½ tsp daily in water.

Zingiber officinale
GINGER

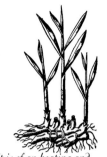

"...it is of an heating and digesting qualitie, and is profitable for the stomacke."
John Gerard, 1597.

ORIGINALLY FROM TROPICAL ASIA, ginger has been used as a medicinal herb in the West for at least 2,000 years. It was introduced into the Americas by the Spaniards, and is now cultivated extensively in the West Indies. As a hot, dry herb, ginger was traditionally used to warm the stomach and dispel chills. In the 18th century, it was added to remedies to modify their action and reduce the irritant effects on the stomach. Ginger is still used in this way in China to reduce the toxicity of some herbs.

Character
Pungent, hot, dry.
Constituents
Volatile oil (inc. borneol, citral), phenols, alkaloid, mucilage.
Actions
Circulatory stimulant, relaxes peripheral blood vessels, promotes sweating, expectorant, prevents vomiting, antiseptic, antispasmodic, carminative, antibacterial.
Topical: increases blood flow to an area.

Parts used

FRESH ROOT
In China, the fresh root, *sheng jiang*, is mainly used to promote sweating and as an expectorant for colds and chills. It is also roasted in hot ashes and used for diarrhea or to stop bleeding, and has been used in trials to combat dysentery. As well as prescribing the fresh root for chills, Western herbalists regard it as a good circulatory stimulant.

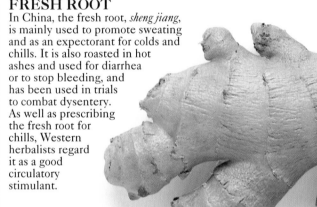

Sliced fresh root

Fresh root

DRIED ROOT
Called *gan jiang* in China, the dried root is used to warm and stimulate the stomach and lungs. In the West, it is used for motion sickness, and in trials has been used successfully for severe sickness in pregnancy and postoperatively.

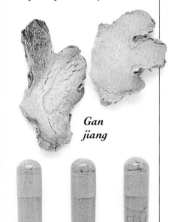

Gan jiang

Capsules

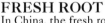

Peeled root skin, or jiang pi, *is used in China for edema and abdominal bloating.*

ESSENTIAL OIL
Ginger oil has been used in both East and West for at least 400 years. In France, it is still prescribed in drop doses on sugar cubes for flatulence and fevers, and to stimulate the appetite. The oil can be added to massage rubs for rheumatic pains and bone injuries.

Applications

FRESH ROOT
 DECOCTION For chills and catarrhal colds, use 1-2 slices to a mug of water and simmer for 10 minutes. A pinch of cinnamon can be added.

 TINCTURE Use 2-10 drops per dose as a warming circulatory stimulant; also use for flatulence, indigestion, and nausea.

DRIED ROOT
 CAPSULES Take 1-2 x 200 mg capsules before a journey for motion sickness. Use up to 1 g doses for morning sickness in pregnancy.

 DECOCTION The Chinese use dried ginger in combination with other herbs as a restorative for *yang* or spleen energies, and for abdominal fullness, nausea and excess phlegm.

ESSENTIAL OIL
 MASSAGE OIL Add 5-10 drops ginger oil to 25 ml almond oil for rheumatism or lumbago. Combines well with juniper or eucalyptus oil.

 OIL Use 1-2 drops on a sugar lump or in ½ teaspoon of honey for flatulence, menstrual cramps, nausea, or stomach upsets.

CAUTIONS
• Avoid excessive amounts of ginger if the stomach is already hot and overstimulated, as in peptic ulceration.
• Use ginger with respect in early pregnancy, although it can be safely taken for morning sickness in the doses described.

AYURVEDIC HERBS
Out of India

THE AYURVEDIC healing tradition in India dates back to the *Rigveda*, an ancient holy book of the Hindus, written between 3500 and 1800 BC. Later theories have also influenced the therapeutic uses of the many thousands of medicinal herbs used on the subcontinent. The *Siddha* system, which attains spiritual perfection through meditation, for example, started around 2000 BC among the Dravidian people of southern India and was believed to originate directly from the Hindu deity Shiva and his wife Parvati. Later, Arab traders brought the Unani-Tibb tradition (based on ancient Greek theories), which was a favorite with the Mogul emperors from the 14th century. Many plants are common to all

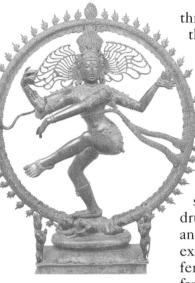

"The essence of all beings is Earth. The essence of the Earth is Water. The essence of Water is plants. The essence of plants is the human being.
Chandogya
Upanishad 1, i 2

three of these systems, although there are often subtle differences that can make the interpretation of Indian plant therapeutics complex. India's many languages also mean that the same plant can be known by a dozen different names.

Around 75 percent of the population of India still uses traditional medicines, which significantly outsell conventional drugs. Many products are complex and adulteration is common, for example *ashtavarga*, used as a fertility tonic, should be made from eight herbs, but analysis has shown that at least 42 different plants have been found in samples. Many prepared remedies contain heavy metals and gemstones and are regarded suspiciously by Western medicine regulators.

Picrorrhiza kurroa
KATUKA

Katuka is an important bitter digestive remedy used in India to stimulate the digestion, improve appetite, and treat jaundice, diarrhea, and constipation. Modern research has confirmed that it acts to protect the liver from toxins, and in some studies it has proved to be more effective than silymarin from milk thistle (see p. 120). In India, *katuka* is also used in *ayush-64*, a traditional remedy taken for malaria.

USES
Katuka is used in the West to stimulate the immune system in acute and chronic infections and in cases of weakened immunity. It has also been used to combat autoimmune disorders such as rheumatoid arthritis and vitiligo. As a bile stimulant, *katuka* can be helpful in the treatment of gall bladder disorders. Typical dose is 500-2000 mg daily. High doses of *katuka* may cause diarrhea. Cases of allergic skin reactions have also been reported.

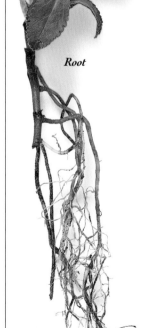

Root

Commiphora mukul
GUGGUL

A close relative of myrrh, guggul (*guggula*) is regarded as purifying and rejuvenating and is the basis of a series of Ayurvedic remedies known as *gugguls*. Traditionally it was used in bandages for aches and pains and added to gargles for sore throats. Research suggests that guggul reduces high cholesterol – in ancient sanskrit texts the herb is recommended for obesity and lipid disorders.

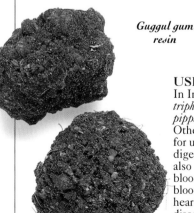

Guggul gum resin

USES
In India, *guggul* is used with *triphala* (see p. 126) and *pippali* for ulcers and arthritis. Other combinations are used for urinary problems and digestive upsets. Extracts are also used to stimulate white blood cell production, reduce blood clotting, and protect the heart from degenerative diseases. Avoid in pregnancy and when breast-feeding.

Santalum album
SANDALWOOD

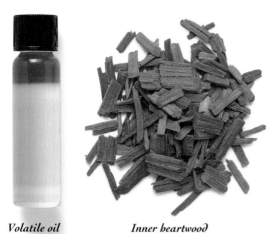

Volatile oil · *Inner heartwood*

Traditionally, sandalwood (*chandana*) is used to cool and calm the body and mind, awaken intelligence, and open the "third eye" to increase devotion and meditation. Aromatherapists use the oil with rose, neroli or benzoin as a calming sedative and antidepressant massage. The wood is used in decoctions for fevers, inflammations, and as a circulatory stimulant.

USES
This herb is antiseptic and antibacterial and can be used as a wash or made into a paste for external sores. The oil is used in massage for urinary problems and digestive upsets with abdominal discomfort, added to warm compresses for dry skin, itching and irritation, and to rosewater for acne. Do not take the oil internally.

Tinospora cordifolia
GUDUCHI

Guduchi powder is used in India as a popular remedy for liver problems, malaria, urinary disorders, and as a tonic for convalescence. It is taken in *ghee* (clarified butter) twice a day as a bitter tonic. The root is used for diarrhea and dysentery, and the leaves are cooling for fevers.

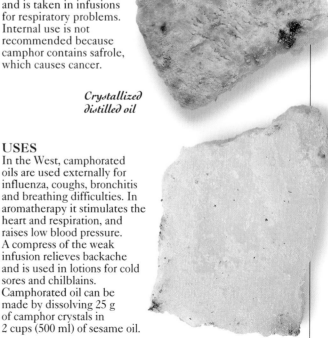

Leaf

Root

USES
Guduchi is used mainly as a bitter digestive tonic for jaundice and liver congestion; it is also a cooling remedy for headaches and fevers, and is used in poultices for fractures. Typical dose is 1-2 g, twice a day.

Cucurma longa
TURMERIC

Turmeric (*haridra*, or *haldi*) is a very popular Indian spice used in cooking to provide flavor and color. It is traditionally used in Ayurvedic medicine as a digestive, circulatory and respiratory stimulant, and in folk medicine for scabies, poor eyesight, to encourage milk flow in breast-feeding, and for rheumatic pains. It is also used externally with honey for sprains and bruises, or as a milk decoction to cleanse the skin.

USES
Turmeric is taken as a digestive stimulant and to combat gastric infections. It is also used as an anti-flammatory for arthritic conditions. Typical dose is 250-1000 mg daily.

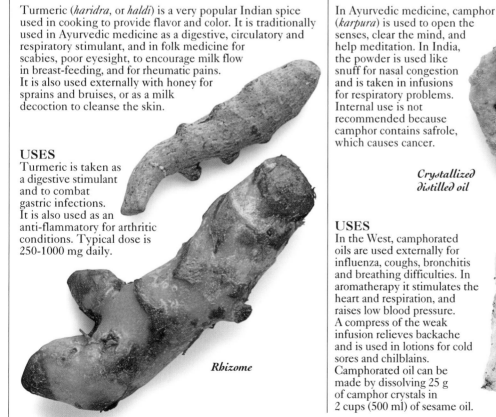

Rhizome

Cinnamomum camphora
CAMPHOR

In Ayurvedic medicine, camphor (*karpura*) is used to open the senses, clear the mind, and help meditation. In India, the powder is used like snuff for nasal congestion and is taken in infusions for respiratory problems. Internal use is not recommended because camphor contains safrole, which causes cancer.

Crystallized distilled oil

USES
In the West, camphorated oils are used externally for influenza, coughs, bronchitis and breathing difficulties. In aromatherapy it stimulates the heart and respiration, and raises low blood pressure. A compress of the weak infusion relieves backache and is used in lotions for cold sores and chilblains. Camphorated oil can be made by dissolving 25 g of camphor crystals in 2 cups (500 ml) of sesame oil.

BUSH HERBS
Remedies Down Under

THE AUSTRALIAN ABORIGINES believed that illnesses that did not have any obvious cause were likely to be the result of a curse formed by placing a ritual drawing on a tree. Recovery was only certain if the offending image was found and destroyed. In New Zealand, the warlike Maori focused mainly on wound herbs and external remedies, and used only a limited range of remedies to treat internal complaints such as fevers and digestive upsets. Before the arrival of European settlers, life expectancy barely reached the mid-20s, and many degenerative diseases common to old age in the West were unknown. Knowledge of healing herbs tended to be highly regionalized and specific

"Herbal treatment did not have to work miracles because the Aborigines only experienced simple disorders."
Geoffrey Vaughan, 1985

to indigenous groups. European settlers took little interest in these native remedies, preferring to cultivate familiar Old World species, which still dominate herbal traditions in both countries.

Over the past few years interest has been revived in native healing arts and several traditional remedies are being tested. Eucalyptus (see p. 61) and tea tree (see p. 89) are probably the best known. The kangaroo apple (*Solanum aviculare*) is proving to be a significant source of synthetic sex hormones and corticosteroids, and the bark of the Moreton Bay chestnut (*Castanospermum australe*), known as a native poison, has recently been used in AIDS treatments and has shown strong antiviral activity to the HIV virus.

Pittosporum spp.
LEMONWOOD

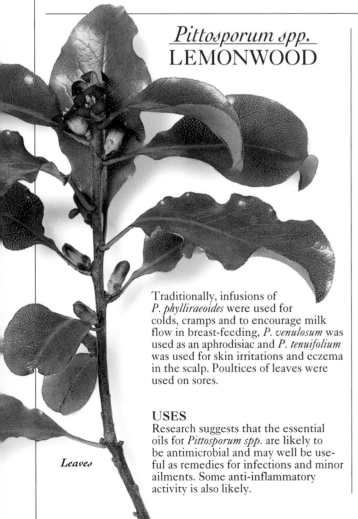

Leaves

Traditionally, infusions of *P. phylliraeoides* were used for colds, cramps and to encourage milk flow in breast-feeding, *P. venulosum* was used as an aphrodisiac and *P. tenuifolium* was used for skin irritations and eczema in the scalp. Poultices of leaves were used on sores.

USES
Research suggests that the essential oils for *Pittosporum spp.* are likely to be antimicrobial and may well be useful as remedies for infections and minor ailments. Some anti-inflammatory activity is also likely.

Melaleuca spp.
PAPERBARKS

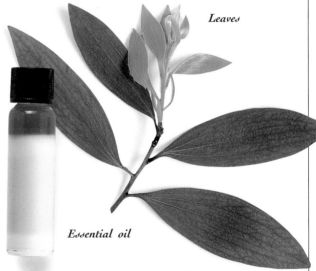

Leaves

Essential oil

As well as tea tree (*Melaleuca alternifolia*, p. 89) Australian Aborigines used other genus members for illness and colds. *M. symphocarpa* was used to treat respiratory problems and headaches, *M. viridiflora* was used for coughs, and *M. leucadendron* for coughs, stomach upsets, and rheumatic aches.

USES
In the West, cajeput and niaouli oils (from *M. cajeputi* and *M. viridiflora*) are used in chest rubs for coughs and colds (5 drops per 5 ml almond or vegetable oil), or in steam inhalants for nasal catarrh and sinus headaches. Do not take internally – they can irritate sensitive skin.

Acacia spp.
AUSTRALIAN WATTLE

Various acacia or wattle trees were an important source of Aboriginal medicines. *A. ancistrocarpa* was used to treat headaches, *A. holosericea* was used for coughs, colds, and laryngitis, and *A. decurrens* was used as an astringent for bleeding and mucous discharges. Ashes of certain acacias were also used as a poultice for arthritic pains.

USES
Acacia extracts can be used in infusions and decoctions for a wide range of common ailments, including common colds, diarrhea, and sore throats.

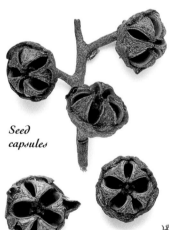

Bark

Leaves

Euphorbia spp.
SPURGE

Several varieties of spurge are used throughout the South Pacific, mainly for respiratory problems and skin sores. *E. hirta* was used in Australia for coughs and bronchial disorders, and *E. glauca*, Maori spurge, was used in infusions for skin sores.

USES
In the West, pill-bearing spurge is used in infusions and decoctions as an asthma remedy. The infusion is also worth trying as a wash for skin sores.

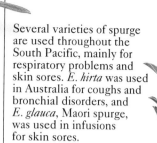

Aerial parts

Leptospermum scoparium/ Kunzea ericoides
NEW ZEALAND TEA TREE

The leaves of *manuka* (*L. Scoparium*) and *kanuka* (*K. ericoides*, formerly *L. ericoides*) were once used as substitutes for tea. The seeds were used in Hawaii for diarrhea, the bark infusion of *kanuka* was taken as a calming sedative, and the bark decoction and seed capsules were given for diarrhea and dysentery.

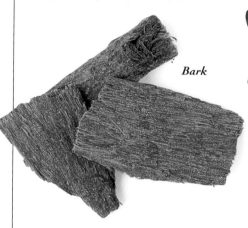

Seed capsules

USES
New Zealand tea trees are astringent and antimicrobial (including *Heliobacter pylori*, which is thought to cause gastric ulcers). *L. scoparium* contains an insecticide that is used to expel intestinal worms. Extracts can also be used as a treatment for sores, infections and fevers.

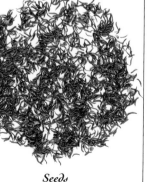

Seeds

Grewia retusifolia
EMU BERRY

Several members of the *Grewia* genus were used by Australian Aborigines, both as food sources and medicine. The emu berry provided fruits to be eaten as food, while its root and bark were used medicinally as astringents and anti-inflammatories.

USES
Use decoctions and macerations for diarrhea, discharges and inflammations.

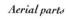

Leaves

Fruit

FUNGI
Medicinal Mushrooms

ALTHOUGH WE TEND to associate healing, fungi-based remedies with modern antibiotic molds such as penicillin – identified in 1928 by Sir Alexander Fleming – they have been used medicinally since ancient times. Bracket fungi, such as agaric (*Polyporus officinalis*), collected from larch trees, were used by Dioscorides for a lengthy list of ills ranging from ague and "falling sickness" (epilepsy) to consumption, asthma, digestive upsets and "the stinging of serpents and the biting of the same". Hoof fungus (*Fomes fomentarius*), another bracket variety that is most common on birch and beech trees, makes an effective emergency styptic poultice for cuts and scrapes. Many mushrooms, such as fly agaric (*Amanita muscaria*), have been used

"... few of them are good to be eaten ... Therefore I give my advice unto those that love such strange and new fangled meates, to beware of licking honey among thornes, lest the sweetnesse of the one do countervaile the sharpness and pricking of the other.
John Gerard, 1597

for their psychoactive properties: fly agaric extracts were eaten by Siberian shamans to induce the trance-like state needed for spirit traveling.

The edible wild mushrooms that appear seasonally on supermarket shelves also have their therapeutic properties. Wood blewits (*Lepista nuda*), for example, have shown antitumor activity in trials, and they also help to regulate sugar metabolism, so may be helpful in treating late-onset diabetes. St. George's mushroom (*Calocybe gambosa*) is also effective for some diabetic conditions. It appears around St. George's Day (April 23) in many parts of Europe, and can be found in fields and downland in late spring and early summer.

WILD MUSHROOMS

The edible wild mushrooms used in cooking also have many therapeutic uses. Wild porcini, used in Chinese medicine in remedies for lumbago, leg pains, and aching bones and tendons, are known to contain the eight essential amino acids. Chanterelles contain a similar mix of amino acids and are also rich in vitamin A. Morels are used in China as a digestive tonic. Oyster mushrooms are a rich source of amino acids and B-vitamins, and in laboratory studies also display antitumor properties and lower cholesterol levels.

USES
Porcini, chanterelles, morels, and oyster mushrooms are a seasonal autumn tonic for combating colds and infections.

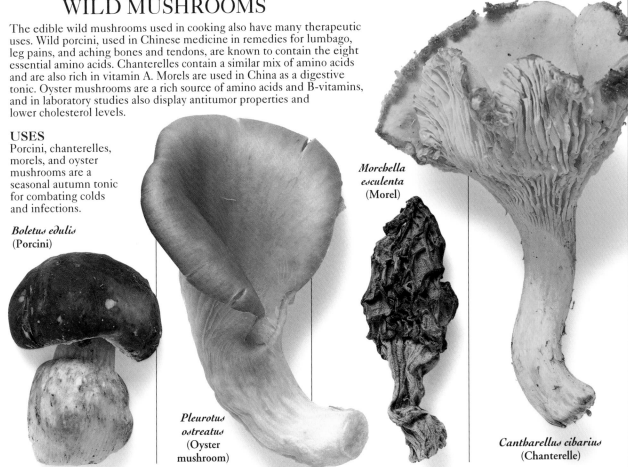

Morchella esculenta
(Morel)

Boletus edulis
(Porcini)

Pleurotus ostreatus
(Oyster mushroom)

Cantharellus cibarius
(Chanterelle)

Wolfiporia cocos
TUCKAHOE

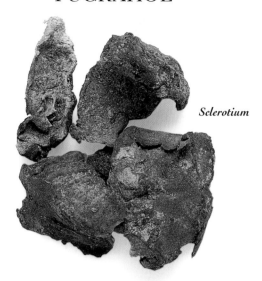

Sclerotium

Tuckahoe (*fu ling*) grows on the roots of pine trees and is known in Native American and Chinese medicine. In China, parts of the fungus are used as a tonic for the spleen and stomach, to clear phlegm, or "calm the spirit" and dispel inappropriate behavior related to spiritual imbalance. In America it is known as Indian bread, an important staple food.

USES
Studies show tuckahoe to be antitumor, antiviral, an immune stimulant, sedative, and analgesic. It is a diuretic used for such problems as diminished urination, edema, or painful urinary dysfunction, and is useful for palpitations and insomnia. Dose is 9-15 g by decoction, or 3-5 ml of tincture. Avoid if there is excessive urination.

Lentinus edodes
SHIITAKE

The shiitake is the second most commonly produced mushroom in the world. Research has shown that it is an effective tonic for the immune system and is strongly antiviral, combatting polio, mumps, measles, and *Herpes simplex*.

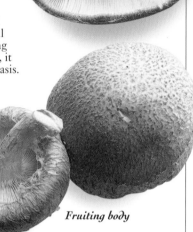

USES
Shiitake can be used in cooking to help stimulate the immune system, to combat common colds, influenza, and other viral infections, and as a useful addition to cancer fighting diets. Unlike some fungi, it can be helpful in candidiasis. Dose is 15 g of dried mushroom daily.

Fruiting body

Cordyceps sinensis
CATERPILLAR FUNGUS

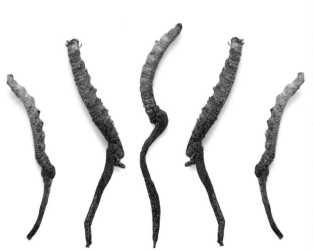

Whole fungus on caterpillars

Caterpillar fungus (*dong chong xia cao*) is a parasite that grows on the caterpillars of an oriental moth. The traditional remedy included the dead larva, although in the West it is now grown on grain. Traditionally the fungus was cooked with duck to add to its potency as an energy tonic to strengthen lungs and kidney.

USES
The fungus is used for asthma, bronchitis, persistent coughs, and other lung diseases. It is also taken in China with chicken or duck soup for irregular menstruation, and used as a tonic in debility, weakness and exhaustion. Dose is 1 g of extract twice a day.

Ganoderma lucidem
REISHI

Known as *ling zhi* in China, reishi was used as a major spiritual tonic by the ancient Taoists. It is now known to stimulate the immune system, lower blood sugar and cholesterol levels, and is sedative and expectorant.

USES
Reishi is a valuable sedative and energy tonic and has been used in AIDS therapy. It can also help degenerative diseases, including heart disease and cancer. Dose is up to 1 g daily.

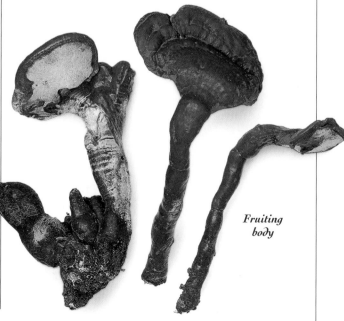

Fruiting body

SOUTH AMERICAN HERBS
Rainforest Remedies

HEALING PLANTS FROM South America have been brought to Europe since the 15th century. Many rapidly gained "cure-all" status, and several have proved to be important sources of powerful drugs. Jesuit's bark *(Cinchona pubescens)* was discovered by missionaries in Lima, Peru, in the 1630s and became an important remedy for malaria and the original source of the drug quinine. Lignum vitae *(Guaiacum officinalis)* was introduced by the Spaniards in 1508 as a remedy for syphilis, and is used by modern herbalists for treating gout and arthritis. Cocaine *(Erythroxylum coca)* was used as a ritual narcotic by South American tribes from at least AD 500, before finding its way to the West, first as an anesthetic

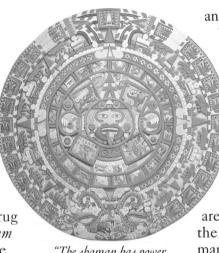

"The shaman has power depending on his knowledge of the medicinal value of herbs ... the importance of the shaman is that he deals both with body and with spirits, that he is both doctor and priest."
Everard Im
Thurn, 1883

and later as a frequently abused "recreational" drug. Chocolate *(Theobroma cacao)* was highly prized by the Aztecs and the beans were used as currency. Cocoa powder was used for treating high blood pressure and angina pectoris, and cocoa butter is still used for burns and skin sores and as a base for vaginal suppositories.

Today, new wonder drugs are still being discovered in the jungles of South America: many have been investigated by pharmaceutical companies in the hope of finding new chemicals, while the plants often become fashionable in the health food market. Many recently introduced South American plants have yet to be fully researched, and it is best to avoid them in pregnancy.

Uncaria tomentosa
PERUVIAN CAT'S CLAW

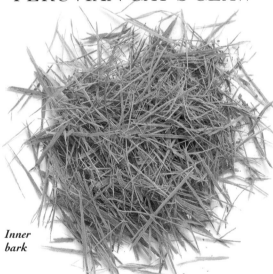

Inner bark

Cat's claw, a woody vine-like plant covered with thorns that resemble the claws of a cat, has been used by Peruvian tribes for centuries. It was first identified by Western researchers in the 1970s and is now widely available. Traditionally regarded as a cure-all, research now focuses on its use as a cancer preventative.

USES
Traditionally used to treat arthritis, asthma, gastritis, diabetes, liver disease, and in contraception, the finely powdered bark should be decocted for at least 45 minutes, using 20 g of the herb to a quart (1 liter) water taken in 60 ml doses. It should be avoided by women who are trying to conceive.

Paullinia cupana
GUARANA

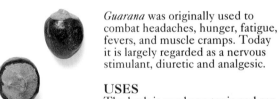

Seeds

Guarana was originally used to combat headaches, hunger, fatigue, fevers, and muscle cramps. Today it is largely regarded as a nervous stimulant, diuretic and analgesic.

USES
The herb is used as a tonic and can help in chronic fatigue syndrome and seasonal affective disorder (SAD). Dose is 1-2 g daily. Avoid in high blood pressure and heart disease.

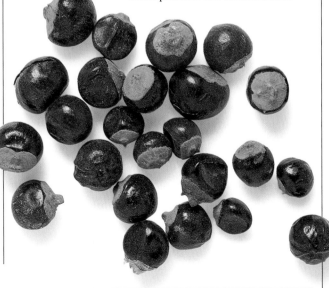

Anemopaegma arvense
CATUABA

Catuaba may be *Erythroxylum catuaba*, or *Anemopaegma arvense*, depending on where it originates. The plant is regarded as an aphrodisiac: in Brazil it is said that "until a father reaches 60, the son is his, after that he is *catuba*'s". A World Health Organization survey has identified the plant as worthy of study as an anti-depressant. It is traditionally used in a decoction sweetened with extracts of *Stevia rebaudiana* – a natural sweetener used in Brazil.

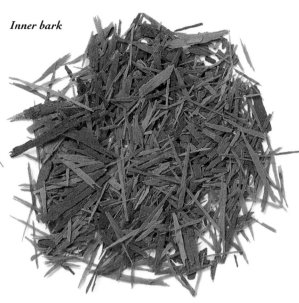

Bark

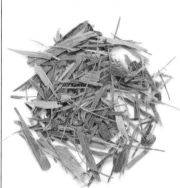

Shredded bark

USES
Catuaba is regarded in the West as a dubious aphrodisiac, but recent research has confirmed its effectiveness in treating impotence. The Tupi Indians also use it as a stimulant for the nervous system and a reproductive organ tonic for men and women. In the West it is marketed in capsules, with a dose of 1 g morning and evening.

Tabebuia impetiginosa
PAU D'ARCO

Inner bark

Pau d'arco has been known as an antimicrobial and antitumor remedy since the 1860s. Research in the early 1990s confirmed that *pau d'arco* extracts are effective for cancer and candida, and Japanese studies suggest that it effectively treats stomach cancer and leukemia.

USES
In the West *pau d'arco* is known as a remedy for candida infections, but is also used for rheumatism, skin infections, ulcers, high blood pressure, colds, and fevers. Typical dose is 2-3 g daily.

Persea americana
AVOCADO

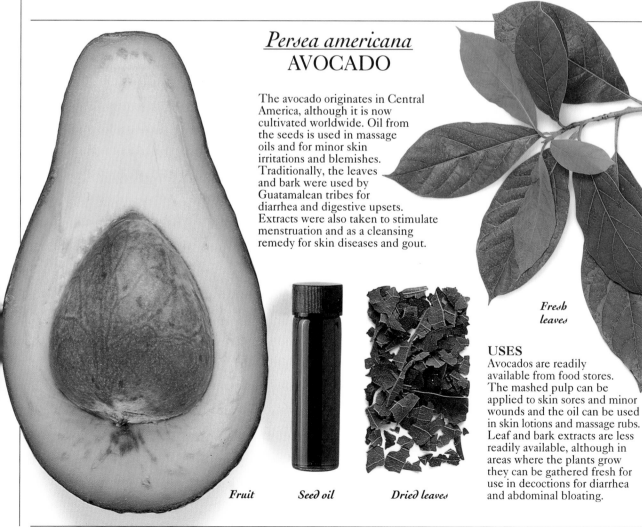

The avocado originates in Central America, although it is now cultivated worldwide. Oil from the seeds is used in massage oils and for minor skin irritations and blemishes. Traditionally, the leaves and bark were used by Guatamalean tribes for diarrhea and digestive upsets. Extracts were also taken to stimulate menstruation and as a cleansing remedy for skin diseases and gout.

Fresh leaves

Fruit   *Seed oil*   *Dried leaves*

USES
Avocados are readily available from food stores. The mashed pulp can be applied to skin sores and minor wounds and the oil can be used in skin lotions and massage rubs. Leaf and bark extracts are less readily available, although in areas where the plants grow they can be gathered fresh for use in decoctions for diarrhea and abdominal bloating.

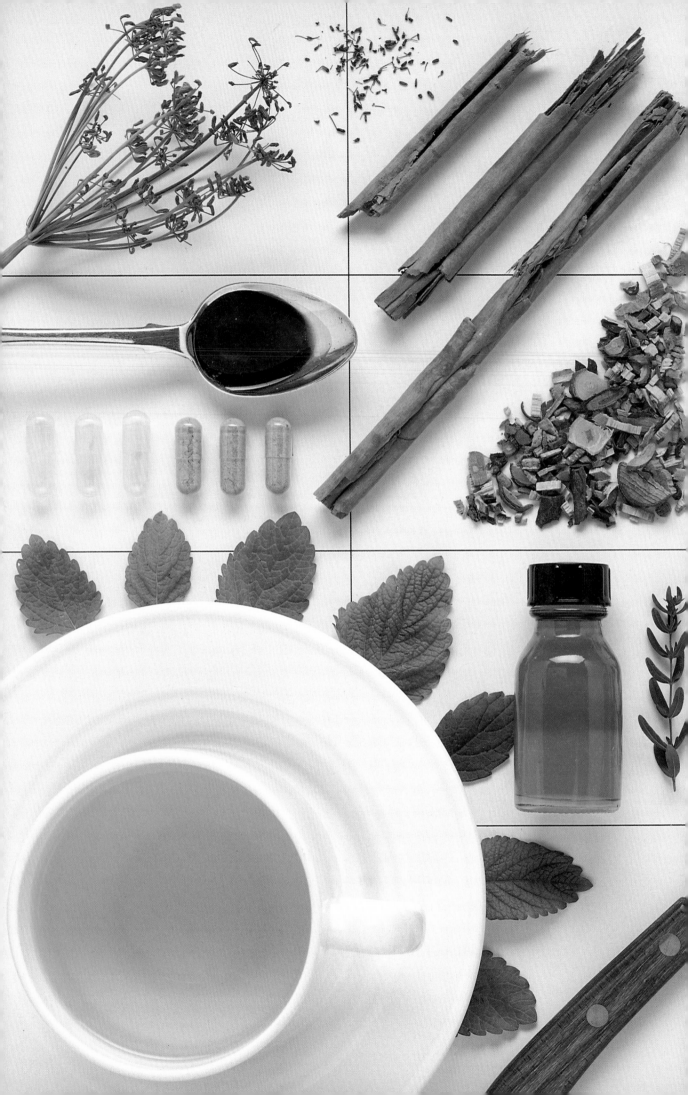

HERBAL REMEDIES

In many parts of the world, herbs are the only option
for all types of health problems. While professional
herbalists in the West may use herbs for severe health
disorders, there is also a wide range of gentler remedies
suitable for home treatment of common complaints.
This section includes instructions on preparing
remedies and an ailment-by-ailment guide.
The focus is on herbs that can be safely used at
home as an alternative to over-the-counter drugs.
Other herbs that are commonly prescribed
are included where appropriate.

HARVESTING & DRYING HERBS

THE CONSTITUENT CHEMICALS and thus the therapeutic properties of herbs can be affected by exactly when they are gathered. Harvest herbs on a dry day, when they are at the peak of maturity and the concentration of active ingredients is highest. Dry them quickly, away from bright sunlight, to preserve the aromatic ingredients and prevent oxidation of other chemicals. To ensure good air circulation, leave in a dry, airy, warm place. An airing cupboard with the door open is ideal, or a sunny room. A damp-free garden shed with a low-powered fan running can also be effective. Avoid using a garage, because herbs become contaminated with gasoline fumes. It is possible to dry herbs completely within six days; the longer it takes the more likely the plant is to discolor and lose its flavor. Keep the drying room between 70-90°F/20-32°C. When the herbs are dry, store in clean, dry, dark glass or pottery containers, with an airtight lid, out of direct sunlight. If stored when damp, the herbs will turn moldy. Label dried herbs with the variety, source, and date: most will keep for 12-18 months.

Flowers _____

Harvest after the morning dew has evaporated, when fully open. Handle carefully, as they are easily damaged. Cut flower heads from the stems and dry whole on trays. Treat small flowers, such as lavender, like seeds; pick before the flowers wither completely. If the stem is large or fleshy, like mullein, remove the individual flowers and dry them separately.

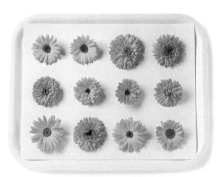

1 Remove obvious dirt, grit, and insects. Spread the flowers on a paper-lined tray or newspaper to dry.

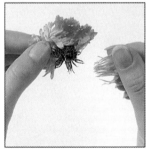

2 When dry, store whole in a dark, airtight container. If using marigolds, as shown here, remove the dried petals and store individually, discarding the central part of the flower.

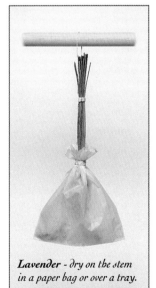

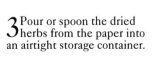
Lavender - dry on the stem in a paper bag or over a tray.

Aerial parts and leaves

Large leaves, such as burdock, can be harvested and dried individually; smaller leaves, such as lemon balm, are best left on the stem. Gather leaves of deciduous herbs just before flowering and evergreen herbs, such as rosemary, throughout the year. If using all the aerial parts, harvest in mid-flowering, giving a mixture of leaves, stem, flowers, and seed head.

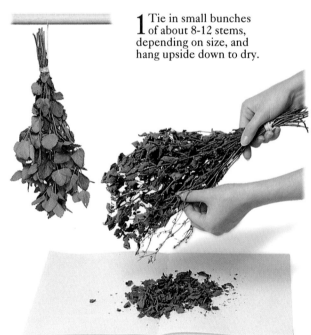

1 Tie in small bunches of about 8-12 stems, depending on size, and hang upside down to dry.

2 When the leaves are brittle to the touch, but not so dry that they turn to powder, rub them from the stem onto paper and discard the larger pieces. If all aerial parts are being used, crumble together.

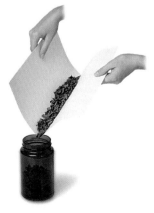

3 Pour or spoon the dried herbs from the paper into an airtight storage container.

Seeds

Harvest entire seed head with about 6-10 in of stalk when the seeds are almost ripe, before too many have been dispersed by the wind or eaten by birds. Hang upside down over a paper-lined tray or in a paper bag, away from direct sunlight; seeds will fall off when ripe.

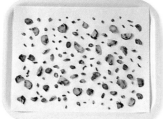

Hang seed heads upside down in small bunches; seeds will usually dry within two weeks.

Roots

Harvest most roots in autumn, when the aerial parts of the plant have wilted and before the ground becomes too hard to make digging difficult. An exception is dandelion where the roots should be gathered in spring. Some roots reabsorb moisture from the air so discard if they become soft.

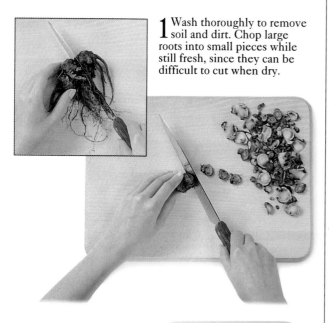

1 Wash thoroughly to remove soil and dirt. Chop large roots into small pieces while still fresh, since they can be difficult to cut when dry.

2 Spread the pieces of root on a tray lined with paper and dry for 2-3 hours in a cooling oven (or 4-6 hours for larger roots). Transfer to a warm, sunny room to complete drying.

Sap and resin

Harvest from the tree in autumn when the sap is falling by making a deep incision in the bark or drilling a hole and collecting the sap in a cup tied to the tree. Sometimes a sizable bucket is needed: a large amount of birch sap, for example, can be collected overnight at certain times of year. Squeeze sap from latex plants such as wild lettuce over a bowl. Many saps can be corrosive, so wear protective gloves.

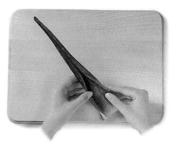

1 For aloe, carefully slice along the center of a leaf and peel back the edges.

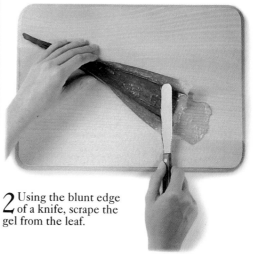

2 Using the blunt edge of a knife, scrape the gel from the leaf.

Fruit

Harvest berries and other fruits when just ripe, before the fruit becomes too soft to dry effectively. Spread on trays to dry. Turn fleshy fruit frequently to ensure even drying. Discard fruit with any signs of mold.

Bark

Harvest in autumn when the sap is falling to minimize damage to the plant. Never remove all the bark – or a band of bark completely surrounding a tree – unless you want to sacrifice the plant to herbal medicine. Dust or wipe bark to remove moss or insects: avoid oversoaking in water. Break into manageable pieces (1-2 inches square), spread on trays, and leave to dry.

Bulbs

Harvest after the aerial parts have wilted. Collect garlic bulbs quickly as they tend to sink downward once the leaves have wilted and are difficult to find.

MAKING HERBAL REMEDIES

THE INSTRUCTIONS GIVEN here use standard quantities of herbs. Throughout the book, all quantities and doses are standard, unless otherwise specified. For combinations of herbs, the total amount in any given remedy should not exceed the standard quantity. For example, an infusion for colds and influenza could contain 10 g each of yarrow, elderflower, and peppermint to give the required proportion of 30 g dried herb to 2 cups (500 ml) water.

MEASURING REMEDIES

You can use standard spoons, droppers, or measuring cups for doses. Quantities for infusions and decoctions should be divided into three equal doses.

drop doses = 5-10 drops depending on age and/or condition

1 ml = 20 drops	65 ml = 1/4 cup
5 ml = 1 teaspoon	130 ml = 1/2 cup
20 ml = 1 tablespoon	

IMPORTANT:
For children and the elderly, doses should be reduced depending on age and/or bodyweight (see pp. 212-13, 216-21). If pregnant, or suffering from gastric or liver inflammation, or when treating children, use nonalcoholic tinctures (see p. 157).

Infusion

A very simple way of using herbs, an infusion is made in much the same way as tea. The water should be just off the boil since vigorously boiling water disperses valuable volatile oils in the steam. Use this method for flowers and the leafy parts of plants. The standard quantity should be made fresh each day and is sufficient for three doses. Drink hot or cold.

Standard quantities
30 g dried herb or 75 g fresh herb to 2 cups (500 ml) water

•

Standard dose
One half-cup
three times a day

•

Equipment
Kettle
Teapot
Nylon sieve or strainer
Teacup
Covered pitcher for storage

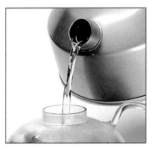

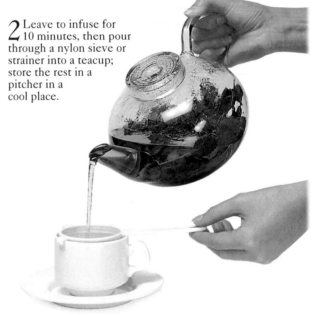

1 Put the herb in a pot with a tight-fitting lid – a teapot is ideal. Pour hot water over the herb.

2 Leave to infuse for 10 minutes, then pour through a nylon sieve or strainer into a teacup; store the rest in a pitcher in a cool place.

Decoction

This method involves a more vigorous extraction of a plant's active ingredients than an infusion and is used for roots, barks, twigs, and some berries. Heat the herb in cold water and simmer for up to 1 hour. As with infusions, the standard quantity should be made fresh each day and is enough for 3 doses. Drink hot or cold.

Standard quantities
30 g dried herb or 60 g fresh herb to 3 cups (750 ml) water, reduced to around 2 cups (500 ml) with simmering

•

Standard dose
One half-cup
three times a day

•

Equipment
Saucepan
(preferably enamel)
Nylon sieve or strainer
Covered pitcher for storage

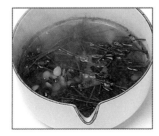

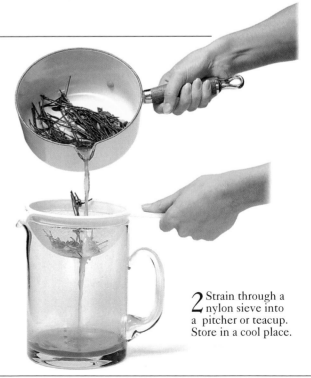

1 Place the herb in a saucepan and add cold water. Bring to boil, then simmer for up to 1 hour until the volume has been reduced by one-third.

2 Strain through a nylon sieve into a pitcher or teacup. Store in a cool place.

Tincture

This is made by steeping the dried or fresh herb in a 25% mixture of alcohol and water (see right). Any part of the plant may be used. Besides extracting the plant's active ingredients, the alcohol acts as a preservative, and tinctures will keep for up to two years. Tinctures should be made from individual herbs; combine prepared tinctures as required. Commercial tinctures use ethyl alcohol, but diluted spirits are suitable for home use. Vodka is ideal, since it contains few additives, although rum helps to disguise the flavor of less palatable herbs.

Standard quantities
200 g dried herb or 600 g fresh herb to 4 cups (1 liter) 25% alcohol/water mixture (e.g. dilute a 75 cl bottle of 37.5% vodka with 37.5 cl water)

•

Equipment
Large screw-top jar
Jelly bag or cheesecloth
Wine press
Large jug or pitcher
Dark glass bottles with screw caps for airtight storage
Funnel (optional)

Standard dose
5 ml three times a day. Tinctures should be taken diluted in water (a little honey or fruit juice can often improve the flavor); for nonalcoholic tinctures see p. 157.

CAUTION
Do not use industrial alcohol, methylated spirits (methyl alcohol), or rubbing alcohol (isopropyl alcohol) in tincture making: all are extremely toxic.

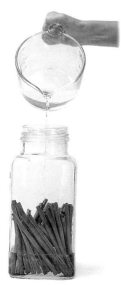
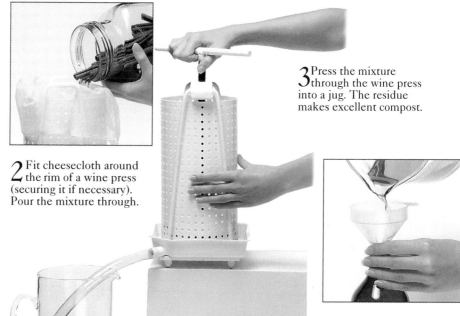

3 Press the mixture through the wine press into a jug. The residue makes excellent compost.

2 Fit cheesecloth around the rim of a wine press (securing it if necessary). Pour the mixture through.

1 Put the herb into a large jar and cover with the vodka/water mixture. Seal the jar, store in a cool place for two weeks, and shake it occasionally.

4 Pour the strained liquid into clean, dark glass bottles, using a funnel if necessary.

Syrup

Honey or unrefined sugar can be used to preserve infusions and decoctions, and syrup makes an ideal cough remedy; honey is particularly soothing. The added sweetness also disguises the flavor of more unpleasant-tasting herbs, such as motherwort. Syrups can also be used to flavor medicines for children.

Standard quantities
2 cups (500 ml) infusion or decoction
500 g honey or unrefined sugar

•

Standard dose
5-10 ml three times a day

•

Equipment
Saucepan
Wooden spoon
Dark glass bottles with cork stoppers for storage
Funnel (optional)

1 Heat 2 cups (500 ml) standard infusion or decoction in a saucepan. Add 500 g honey or unrefined sugar and stir constantly until dissolved.

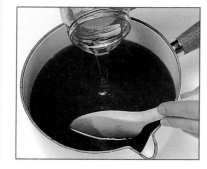
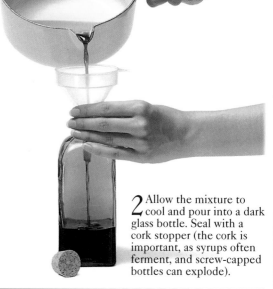

2 Allow the mixture to cool and pour into a dark glass bottle. Seal with a cork stopper (the cork is important, as syrups often ferment, and screw-capped bottles can explode).

Infused oils

Active plant ingredients can be extracted in oil, for external use in massage oils, creams and ointments. Infused oils will last up to a year if kept in a cool, dark place, although smaller amounts made fresh are more potent. There are two techniques: the hot method is suitable for comfrey, chickweed, or rosemary, and the cold method for marigold and St. John's wort. If possible, repeat the process for cold infused oil using new herb and the once-infused oil, leaving to stand for a further few weeks before straining.

HOT INFUSION

Standard quantities
250 g dried herb or 750 g fresh herb to 2 cups (500 ml) sunflower oil
•
Equipment
Glass bowl and saucepan or double saucepan
Wine press
Jelly bag or cheesecloth
Large jug or pitcher
Airtight, glass storage bottles

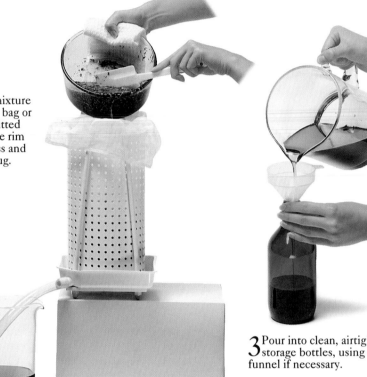

2 Pour the mixture into a jelly bag or cheesecloth fitted securely to the rim of a wine press and strain into a jug.

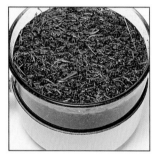

1 Put the oil and the herb in a glass bowl over a pan of boiling water or in a double saucepan and heat gently for about three hours.

3 Pour into clean, airtight storage bottles, using a funnel if necessary.

COLD INFUSION

1 Pack a large jar tightly with the herb and cover completely with oil. Put the lid on and leave on a sunny windowsill or in the greenhouse for two to three weeks.

Standard quantities
Enough flower heads to pack a storage jar
4 cups (1 liter) cold pressed oil, depending on size of jar

Equipment
Jelly bag/cheesecloth or wine press
Large jug or pitcher
Airtight, glass storage bottles

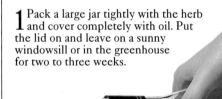

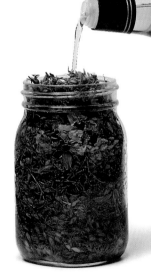

2 Pour the mixture into a jelly bag (shown here) or cheesecloth, fitted securely with string or elastic band to the rim of a jug.

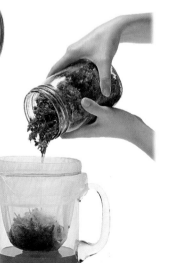

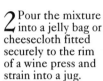

3 Squeeze the oil through the bag. Repeat steps 1 and 2 with new herb and the once-infused oil: after a few weeks, strain again and store.

Cream

A cream is a mixture of water with fats or oils, which softens and blends with the skin. It can be easily made using emulsifying ointment (available from most pharmacies), which is a mixture of oils and waxes that blends with water. Homemade creams will last for several months, but the shelf-life is prolonged by storing the mixture in a cool place or refrigerator or adding a few drops of benzoin tincture as a preservative. Creams made from organic oils and fats deteriorate more quickly (see p. 157). The method shown below is suitable for most herbs.

Standard quantities
150 g emulsifying ointment
70 ml glycerine
80 ml water
30 g dried herb
•
Equipment
Glass bowl and saucepan or
double saucepan
Wooden spoon or spatula
Wine press
Jelly bag or muslin bag
Bowl
Small palette knife
Small, airtight storage jars

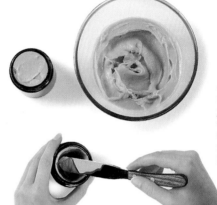

1 Melt the fats and water in a bowl over a pan of boiling water or in a double saucepan, add the herb and heat gently for three hours.

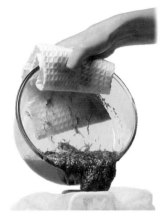

2 Fit a jelly bag around the rim of a wine press. Strain the mixture into a bowl. Stir constantly until cold.

3 Use a small palette knife to fill the storage jars. Put some cream around the edge of the jar first, and then fill the middle.

Ointment

An ointment contains only oils or fats, but no water, and unlike cream it does not blend with the skin but forms a separate layer over it. Ointments are suitable where the skin is already weak or soft, or where some protection is needed from additional moisture, as in diaper rash. Ointments were once made from animal fats, but petroleum jelly or paraffin wax is suitable.

Standard quantities
500 g petroleum jelly or soft
paraffin wax
60 g dried herb

Equipment
Glass bowl and saucepan or
double saucepan
Wooden spoon
Jelly bag or cheesecloth
Jug
Glass jars with lids

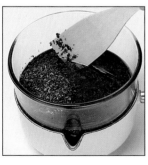

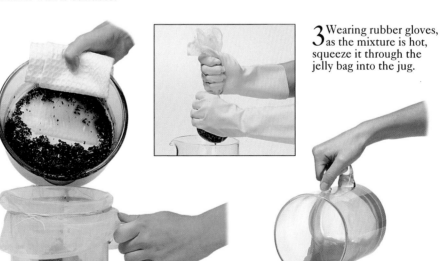

1 Melt the wax or jelly in a bowl over a pan of boiling water or in a double saucepan, stir in the herbs, and heat for about two hours or until the herbs are crisp.

2 Pour the mixture into a jelly bag or cheese-cloth, fitted securely with string or an elastic band to the rim of a jug.

3 Wearing rubber gloves, as the mixture is hot, squeeze it through the jelly bag into the jug.

4 Quickly pour the strained mixture, while still warm and molten, into clean glass storage jars.

Powders and capsules

Herbs can be taken as powders stirred into water, or sprinkled on food, or made into capsules (these are preferable for more unpalatable herbs and are convenient for carrying around). It is best to use commercially prepared powders, which are available from specialist suppliers. Grinding herbs in a domestic grinder generates heat, which can cause chemical changes in the herbs, and hard roots can damage the grinder. Two-part gelatin or vegetarian capsule cases are available from specialist suppliers, see p. 240.

Standard quantities
Size 00 capsule case holds
200-250 mg powdered herb
•
Standard dose
Generally 2-3 capsules two
to three times a day
$\frac{1}{2}$-1 tsp powder in half
a glass of water three
times a day
•
Equipment
Saucer or flat dish
Capsule cases
Dark glass storage jars

1 To fill capsules, pour the powdered herb into a saucer, separate the two halves of a capsule case and slide them together through the powder, scooping it into the capsule.

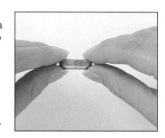

2 Fit together the two halves of the capsule. Store in a dark glass jar in a cool place.

Compress

Often used to accelerate healing of wounds or muscle injuries, a compress is simply a cloth pad soaked in a hot herbal extract and applied to the painful area. A cold compress is sometimes used for headaches. Infusions, decoctions, and tinctures diluted with water can all be used for a compress, and the pad can be soft cotton or linen, cotton ball, or surgical gauze.

1 Soak a clean piece of soft cloth in a hot infusion or other herbal extract. Squeeze out the excess liquid.

Standard application
Use a standard infusion,
decoction or 5-20 ml tincture
in 2 cups (500 ml) hot water
(as specified)
•
Equipment
Cloth pad
Bowl

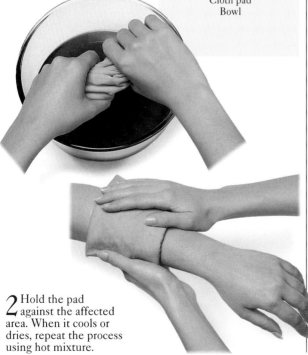

2 Hold the pad against the affected area. When it cools or dries, repeat the process using hot mixture.

Poultice

This has a similar action to a compress, but the whole herb rather than a liquid extract is applied. Poultices are generally applied hot (as shown below), but cold, fresh leaves can be just as suitable. Chop fresh herbs in a food processor for a few seconds or boil in a little water for 2-5 minutes. Dried herbs can be decocted or powders mixed with a little water to make a paste.

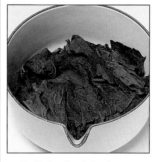

Standard application
Use sufficient herb to cover
the affected area
Replace the poultice every
2-4 hours or earlier
as need be
•
Equipment
Saucepan
Gauze/cotton strips

1 Boil the fresh herb, squeeze out any surplus liquid and spread it on to the affected area. Smooth a little oil on the skin first, to prevent the herb from sticking.

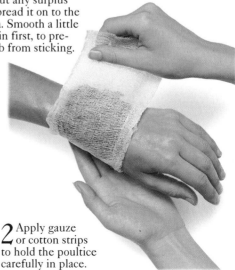

2 Apply gauze or cotton strips to hold the poultice carefully in place.

OTHER HERBAL REMEDIES

Massage oils

Most essential oils irritate the skin and should be diluted before using for massage. Almond or wheatgerm is best as a carrier oil, but sunflower oil can be used if that is all you have available. In general, 5-10 drops essential oil to 20 ml (1 tbsp) carrier oil is adequate. Once diluted in this way, essential oils soon deteriorate, so prepare mixtures as required. Good massage needs skill and practice, but in home use the oil can be suitable for localized problems such as aching joints or chest coughs. Pour about 2-5 ml massage oil on your hand and rub gently into the affected area. An infused oil can also be suitable in some circumstances, for example, comfrey for strains and sprains, St. John's wort for inflammations, and bladderwrack for arthritic conditions.

Creams and ointments from infused oils

Hot or cold infused oils can be thickened with beeswax and water-free lanolin to make ointments, or with beeswax, water-free lanolin, and herbal tinctures to make creams. For a cream, melt 25 g beeswax with 25 g water-free lanolin, add ½ cup (100 ml) infused oil and 50 ml herbal tincture, then strain, stir, and store as shown on p. 155. For an ointment, melt 25 g beeswax with 25 g water-free lanolin, then add ½ cup infused oil. Pour into clean, dark glass jars while still warm, and allow to cool.

Organic alternative to emulsifying ointment

Instead of using emulsifying ointment for making cream, a combination of organic oils and waxes can be used. Follow the instructions given on p. 155, but melt 25 g white beeswax and 25 g water-free lanolin instead of the emulsifying ointment and then add ½ cup (100 ml) sunflower oil, 25 ml glycerine, 75 ml water, and 50 g dried herb. Heat and strain as before, but stir 5 drops of benzoin tincture into the cooling mixture as a preservative.

Steam inhalants

These are ideal for conditions such as mucus, asthma, or sinusitis. Place 1-2 tbsp dried herb in a bowl and pour boiling water over it. Lean over the bowl with a towel draped over your head and the bowl, and inhale for as long as you can bear the heat or until the mixture cools. Avoid going into a cold atmosphere for at least 30 minutes.

Nonalcoholic tinctures (hot water method)

In some cases a tincture made from ethyl alcohol is unsuitable as a herbal remedy, for example, in pregnancy, in gastric or liver inflammation, or when treating children or recovering alcoholics. Adding a small amount (25-50 ml) of almost boiling water to the tincture dose (usually 5 ml) in a cup and allowing it to cool effectively evaporates most of the alcohol.

Tincture ratios

Tinctures are sometimes recommended for use in ratio form, for example, "take 5 ml of a 1:4 tincture." When taking a tincture in ratio form, the proportion used is weight to volume. A 1:4 tincture could be made with 1 lb or 1 kg herb to 4 pints or 4 liters alcohol/water mix, or 100 g herb to 1¾ cups (400 ml) alcohol/water mix. The units used are immaterial and can be large or small accordingly.

Fluid extracts

Fluid extracts are available commercially and generally not made at home as they are measured precisely to pharmaceutical grades. They are used to increase the strength of a herbal mixture when additional action is needed.

Tonic wines

This simple method yields a mixture that is a pleasure to take. It is especially suitable for roots such as *he shou wu*, *dang gui*, and ginseng. Put 500 g herb in a large jar and pour 2 quarts (2 liters) of good quality, preferably red, wine over it. Ensure the herb is completely covered, or it will turn moldy. Cover the jar and leave for 2 weeks. Take in 1/3-cup doses.

Macerations

Some herbs, like valerian root, are best macerated rather than infused or decocted; use the maceration as an infusion or decoction. Pour 2 cups (500 ml) cold water over 25 g dried herb, and leave the mix in a cool place overnight; strain through a nylon sieve.

Chinese decoctions

In China, herbs are mainly given in decoctions. Much larger quantities are used than in the West, with up to 150 g dried herb in 1 quart (1 liter) of water reduced to 1¼-1¾ cups (300-400 ml) for three doses. The concentrated mixture that results may need to be diluted with water to suit Western palates.

Lotions

A lotion is a water-based mixture that is applied to the skin as a cooling or soothing remedy to relieve irritation or inflammation. Alcohol-based mixtures – such as tinctures – can be added to lotions to increase the cooling effect. Typically, a lotion to relieve skin irritation, for example, might include 40 ml rosewater, 20 ml borage juice, 20 ml distilled witch hazel, and 20 ml chickweed tincture. Apply a little of the lotion with a cotton ball or absorbent gauze two or three times a day. If treating a small area, cover the area with a bandage afterward.

Skin washes

Infusions or diluted tinctures can be used to bathe wounds, sores, skin rashes, ulcers, or other skin conditions. Soak a pad of cotton in the wash and bathe the affected area from the center outward. Alternatively, use a plastic atomizer to spray the herbal mixture on rashes or varicose ulcers.

Suppositories

Steel molds to make up to 24 suppositories, as well as disposable molds, are available from specialist suppliers. A homemade mold can be shaped from cooking foil: press it around a small object about 1/2 inch in diameter and 1 inch in length – a thimble is ideal. First lubricate the mold by filling it with a mixture made from 20 ml soft soap, ½ cup (100 ml) glycerine, and 80 ml industrial alcohol or methylated spirits. After a few minutes, pour off the lubricant and drain well. Fill the mold with a suppository mixture made by melting 20 g cocoa butter in a double saucepan and stirring in 10-20 drops (0.5-1 ml) essential oil. The unused suppository lubricant can be stored in a clean glass bottle for future use. Alternatively, heat 15 g gelatin with 20 ml glycerine and 30 ml infusion or diluted tincture. Pour the mixture into a lubricated mold and leave to set for about two hours; then open the mold and carefully remove the suppositories, and store them in a cool place.

Juices

Herb juices can be prepared using a food processor or a domestic juicer to pulp the plant. Squeeze the pulp through a nylon sieve or jelly bag to obtain the juice. Large quantities of herb are needed – a 10 quart (10 liter) bucket of fresh herb may yield only ½ cup (100 ml) or less of juice.

HERBAL FIRST AID

IN A DOMESTIC EMERGENCY, we are more inclined to reach for nonprescription antiseptics and painkillers than herbal medicines. Yet herbs can provide effective alternatives to many over-the-counter pharmacy offerings and might be available when the standard first aid kit is not – in an emergency in the countryside, for example. For home use, commercial herbal preparations can supplement fresh herbs.

Remedies to buy

Herbal remedies can be bought ready-made in a variety of different forms, including creams, essential oils, and capsules. Shown here are the most useful herbal remedies to keep at home in a first aid kit.

FIRST AID KIT
Keep herbal first aid remedies in a box in a cool place out of the reach of children.

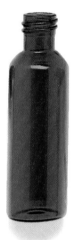

RESCUE REMEDY
The Bach Flower Remedies have a potent effect on the emotions. Rescue Remedy, also available as a cream, is good for shocks and nervous upsets.

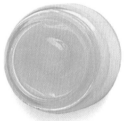

MARIGOLD CREAM
Often sold as *Calendula*, this is antiseptic and antifungal. It is useful for all sorts of cuts and scrapes.

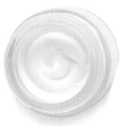

COMFREY OINTMENT
This speeds healing of wounds by encouraging cell growth; use only on clean cuts because the rapidly healing skin may trap dirt.

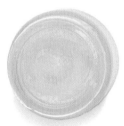

CHICKWEED CREAM
A valuable first aid remedy for drawing stubborn splinters, boils, and insect stings, or for burns and scalds.

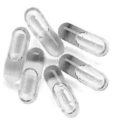

ARNICA CREAM
Effective for bruises and sprains. Do not use on broken skin; it can be an irritant.

ARNICA 6X PILLS
Essential for domestic shocks or accidents, these homeopathic pills can be taken at 30 minute intervals until the patient feels more settled.

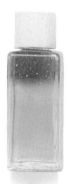

LAVENDER OIL
Add 2-3 drops to a teaspoon of carrier oil and massage into the nape of the neck and temples at the first hint of a headache or migraine. Use the same mix to relieve minor burns, scalds, and sunburn.

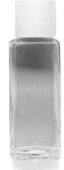

TEA TREE OIL
Highly antiseptic and antifungal for cuts and abrasions, as well as warts and cold sores.

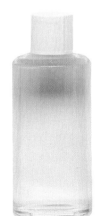

EVENING PRIMROSE CAPSULES
A useful hangover cure. Take a large dose (2-3 g) on "the morning after" to bring rapid relief.

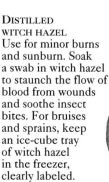

DISTILLED WITCH HAZEL
Use for minor burns and sunburn. Soak a swab in witch hazel to staunch the flow of blood from wounds and soothe insect bites. For bruises and sprains, keep an ice-cube tray of witch hazel in the freezer, clearly labeled.

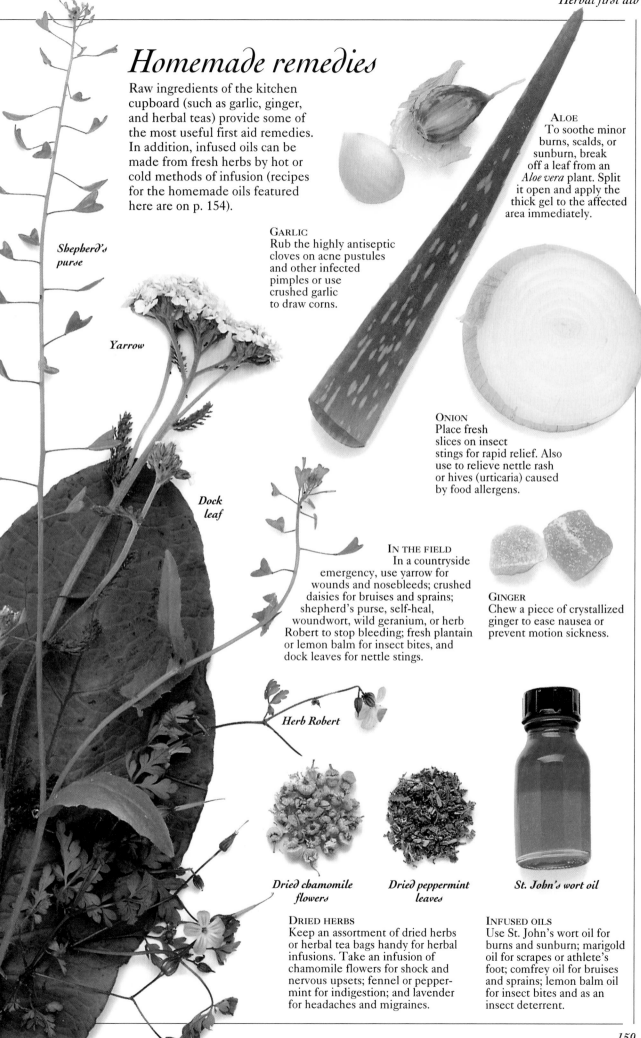

Homemade remedies

Raw ingredients of the kitchen
cupboard (such as garlic, ginger,
and herbal teas) provide some of
the most useful first aid remedies.
In addition, infused oils can be
made from fresh herbs by hot or
cold methods of infusion (recipes
for the homemade oils featured
here are on p. 154).

*Shepherd's
purse*

Yarrow

*Dock
leaf*

Herb Robert

ALOE
To soothe minor
burns, scalds, or
sunburn, break
off a leaf from an
Aloe vera plant. Split
it open and apply the
thick gel to the affected
area immediately.

GARLIC
Rub the highly antiseptic
cloves on acne pustules
and other infected
pimples or use
crushed garlic
to draw corns.

ONION
Place fresh
slices on insect
stings for rapid relief. Also
use to relieve nettle rash
or hives (urticaria) caused
by food allergens.

IN THE FIELD
In a countryside
emergency, use yarrow for
wounds and nosebleeds; crushed
daisies for bruises and sprains;
shepherd's purse, self-heal,
woundwort, wild geranium, or herb
Robert to stop bleeding; fresh plantain
or lemon balm for insect bites, and
dock leaves for nettle stings.

GINGER
Chew a piece of crystallized
ginger to ease nausea or
prevent motion sickness.

*Dried chamomile
flowers*

*Dried peppermint
leaves*

St. John's wort oil

DRIED HERBS
Keep an assortment of dried herbs
or herbal tea bags handy for herbal
infusions. Take an infusion of
chamomile flowers for shock and
nervous upsets; fennel or peppermint for indigestion; and lavender
for headaches and migraines.

INFUSED OILS
Use St. John's wort oil for
burns and sunburn; marigold
oil for scrapes or athlete's
foot; comfrey oil for bruises
and sprains; lemon balm oil
for insect bites and as an
insect deterrent.

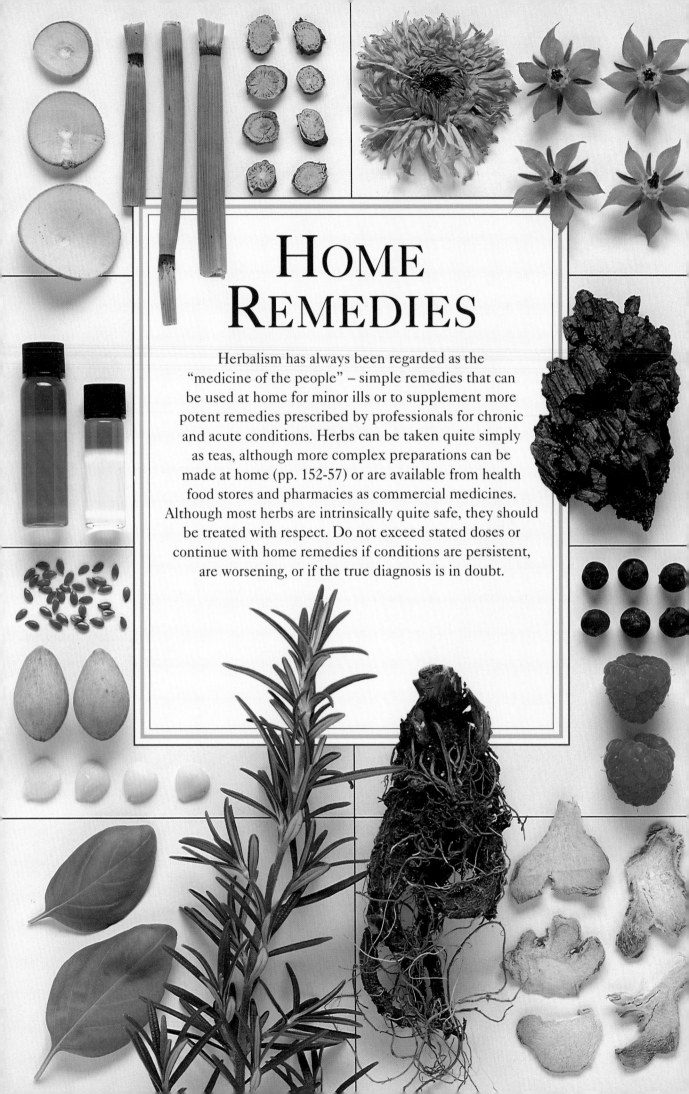

HOME REMEDIES

Herbalism has always been regarded as the "medicine of the people" – simple remedies that can be used at home for minor ills or to supplement more potent remedies prescribed by professionals for chronic and acute conditions. Herbs can be taken quite simply as teas, although more complex preparations can be made at home (pp. 152-57) or are available from health food stores and pharmacies as commercial medicines. Although most herbs are intrinsically quite safe, they should be treated with respect. Do not exceed stated doses or continue with home remedies if conditions are persistent, are worsening, or if the true diagnosis is in doubt.

HOW TO USE THIS SECTION

In this section, ailments are grouped according to body systems, life stages, or action. The complaints covered here are those where home remedies are most appropriate although herbs can, of course, be used for many more ailments. The list of complaints is not intended to be comprehensive and the herbs given for each ailment represent only a small cross-section of the many plants that could be used. Selection of individual remedies will often depend on availability, but choose those that appear to have the most relevant actions. For example, do you need an expectorant for coughs to clear phlegm, a suppressant to ease a persistent tickle, an antibacterial to combat infection, or a tonic to strengthen weak lungs? Herbs can work very quickly, especially for an acute condition. However, long-standing, chronic disorders may require treatment for several months before significant results are achieved. Generally, symptoms will change as the weeks progress, so be prepared to review the remedy at least once a month, and alter it to reflect new conditions. Professional herbalists will often adjust remedies every few weeks as health and energy balance changes. For ailments not covered in this section or for persistent conditions, consult a professional (see p. 230). Details of herbal suppliers are given on p. 240. If gathering herbs in the wild or from gardens, always consult a good plant guide or field herbal to ensure plants are selected correctly.

Sample entry

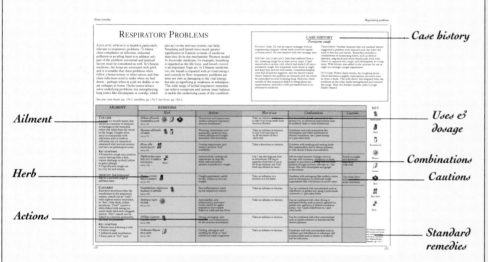

Case history

Ailment

Herb

Actions

Uses & dosage

Combinations

Cautions

Standard remedies

CASE HISTORY Based on a real life case, this shows how herbs are used with other therapeutic approaches such as diet, exercise, or relaxation. Names and circumstances have been changed to preserve anonymity.

AILMENT Brief description of causes and some key symptoms.

HERB Listed in alphabetical order by botanical name, with the most widely used common name. Symbols indicate which part of the plant to use. Before using any herb, refer to the pages shown in brackets.

ACTIONS Major therapeutic effects of the herb relevant to the ailment.

USES & DOSAGE The form in which to take each herb medicinally. Standard adult doses should be assumed unless otherwise specified. Before making or using any remedy, refer to *Making Herbal Remedies*,

pp. 152-57, which provides details of standard formulations and dosages.

COMBINATIONS Most herbs work best in combination, although the exact choice of remedies can vary enormously depending on particular individuals, their symptoms, and constitution. For each ailment, additional herbs are suggested to enhance therapeutic actions. Herbalists rarely combine herbs in equal quantities, because some symptoms may be more acute and specific herbs may be considered more important for treatment. However, the herbs suggested here can be used in equal proportions unless otherwise specified.
  When using a combination of herbs, the total should not exceed the standard adult dose specified in *Making Herbal Remedies*, pp.152-57. For example, a standard infusion

(enough for 3 doses) is made with 30 g dried herb to 2 cups (500 ml) water. If using three herbs in combination, mix 10 g of each to 2 cups (500 ml) water. Make tinctures individually, then combined, to make a specified dose with others.

CAUTIONS Many herbs contain extremely powerful chemicals and overdose can be harmful. Before taking any herbal remedy, check the cautions given here and on the pages shown in brackets in the *Herb* column. Some herbs may, by law, only be prescribed by a qualified practitioner. For herbs used in combinations, check cautions on pp. 228-29 or in the A-Z section (pp. 28-139) as appropriate.

STANDARD REMEDIES All the information in *Uses & dosage* applies to standard recipes and doses listed on pp. 152-57, unless otherwise stated.

IMPORTANT NOTES

• If taking medication for a particular complaint, always consult your doctor or other professional medical practitioner. Some herbs will inter-act with prescription drugs and care is needed. If on prescribed medication, consult a professional before attempting home remedies.

• In any acute condition – fevers, coughs, digestive upsets, severe headaches – seek professional help if there is no improvement within a few days or if the condition appears to be worsening.

• Give children a fraction of an adult dose depending on age (see p. 217).

• In the elderly, metabolism gradually slows down: reduce standard adult doses with increasing frailty and loss of body weight.

• Essential oils are extremely potent and many can irritate mucous membranes. Unless otherwise clearly stated in the remedy charts, *do not* take essential oils internally without professional medical supervision. Before using externally, dilute essential oils in a carrier oil such as wheatgerm, almond, or sunflower. Because essential oils are so expensive, many synthetic chemical substitutes are offered for sale. Always buy a reputable brand, guaranteed to be pure and unadulterated; do not be misled by low-cost products.

MUSCULOSKELETAL PROBLEMS

THE USUAL REACTION to muscular pain is to reach for a painkiller, such as acetaminophen, which quickly lulls the body back into pain-free comfort. Pain, however, is only a symptom of an underlying problem: pulled muscles and strained tendons need restricted movement to heal, and the pain reminds us to keep movement to a minimum. Herbal remedies can do more than just deaden pain; many plants repair the damage of injury or degenerative disease, and provide symptomatic relief; some act as muscle relaxants, others as antispasmodics or anti-inflammatories. A herbal approach to

osteoarthritis, for example, may involve using comfrey ointment to help repair damaged and degenerating bone, with anti-inflammatory herbs such as willow, devil's claw or meadow-sweet to help relieve pain, and cleansing plants such as yellow dock or celery seed to eliminate toxins which can collect in the joints and contribute to discomfort. In Chinese medicine, arthritic and rheumatic pains are attributed to external "evils", such as heat, damp or cold, and are treated with "warming" or "cooling" herbs and energy tonics to combat future attacks by these "evils".

AILMENT	REMEDIES	
	Herb	*Actions*
SPRAINS & STRAINS Injuries to joints and muscles, including back strains. **KEY SYMPTOMS** • Pain following obvious injury or exertion • Swollen joints or limbs • Bruising. *IMPORTANT: If fractures are suspected or if symptoms persist for more than a few days without improvement, seek urgent professional help.*	*Arnica montana* **ARNICA** (see p. 228)	Promotes healing and has an antibacterial action; causes reabsorption of internal bleeding in bruises and sprains.
	Symphytum officinale **COMFREY** (see p. 123)	Encourages cell regrowth in connective tissues and bones; breaks down red blood cells in bruising.
	Thymus vulgaris **THYME** (see p. 127)	Antispasmodic; stimulates blood flow to the tissues, encouraging repair.
ARTHRITIS There are two main types of arthritis: osteoarthritis (OA) is pain and swelling of the joints, generally due to wear and tear; rheumatoid arthritis (RA) is inflammation of many joints, and requires professional treatment. **KEY SYMPTOMS** • Stiffness and joint pain • Creaking sounds in joints • Swollen or deformed joints • Hot or burning joints (RA) • Symmetrical joint swellings (RA) • Often worse in damp, cold weather (OA) • Frozen shoulder (chronic pain and stiffness in the shoulder joint) can be treated as for OA.	*Angelica archangelica* **ANGELICA** (see p. 38)	A warming and stimulating herb, good for "cold" types of osteoarthritis and for rheumatism (see p. 164).
	Harpagophytum procumbens **DEVIL'S CLAW** *(Tuber)* (see p. 72)	Potent anti-inflammatory; action has been compared with cortisone. Better for OA and degenerative conditions than for RA.
	Menyanthes trifoliata **BOGBEAN** (see p. 228)	Cleansing, cooling and anti-inflammatory; a useful herb for "hotter" types of arthritis and muscle pain.
	Salix alba **WILLOW** (see p. 114)	Rich in salicylates (anti-inflammatories that cool hot joints); useful in acute phases and for muscle pains.
GOUT Generally associated with a build-up of uric acid in the joints linked to dietary excess. **KEY SYMPTOM** • Swollen, inflamed, very painful joints; often in the toes or feet.	*Apium graveolens* **CELERY** (see p. 39)	Clears uric acid from the joints, useful for gout and arthritic problems.
	Teucrium chamaedrys **WALL GERMANDER** (see p. 229)	Bitter, digestive tonic and diuretic.

CASE HISTORY
Arthritic pains

PATIENT: Mary, a retired school secretary aged 66, an enthusiastic lacemaker and gardener.

HISTORY AND COMPLAINT: For the past three years Mary had suffered from pain and stiffness in her hands, knees and hips, as well as breathlessness, palpitations, and sore, irritated eyes. Hospital tests ruled out rheumatoid arthritis, but X-rays revealed wear and tear on the joints. Mary had a history of nervous problems and had taken antidepressants and sleeping pills for five years. A recent bereavement had exacerbated her symptoms.

TREATMENT: The antidepressants carried the risk of liver damage, and Mary's symptoms suggested some liver congestion and weakness, so medication included tinctures of *bai shao yao*, *huai niu xi* and bogbean, as well as angelica root, willow bark, and *fang feng* (total 5 ml three times a day). A few drops of the Bach flower remedy, Star of Bethlehem, were added to help her cope with her recent loss. Devil's claw (two capsules up to three times a day) helped while symptoms were acute, and a massage oil containing rosemary and juniper essence in infused bladderwrack oil was useful.

OUTCOME: A month later, Mary's painful joints and sore eyes were back to normal and her hands were no longer stiff. She switched to a herbal remedy for insomnia, and her doctor changed the antidepressants to reduce side effects.

How to use	*Combinations*	*Cautions*
Apply cream to the affected area, or soak a pad in dilute tincture and use as a compress; take homeopathic *Arnica 6x* every 1 to 2 hours.	Use as a simple.	Do not use on broken skin; use homeopathic *Arnica* only internally.
Rub cream or ointment on to the affected area as frequently as required.	Add 5-10 drops essential oils, such as thyme, lavender, or juniper, to 25 ml infused oil to stimulate blood flow and ease pain.	Use only if the injury is clean; not advisable for long-term use.
Add 10 drops oil to 20 ml water and use as a compress; or add 5 drops oil to a hot bath.	Mix with 5-10 drops essential oils such as lavender, rosemary or sage, in 25 ml almond, or sunflower oil as a massage oil to stimulate blood flow and ease pain.	Massage can be damaging if given too soon after injury.
Soak a pad in dilute tincture or decoction and use as a compress; take a decoction, or add 5 drops oil to a bath.	Add celery seed or a little prickly ash to a decoction. Mix angelica and rosemary oil (5-10 drops of each in 25 ml carrier oil) as a massage oil to relieve pain.	Avoid in pregnancy.
Take 1-3 g powder a day in capsule form during the acute phase; take up to 15 ml tincture a day, or use in combinations.	Combine with equal amounts of tinctures of other anti-inflammatories or cleansing herbs, such as angelica, St. John's wort, bogbean, or celery seed.	
Take up to 8 ml tincture three times a day; also use as an infusion or macerate 10 g herb in ½ cup (100 ml) red wine.	Mix black cohosh or celery seed in an infusion, using 2 parts bogbean to 1 part other herbs; or add anti-inflammatories such as meadowsweet to tincture.	
Take up to 5 ml fluid extract three times a day, or use in combination with other tinctures.	Add tinctures of other antirheumatics or cleansing herbs, such as angelica, black cohosh, *lignum vitae*, yellow dock, or burdock.	
Take an infusion of 1 tsp to 2 cups (500 ml) water, or combine with other tinctures.	Add 1 part *lignum vitae* to 2 parts celery seed in an infusion; use diuretics like yarrow or gravelroot in tincture.	Use untreated seeds only; avoid in pregnancy.
Take an infusion or use up to 15 ml tincture a day.	Combine with yarrow and celery seed in an infusion to encourage uric acid excretion.	Do not exceed stated dose.

KEY

Aerial parts

Bark

Essential oil

Flowers

Leaves

Root

Seeds

STANDARD REMEDIES
All recipes and doses are standard unless otherwise specified; see *Making Herbal Remedies, pp. 152-57.*

AILMENT	REMEDIES	
	Herb	*Actions*
RHEUMATISM & MYALGIA Rheumatism describes muscular pains. It can include fibrositis (inflammation of muscle sheath), or may be due to overexertion. **KEY SYMPTOMS** • Painful, sore, aching muscles • May be associated with food intolerance or traumatic injury.	*Cimicifuga racemosa* BLACK COHOSH (see p. 51)	Analgesic, cooling, and soothing; contains salicylic acid to reduce inflammation and ease stiffness.
	Rosemarinus officinalis ROSEMARY (see p. 112)	Stimulating, analgesic, and antirheumatic; warms muscles by encouraging blood flow to the area.
BACKACHE & LUMBAGO Backache may be due to pulled muscles, damaged discs, kidney, or nerve problems. Lumbago is pain in the lower back. **KEY SYMPTOM** • Pain that can be debilitating, chronic and restrictive. *IMPORTANT: Seek professional help for any persistent back pain of unknown cause.*	*Berberis vulgaris* BARBERRY (see p. 228)	Anti-inflammatory, cleansing; can be especially helpful for low back pains.
	Juniperus communis JUNIPER (see p. 78)	Antirheumatic, stimulating; clears excess lactic acid from muscles.
TENNIS ELBOW & TENOSYNOVITIS Tennis elbow is inflammation of the bursa (the elbow joint); tenosynovitis affects tendon sheaths. **KEY SYMPTOMS** • Pain and difficulty in moving the affected joint • Numbness or tingling.	*Achillea millefolium* YARROW (see p. 30)	Reduces inflammation in joints, tendons, and muscles to give pain relief and improve movement.
	Guaiacum officinalis LIGNUM VITAE (see p. 228)	Anti-inflammatory and cooling; suitable for any muscle or joint inflammations, including tendon problems.
REPETITIVE MOTION INJURY (RMI) Painful spasms and weakness in the hands, arms, shoulders, neck, or back, associated with repetitive physical actions. **KEY SYMPTOMS** • Extreme pain • Sudden onset; preceded by numbness and tingling.	*Filipendula ulmaria* MEADOWSWEET (see p. 63)	Contains salicylates to reduce inflammation and ease pain; gentle digestive stimulant to improve metabolism.
	Lentinus edodes SHIITAKE MUSHROOM (see pp. 144-45) *(Fruiting body)*	Tonics like shiitake can help to improve the body's ability to cope with physical stress while reducing the inflammation associated with the symptoms.
SCIATICA Pain caused by irritation or pressure on the sciatic nerve, which runs from the spine along the outer thigh to the foot. **KEY SYMPTOM** • Pain along the path of the nerve.	*Capsicum frutescens* CAYENNE (see p. 50)	Stimulates blood flow, strengthens the nerves and relieves nerve pains.
	Zanthoxylum americanum PRICKLY ASH (see p. 229)	Stimulates circulation to supply nutrients to tissues and help to repair and remove wastes; eases spasmodic pains.
CRAMP Muscle spasm, which may be associated with stress, fatigue or an imbalance of body salts. **KEY SYMPTOMS** • Sharp, severe pain in the legs • Affected muscle feels rigid.	*Dioscorea villosa* MEXICAN WILD YAM (see p. 57) *(Rhizome)*	Muscle relaxant; also relaxes peripheral blood vessels.
	Viburnum opulus GUELDER ROSE (see p. 136)	Effective relaxant for both smooth and skeletal muscles; anti-inflammatory.

How to use	*Combinations*	*Cautions*
Take a decoction or 10-40 drops of tincture per dose, three times daily; take one 200 mg capsule of powder up to three times a day.	Combine with bogbean in decoctions or with anti-inflammatories such as devil's claw in capsules.	
Massage with 10 drops oil in 5 ml infused bladderwrack oil as required. Also helpful for arthritic pains.	Use infused St. John's wort as an alternative base or add additional warming and analgesic essential oils such as eucalyptus, juniper, hyssop or thyme.	
Take in a decoction, half a cup per dose, or up to 5 ml tincture, three times daily.	Use with diuretics such as celery seed, buchu and horsetail for back pain associated with kidney problems; with anti-inflammatories such as black cohosh and devil's claw for muscle or joint inflammations.	Avoid in pregnancy.
Take 10-20 drops tincture per dose; use ½ tsp crushed berries per cup of infusion; use 10 drops essential oil per 5 ml almond oil as an external massage oil.	Use with analgesics and anti-inflammatories such as valerian, devil's claw, white willow, and black cohosh in tinctures or capsules (two 200 mg capsules of powder per dose).	Avoid in pregnancy and kidney disease. Do not take internally for more than six weeks without a break.
Use 10 drops essential oil in 20 ml infused St. John's wort oil for a massage; use a cold infusion to soak a compress to relieve pain and stiffness.	Use with lavender oil in external massage or combine with stinging nettle and arnica infusions in a compress.	Prolonged use may cause skin rashes or, rarely, increase photosensitivity.
Take half a cup of decoction made from ½ tsp chippings per cup; take up to 10 ml tincture per day.	Use with antispasmodics and anti-inflammatories such as guelder rose, prickly ash bark, and black cohosh in tinctures or decoctions.	
Use in an infusion or tincture.	Use with nervines such as St. John's wort and vervain in infusions; with white willow and valerian in tinctures.	Avoid in cases of salicylate allergy.
Take up to 10 g dried shiitake powder per dose with water; for a decoction use 90 g fresh mushrooms in a daily soup.	Add Siberian ginseng or *huang qi* powders, or add a piece of either root, to the soup and simmer for at least 50 minutes to increase resistance to stress and tonify the system.	
Use the infused oil in a massage or take 5 drops tincture in water per dose.	Add 2-5 drops juniper or rosemary oil to the infused oil as additional circulatory stimulants; add up to 5 ml nervines such as St. John's wort or valerian tincture per dose.	Prolonged or excessive topical use may lead to blistering.
Use in decoctions (½ tsp per cup) or take up to 10 ml tincture daily.	Use in decoctions with anti-inflammatories and nervines such as *lignum vitae*, black cohosh and valerian; in tinctures with St. John's wort, white willow and black cohosh.	Avoid in pregnancy unless under professional guidance.
Sip a decoction or take 1 ml tincture; repeat every 15 minutes if symptoms persist.	Use as a simple or with guelder rose tincture.	
Use 25 ml tincture in 75 ml rosewater as a lotion, or in a cream.	Combines well with Indian tobacco in cramp creams; use 10 ml Indian tobacco tincture in 60 ml guelder rose cream.	Internal use of Indian tobacco is restricted.

KEY

Aerial parts

Berries

Essential oil

Heartwood

Root

Stem bark

STANDARD REMEDIES
All recipes and doses are standard unless otherwise specified; see *Making Herbal Remedies, pp. 152-57.*

HEADACHES & MIGRAINES

HEADACHES ARE NOT illnesses in their own right, but symptoms of underlying "dis-ease". Tension headaches, for example, respond to calming herbs, but persistent ones may indicate a need for relaxation, stress-release techniques, or a radical appraisal of lifestyle. Headaches due to catarrh or sinusitis are eased by decongestant herbs, fresh air, and a diet free from mucus-forming foods such as dairy produce. Migraines can be related to food intolerance or pollutants. "Hot" migraines, associated with dilated blood vessels, are relieved by ice packs and cooling remedies; "cold" ones, related to constricted blood vessels, respond to a hot towel on the forehead and warm, stimulating, herbs. Some women find that migraines are linked to their menstrual cycle, and hormonal herbs may help. Digestive remedies, especially liver-cleansing herbs such as agrimony, can also alleviate headaches. In Chinese medicine, the eyes are associated with the liver, and migraine can be identified with overexuberant liver *qi* (energy).

IMPORTANT: *Seek professional advice for sudden, persistent headaches.*

See also: sinusitis, pp. 172-73; anxiety and tension, pp. 196-97; PMS, pp. 202-03.

AILMENT	REMEDIES	
	Herb	*Actions*
TENSION HEADACHES May be caused by tense neck muscles due to stress. Symptoms resolve with relaxation. **KEY SYMPTOM** • Pain, usually frontal.	*Scutellaria lateriflora* **SKULLCAP** (see p. 118)	Relaxant and restorative for the central nervous system; sedative; antispasmodic.
	Stachys officinalis **WOOD BETONY** (see p. 121)	Sedative; stimulates cerebral circulation; useful nervine for anxiety and worries.
MIGRAINE Severe headache, which can be linked to food sensitivity, pollutants, menstrual cycle, or stress. It is associated with changes in tension within the arteries of the brain. Untreated symptoms may last for a few minutes or several days. **KEY SYMPTOMS** • Visual disturbances preceding pain • Pins and needles in limbs • Nausea and vomiting • Light sensitivity.	*Gelsemium sempervirens* **YELLOW JASMINE** (see p. 229)	Potent analgesic and sedative; useful for migraines and neuralgia.
	Lavandula spp. **LAVENDER** (see p. 81)	Sedative; analgesic with antispasmodic action; cooling, bitter remedy useful for "hot" migraines.
	Tanacetum parthenium **FEVERFEW** (see p. 124)	Anti-inflammatory; dilates the cerebral blood vessels, easing "cold" migraines associated with constricted blood vessels.
NEURALGIA Severe burning or stabbing pain often felt along the course of facial nerves. Can follow injury or exposure to cold and drafts. **KEY SYMPTOMS** • Severe, very localized pain • Related areas of skin highly sensitive to touch • Regular recurrences.	*Citrus limon* **LEMON** (see p. 229)	Cooling, astringent; reputed nerve tonic; anti-inflammatory.
	Hypericum perforatum **ST. JOHN'S WORT** (see p. 75) *(Flowering Tops)*	Repairs and restores the nervous system; anti-inflammatory.
	Verbena officinalis **VERVAIN** (see p. 135)	Sedative; antispasmodic; restorative for the nervous system.

CASE HISTORY
Tension headaches

PATIENT: Vera, a married secretary of 45, with two teenage daughters and a live-in mother-in-law.

HISTORY AND COMPLAINT: Vera suffered from headaches once or twice a week, for which she took over-the-counter analgesics. The pain was always localized over her right eye and often persisted for two or three days. Vera also complained of frequent bouts of diarrhea. She had a tendency to depression and extreme fatigue, and never managed to find time for herself. Medical tests detected no abnormalities. She found her daughters difficult, and the constant presence of her elderly mother-in-law annoying. Shortage of money was a continual worry.

TREATMENT: A little self-indulgence was called for: lavender oil for the bath and five minutes to herself after work. Medication for stress intolerance and depression featured relaxing and tonic nervines, which also eased stomach tensions. Bach flower remedies (Impatiens, Willow, and Beech) were added to encourage tolerance. Tinctures of wood betony, vervain, lemon balm, oats, and pasque flower were taken in 5 ml doses three times a day, with ginseng as a general tonic.

OUTCOME: Over two months Vera's headaches became less frequent and severe. A bout of family arguments brought them back, but Vera realized how closely they were linked to stress at home and to her emotions – when her mother-in-law went away for two weeks Vera was pain-free. A residential home might have solved the problem, but Bach flower remedies had to do the job instead.

KEY

Aerial parts

Essential oil

Flowers

Fruit

Root

How to use	*Combinations*	*Cautions*
Take an infusion or tincture.	Mix 45 ml skullcap tincture and 5 ml lemon balm and take up to four 5 ml doses a day as a calming nervine.	
Take an infusion or tincture.	Add sedative nervines such as lavender, vervain, St. John's wort and skullcap to the infusion or tincture.	Avoid high doses in pregnancy.
Use restricted to professional practitioners in UK, Australia, and New Zealand; maximum safe dose in UK is 5 drops 1:10 tincture in water up to 4 times. Maximum dose 5 ml per week.	Prescribed as a simple in acute phases, but can be prescribed in conjunction with drops of Jamaican dogwood tincture (up to 20 drops three times a day) and either lavender tea for "hot" migraines or rosemary for "cold" conditions.	Use only as prescribed; overdose can cause nausea and double vision.
Dilute 10 drops lavender oil in 25 ml carrier oil and massage into the temples at the first hint of symptoms; take an infusion of the flowers.	After the massage, drink an infusion of lavender flower and vervain (total of 30 g herb to 2 cups [500 ml] water) in wineglass doses.	Avoid high doses in pregnancy.
Eat one leaf a day as a prophylactic, or take 5-10 drops tincture every 30 minutes while symptoms persist.	Combine with other tranquilizers and analgesics, such as valerian or Jamaican dogwood tincture, taking up to 20 drops three times a day.	Avoid if taking warfarin; side effects of eating leaves can include mouth ulcers.
Gently rub a slice of fresh lemon or a little juice on the affected area, or use well-diluted lemon oil.	For symptomatic relief use as a simple.	Oil can irritate: use no more than 5 drops in 25 ml carrier oil.
Take an infusion; apply the infused oil externally to the affected area.	Add lavender and skullcap to the infusion as calming nervines.	Can cause dermatitis if skin is exposed to sunlight after taking internally.
Soak a pad in a decoction for a compress; use ointment; take infusion or 5 ml tincture.	Add lavender or St. John's wort to tincture or infusion, or up to 20 drops Jamaican dogwood tincture.	Avoid therapeutic doses in pregnancy.

STANDARD REMEDIES
All recipes and doses are standard unless otherwise specified; see *Making Herbal Remedies, pp. 152-57.*

INFECTIONS

MODERN SCIENCE attributes infections to bacteria and viruses. Previous generations blamed flying venom, "elf-shot" or the evil eye, while Chinese medicine attributes chills and fevers to "six evils" related to climatic factors – wind, cold, heat, dampness, dryness, and fire – and blames "pestilence" for severe epidemics. Many herbs traditionally used to fight infections have been identified as potent antibiotics and immune system stimulants. Unlike wide-spectrum conventional antibiotics, they are specific in the microbes they attack,

so have less impact on the friendly bacteria in the gut, making the digestive upsets that can follow conventional medication less likely. Herbs can help to control the course of an illness as the body works to restore balance. Common colds, for example, may be "hot" or "cold" in character, or alternate between the two as the illness progresses. "Cold" conditions need warming herbs such as ginger, *gui zhi* or angelica; "hot" infections can be cooled with herbs that promote sweating, such as boneset, catmint, peppermint or mulberry leaf.

See also: catarrh, pp. 170-71; coughs, pp. 170-71; fungal infections, pp. 180-81; candidiasis, pp. 192-93.

AILMENT	REMEDIES	
	Herb	*Actions*
COLDS & INFLUENZA Generally considered to be due to viral or bacterial infections, colds and influenza are often associated with stress, fatigue, depression, and excess cold or heat. **KEY SYMPTOMS** • Fever • Muscle pain and/or headache • Nasal catarrh or stuffiness • Cough • Sore throat.	*Allium sativum* GARLIC (see p. 33) *(Bulb)*	Antimicrobial; antifungal; suitable for a wide range of infectious conditions.
	Cinnamomum cassia GUI ZHI (see p. 52)	Warms "cold" conditions; promotes sweating; antibacterial.
	Eupatorium perfoliatum BONESET (see p. 228)	Promotes sweating; reduces fever; expectorant; good for hot feverish colds and influenza with muscle pain.
	Nepeta cataria CATMINT (see pp. 228)	Cools fevers, promotes sweating; astringent in catarrhal congestion.
BOILS & ABSCESSES Localized infections often due to bacteria entering a hair follicle or wound. May indicate a weakened immune system. **KEY SYMPTOMS** • Tender, inflamed area of skin • Obvious pus in boils • Pain.	*Forsythia suspensa* LIAN QIAO (see p. 229)	Antibacterial, anti-inflammatory; reduces heat; resolves abscesses and boils; cools fevers.
	Scrophularia spp. FIGWORT AND XUAN SHEN (see p. 117)	Anti-inflammatory, antibacterial; cleansing for toxic conditions.
WEAK IMMUNE SYSTEM Associated with exhaustion, food allergy, or depression, this leaves the body vulnerable to infection. It could signify a more serious underlying disorder. **KEY SYMPTOMS** • Persistent colds or influenza • Frequent skin infections • Chronic fatigue.	*Astragalus membranaceus* HUANG QI (see p. 224-5) *(Rhizome)*	Increases production of white blood cells and strengthens the immune response; anti bacterial; energy tonic; strengthens *wei qi*, or defence energy.
	Echinacea spp. ECHINACEA (see p. 58)	Antibacterial, antiviral; strengthens resistance to infections; useful for all septic or infectious conditions.

CASE HISTORY
Exhaustion leading to a weak immune system

PATIENT: Lucy, aged 35, the mother of an active three year old, busily at work renovating an old farmhouse with her husband.

HISTORY AND COMPLAINT: For the past four years, Lucy had suffered constant colds and miscellaneous viruses. Problems started during pregnancy, as Lucy used up her energies coping with a high-powered job in publishing and making the transition to full-time mother. Although her diet was good and she regularly exercised, repeated infections left her exhausted, lethargic, and feeling down. For two years, her doctor prescribed antidepressants as well as continual courses of antibiotics. The colds had increased since her daughter had started preschool.

TREATMENT: Herbal remedies focused on immune stimulants and uplifting tonic herbs: *ling zhi, huang qi,* vervain, lemon balm, and echinacea, with echinacea capsules as an extra boost when cold symptoms began. Supplements of *Lactobacillus acidophilus* and other friendly bacteria helped the digestive system recover from excessive antibiotics. Cold symptoms were treated with elderflower, yarrow, and peppermint tea, sage gargles, and white horehound, thyme, and liquorice cough syrups.

OUTCOME: After four months the recurrent colds had disappeared and Lucy began to feel more energetic and enthusiastic about life. After discussion with her doctor the antidepressants were gradually stopped.

KEY

Aerial parts

Fruit

Leaves

Root

Twigs

How to use	Combinations	Cautions
Eat up to six fresh cloves a day in acute conditions, or take proprietary capsules.	Best as a simple; limit the odor by eating parsley.	If it irritates the stomach, take ginger or fennel tea. Avoid therapeutic doses during pregnancy and lactation.
Take a decoction or tincture; use bark (*rou gui*) if *gui zhi* is unavailable.	For chills, mix with a little fresh ginger root.	Avoid in pregnancy. Not suitable for "hot" feverish colds.
Take an infusion or tincture three to four times a day.	For feverish colds and influenza, combine with yarrow, elderflower, and peppermint.	High doses can cause vomiting.
Take an infusion or tincture three to four times a day.	For feverish colds, mix with yarrow, elderflower, boneset, ground ivy, angelica, or mulberry leaf to enhance specific actions.	
Take a decoction.	Combine with cooling herbs such as *jin yin hua,* burdock seeds or *huang qin,* or antibacterials such as echinacea in capsules.	Use before boils start to discharge pus. Avoid in diarrhea.
Make a poultice from figwort leaves; take a decoction of xuan shen or a tincture.	Add cooling herbs such as *lian qiao, jin yin hua,* goldenseal or *huang qin* to the decoction, and take antibacterials like echinacea in capsules.	Heart stimulant, so avoid in heartbeat abnormalities (tachycardia).
Take a decoction or tincture.	For debilitated conditions, add other energy tonics such as licorice, *dang gui* and *bai zhu.*	Avoid if condition involves excess "heat" or *yin* deficiency.
Take 500 mg powdered root in capsules or 10 ml tincture. Repeat up to four times a day.	Use as a simple, or add anticatarrhal remedies such as elderflower and catmint, or fever herbs such as yarrow or boneset, depending on symptoms.	High doses can occasionally cause nausea and dizziness.

STANDARD REMEDIES All recipes and doses are standard unless otherwise specified; see *Making Herbal Remedies, pp. 152-57.*

RESPIRATORY PROBLEMS

A HOLISTIC APPROACH to health is particularly relevant to respiratory problems. To blame chest complaints on infection, industrial pollution or an ailing heart is to address only part of the problem: emotional and spiritual factors must be considered as well. In Chinese medicine, the lungs are associated with grief, and it is notable that chest problems often follow a bereavement or other sorrow, and that chest infections tend to strike when we feel down – perhaps when in a job we dislike or if we are unhappy at home. Herbs cannot always solve underlying problems, but strengthening lung tonics like elecampane or cowslip, which also act on the nervous system, can help. Breathing and breath have much greater significance in Eastern systems of medicine than they do in the mechanistic Western model. In Ayurvedic medicine, for example, breathing is regarded as the life force, and breath control is an important Yogic art. In Chinese medicine too, the breath is equated with *qi* (vital energy) and controls its flow: respiratory problems are seen not only as damaging to the vital energy, but also as signifying *qi* weakness or imbalance. The wide range of herbal respiratory remedies can relieve symptoms and restore inner balance to tackle the underlying cause of the condition.

See also: sore throat, pp. 176-77, tonsillitis, pp. 176-77; hay fever, pp. 192-93.

AILMENT	REMEDIES	
	Herb	*Actions*
COUGHS A cough is a muscle spasm that occurs as a reaction to irritation or blockage in the bronchial tubes (the tubes from the throat to the lungs). Coughs often occur in conjunction with infections such as colds or influenza, but are sometimes associated with nervous tension and have no pathological cause. **KEY SYMPTOMS** • Productive cough may produce mucus varying from a thin, watery discharge to thick yellow or green phlegm • Unproductive cough can be very dry and irritating. *IMPORTANT: Seek professional help for a persistent cough of unknown cause.*	*Althaea officinalis* **MARSHMALLOW** (see p. 36)	Demulcent and expectorant; soothes inflamed respiratory mucous membranes.
	Hyssopus officinalis **HYSSOP** (see p. 76)	Warming, expectorant, anti-spasmodic; useful for thin, watery phlegm and coughs associated with bronchitis.
	Morus alba **SANG BAI PI** (see p. 92)	Cooling expectorant, antitussive; good for "hot" conditions.
	Phyllostachys nigra **ZHU RU/ VAMSHA ROCHANA** (see p. 100) *(Resin)*	Antimicrobial, cooling and expectorant to clear the thick, infected yellow phlegm or productive coughs.
	Prunus serotina **WILD CHERRY** (see p. 107)	Cough suppressant; useful for dry, irritant or nervous coughs.
CATARRH Excessive secretions from the membranes in the respiratory system, catarrh can be "cold", with copious watery secretions, or "hot", with thick, yellow secretions. "Cold" catarrh is often linked with eating too much sweet food and a sluggish system. "Hot" catarrh can be linked to a nervous personality, and may be persistent. **KEY SYMPTOMS** • Runny nose following a cold • Irritant cough • Inflamed nasal membranes • Sinus pain in "hot" type.	*Gnaphthalium uliginosum* **MARSH CUDWEED** (see p. 229)	Anti-inflammatory; tones up the respiratory system.
	Sambucus nigra **ELDER** (see p. 116)	Anticatarrhal, anti-inflammatory and expectorant; useful for upper respiratory tract catarrh linked to colds and hay fever.
	Solidago virgaurea **GOLDEN ROD** (see p. 228)	Drying, astringent, anti-catarrhal; anti-inflammatory for the mucous membranes.
	Verbascum thapsus **MULLEIN** (see p. 134)	Cooling, astringent and soothing for thick or "hot" catarrh and nasal congestion.

CASE HISTORY
Persistent cough

PATIENT: John, 52, was an export manager with an engineering company whose work involved regular overseas travel. He was married with two teenage sons.

HISTORY AND COMPLAINT: John suffered from a dry, irritating cough for at least seven years. It started after a severe cold, which had trailed off into a persistent cough. His symptoms were worse at night and kept him and his wife awake. Countless hospital tests all proved negative, and the doctor's latest theory blamed the problem on stomach acid, for which he prescribed an acid reducing drug. However, three months of this treatment failed to bring about any improvement, and John's wife persuaded him to try alternative medicine.

TREATMENT: Neither hospital tests nor medical history suggested a problem with stomach acid, but John did tend to feel hot and thirsty. Remedies included a combination of moistening herbs, such as ribwort plantain, *sang bai pi*, and white horehound, with wild cherry to suppress the cough, and elecampane as a lung tonic. Wild lettuce was added to the mixture for use at night as a stronger cough suppressant.

OUTCOME: Within three weeks, the coughing bouts, which had been a nightly interruption, occurred only once or twice a week. The wild cherry was dropped from the medicine as the other herbs strengthened and restored the lungs. After two more months, John's cough finally cleared.

How to use	*Combinations*	*Cautions*
Take an infusion or tincture, or take 5 ml syrup made from leaves or flowers.	Can be combined with anticatarrhals like ground ivy, or additional expectorants such as mulberry bark or white horehound.	
Take an infusion or tincture, or mix 5 ml essential oil in 20 ml carrier oil for a chest rub.	Combines well with restoratives like elecampane and white horehound in chronic conditions: use 2 parts hyssop to 1 part other herb.	
Take a decoction or tincture.	Combine with soothing and cooling herbs like marshmallow leaf or ribwort plantain, or with thyme if there is an infection.	
Use 1 tsp shavings per dose in decoctions; 250 mg in capsules of powder or up to 50 drops tincture; use 5 ml fresh sap diluted in water.	Add an equal amount of ginger juice to the sap; add cinnamon, cardamom, or black pepper to powdered shavings with an equal amount of sugar or honey and take in 1 tsp doses. Mix *zhu ru* with elecampane and ginger in decoctions.	Avoid in coughs and diarrhea associated with cold.
Take an infusion, or a tincture in 2 ml doses.	Combine with astringents like mullein, tonics such as elecampane or additional cough suppressants like wild lettuce in severe cases.	Can cause drowsiness; avoid in acute infections.
Take an infusion or tincture.	Can be combined with anticatarrhals such as elderflower or golden rod, using 2 parts marsh cudweed to 1 part other herbs.	
Take an infusion or tincture.	Can be combined with other drying or astringent herbs, such as yarrow, ground ivy, golden rod, agrimony, or bistort to enhance action. Use 3 parts elderflower to 1 part other herbs.	
Take an infusion or tincture.	Can be combined with other anticatarrhals such as marsh cudweed or demulcents like ribwort plantain.	
Take an infusion or tincture.	Combines well with anticatarrhals such as coltsfoot and elderflowers in infusions; add antimicrobials such as thyme or mulberry leaf for infections.	

KEY

Aerial parts

Bark

Essential oil

Flowers

Leaves

Root

Root bark

Stem

STANDARD REMEDIES
All recipes and doses are standard unless otherwise specified; see *Making Herbal Remedies, pp. 152-57.*

AILMENT	REMEDIES	
	Herb	*Actions*
SINUSITIS This is inflammation or infection of the sinus cavities in the skull. It often follows a cold but may be associated with dental problems, such as a deep-seated root abscess. **KEY SYMPTOMS** • Pain affecting sinus areas • Headaches, which may be severe • Sinuses tender to the touch • Nasal discharge, often streaked with blood.	*Glechoma hederacea* GROUND IVY (see pp. 228)	Anticatarrhal and astringent; suitably drying for catarrh in the sinuses and bronchi.
	Hydrastis canadensis GOLDENSEAL (see p. 74) *(Rhizome)*	Powerful, cooling, astringent and anticatarrhal.
	Myrica cerifera BAYBERRY (see pp. 228)	Warming and astringent; stimulates the circulatory system.
	Piper longum PIPPALI or LONG PEPPER (see p. 102)	Warming anticatarrhal; useful for sinus headaches and allergic rhinitis.
BRONCHITIS Bronchitis is inflammation of the bronchi, which may be due to infection. Chronic conditions are often exacerbated by common colds or associated with smoking and pollution. *NOTE: All herbs listed for bronchitis are also suitable for asthmatic conditions.* **KEY SYMPTOMS** • Productive cough, often pus-containing phlegm • Elevated temperature • Chest pains and breathlessness if the condition is chronic.	*Inula helenium* ELECAMPANE (see p. 77)	Lung tonic and expectorant; restorative and warming; good for weakened lungs and stubborn coughs.
	Marrubium vulgare WHITE HOREHOUND (see pp. 229)	Antispasmodic, demulcent, and expectorant; relaxes the bronchi and eases congestion.
	Primula veris COWSLIP (see p. 105)	Potent expectorant, good for loosening old phlegm and easing stubborn, dry coughs.
	Thymus vulgaris THYME (see p. 127)	Antiseptic and expectorant; useful for thick, infected phlegm and dry, difficult coughs.
ASTHMA Asthma is a spasm of the bronchi (bronchospasm) leading to wheezing and breathlessness. It may be associated with other allergic symptoms such as hay fever or eczema, and can run in families. Chinese medicine often associates asthma with weak kidney energy and a failure of correct *qi* circulation. Kidney tonics such as *gui zhi* could be appropriate in treatment. *NOTE: All herbs listed for bronchitis are also suitable for asthmatic conditions.* **KEY SYMPTOMS** • Wheezing on breathing out • Great difficulty in breathing. *IMPORTANT: Severe asthma can be life-threatening and require professional medical help. Chronic asthmatics should seek professional medical advice before interrupting conventional treatment.*	*Ephedra sinica* MA HUANG (see p. 59)	Bronchial relaxant; relaxes blood vessels; warming for all "cold" conditions of the chest.
	Eucalyptus globulus EUCALYPTUS (see p. 61)	Antiseptic, antispasmodic, and expectorant.
	Grindelia camporum GUMPLANT (see pp. 228)	Antispasmodic and expectorant; eases bronchospasm.
	Matricaria recutita GERMAN CHAMOMILE (see p. 88)	Antiallergenic, anti-inflammatory, and antispasmodic; useful for allergic asthma.

How to use	*Combinations*	*Cautions*
Take an infusion or tincture.	Can be used with other anticatarrhals like elderflower or ribwort plantain. Use 2 parts ground ivy to 1 part additional herbs.	
Take one or two 200 mg capsules of powder or 1 ml tincture three times a day.	Add eyebright powder to capsules.	Avoid in pregnancy or high blood pressure.
Use powder as a snuff, or add 5 ml tincture to 20 ml emulsifying ointment and use as a sinus massage.	Add 2-3 drops eucalyptus oil to ointment as an antiseptic and antispasmodic.	Avoid in very "hot" conditions.
Take in milk infusion or as capsules (1-2 200 mg capsules of powder per dose), or up to 40 drops tincture per dose.	Generally used as a simple with milk, but support with antibacterials such as thyme, *lian qiao* or echinacea in tinctures or capsules where there is infection.	
Take a decoction, tincture or syrup.	Use as a simple, or add 10 ml horsetail juice to heal lung damage; other restorative lung herbs that can be added include hyssop or white horehound.	
Take an infusion, tincture or syrup; suck horehound candy (available commercially).	Can be combined with tonics like elecampane or hyssop, or warming expectorants like angelica. Use 2 parts white horehound to 1 part additional herbs.	
Take a decoction, tincture or syrup.	Can be combined with strong expectorants like gumplant and soothing demulcents such as ribwort plantain or liquorice. Use 2 parts cowslip to 1 part additional herbs.	Do not take high doses in pregnancy. Avoid if taking warfarin.
Take an infusion, tincture or syrup; for a chest rub, mix 10 drops essential oil in 20 ml almond oil.	Can add additional expectorants such as mulberry bark or healing herbs like horsetail for damaged lungs; the chest rub can be enhanced with 5 drops hyssop or peppermint essential oil.	Avoid therapeutic doses in pregnancy.
In UK, Australia and New Zealand use is restricted to professional practitioners. Maximum permitted dose in UK is 2.5 ml of 1:4 tincture three times a day.	Can be prescribed in combination with infusions of white horehound or hyssop; pill-bearing spurge and gumplant are often added as additional antispasmodics.	Take only as prescribed. Avoid in hypertension, glaucoma or if taking MAO inhibitors.
Mix 1-2 ml oil in 25 ml carrier oil for a chest rub; place a few drops on a pillow or handkerchief as an inhalant.	Add a total of 10-15 drops thyme, peppermint, lemon balm or fennel essential oils to increase antiseptic and expectorant actions.	Do not take with low blood pressure, since it reduces blood pressure. High doses can irritate kidneys.
Immerse 15 g in 2 cups (500 ml) water for an infusion and take up to 5 ml a day in doses of 1-2 ml.	Can be combined with additional antispasmodics such as pill-bearing spurge (up to 1 ml per dose of tincture), or with other expectorants and lung tonics like cowslip or elecampane.	
Add the essential oil to a chest rub or steam inhalant; immerse 1 tbsp flowers in a bowl of boiling water for a steam inhalant at the first sign of an attack.	Support with internal medication as for bronchitis, above.	Do not exceed stated dose. Do not use essential oil in pregnancy.

KEY

 Aerial parts

 Bark

 Essential oil

 Flowers

 Fruit

 Leaves

 Root

 Twigs

STANDARD REMEDIES
All recipes and doses are standard unless otherwise specified; see *Making Herbal Remedies*, pp. 152-57.

EARS, EYES, MOUTH & THROAT

ALTHOUGH MUCH OF MODERN medical practice tends to isolate sight, hearing and speech from the rest of the body, the health of the eyes, ears and mouth reflects the state of the whole body. It is now recognized that persistent problems in these organs often relate to other systemic disorders: "glue ear" in children is connected with milk allergies, and recurrent cold sores are linked to fatigue, stress and a rundown immune system. In Chinese medicine, eye problems are related to liver imbalance; hearing difficulties and tinnitus can imply kidney weakness; and persistent mouth problems or sore lips may indicate excess "heat" in the spleen. Herbal remedies are ideal for these ailments, offering symptomatic relief as well as tackling the underlying cause. In some instances, changes in diet or lifestyle are a crucial feature of the cure. Tired, strained eyes, for example, can be soothed by eyebaths of rosewater or a weak infusion of eyebright, pot marigold, cornflowers, or strawberry leaves, but better lighting levels and frequent breaks from VDU screens may be the only real solution.

See also: infections, pp. 168-69; candidiasis, pp. 192-93.

AILMENT	REMEDIES	
	Herb	*Actions*
EARACHE This can be associated with catarrhal conditions or infection. **KEY SYMPTOMS** • Pain, often severe, in one or both ears • Blocked sensation in the ears • Buzzing or ringing sounds • Excessive waxy discharge • Fever • Vertigo or nausea if the inner ear is affected. *IMPORTANT: Severe infections can lead to deafness, so seek professional medical help if symptoms persist.*	*Hydrastis canadensis* GOLDENSEAL (see p. 74)	Powerful, cooling astringent with an anticatarrhal action.
	Plantago lanceolata RIBWORT PLANTAIN (see p. 104)	Tonifies mucous membranes and controls catarrh; useful for catarrhal conditions of the middle ear.
	Pulsatilla vulgaris PASQUE FLOWER (see pp. 226-27)	Sedative, analgesic; acts directionally on ears.
	Verbascum thapsus MULLEIN (see p. 134)	Demulcent and mildly sedative wound herb.
CONJUNCTIVITIS & BLEPHARITIS Conjunctivitis is an inflammation of the membrane that covers the eyeball (the conjunctiva). In blepharitis, the edges of the eyelid become inflamed. Both can be caused by infection, allergy, or physical or chemical irritation. **KEY SYMPTOMS:** CONJUNCTIVITIS • "Gritty" feeling in the eye • Increased sensitivity to light • Pain, soreness or swelling • Red or pink eye • Discharge that may be watery or contain pus. **KEY SYMPTOM:** BLEPHARITIS • Red, scaly eyelids.	*Agrimonia eupatoria* AGRIMONY (see p. 31)	Astringent and healing for mucous membranes; liver tonic that may help the eyes.
	Calendula officinalis POT MARIGOLD (see p. 47)	Anti-inflammatory, astringent wound herb, antiseptic; helpful for local irritation.
	Dendranthema x *grandiflorum* JU HUA (see p. 56)	Antibacterial, anti-inflammatory and liver herb; good for persistent eye problems.
	Euphrasia officinalis EYEBRIGHT (see p. 228)	Astringent, anticatarrhal and anti-inflammatory.

CASE HISTORY
Excess catarrh causing deafness

PATIENT: Robert, an active 12 year old, had become withdrawn and was falling behind at school.

HISTORY AND COMPLAINT: Robert had suffered from constant catarrh since babyhood. His ears were always blocked and prone to infection; as a toddler he suffered from persistent "glue ear"; he had gone through three tympanostomies and was now into his third year of T-tubes. His hearing was getting worse, making school work and normal playground conversation difficult and he complained of a constant buzzing in his ears. Whenever he went swimming, earache and infection were sure to follow. His diet was fairly typical of a 12 year old – too few green vegetables and more than 2½ cups of milk a day.

TREATMENT: Herbal medicine included golden rod, echinacea and pasque flower in tincture form, with goldenseal capsules. For a trial month, Robert's mother replaced all milk and milk products in his diet with soy milk, and included more green vegetables and fish to boost mineral and vitamin intake.

OUTCOME: After only two weeks of herbs and a milk-free diet, Robert's hearing had improved. After three months, he had been free of ear infections and catarrh for six weeks, and could swim without getting an ear infection. The herbs were phased out and three months later, after a hospital check-up, the T-tubes were removed. He is happy with a low milk diet, and the occasional ice cream causes few problems.

KEY

How to use	Combinations	Cautions
Take two 200 mg capsules or 20 drops tincture three times a day; as eardrops, use 10 ml tincture in ½ cup (100 ml) water (see mullein caution).	Add eyebright powder to capsules as an additional anticatarrhal.	Avoid in pregnancy or high blood pressure; do not exceed the stated dose.
Take an infusion or tincture.	Combine tincture with elderflower tincture as an anticatarrhal, or 10 drops pasque flower tincture to focus action on the ears.	
Take 1-2 ml tincture three times a day.	Combine with anticatarrhals like goldenseal or eyebright. Use 10 drops goldenseal or up to 5 ml eyebright tinctures per dose.	
Use cold infused oil as eardrops.	Support with antibiotic herbs such as echinacea in capsules, and anticatarrhals such as elderflower infusion or goldenseal capsules.	Do not use eardrops if there is a risk that the ear drum is perforated.
Bathe the eyes in an eyewash of weak, well-strained infusion (10 g herb to 2 cups (500 ml) water).	If there is any infection, support with antibacterials such as echinacea taken internally.	
Soak a pad in a well-diluted tincture and apply to the eyes as a compress; bathe styes with 5 ml tincture in 50 ml water.	Use as a simple.	
Take an infusion or tincture.	Combine with anticatarrhals like eyebright or elderflower, or liver herbs like agrimony or self-heal.	
Soak a pad in an infusion and apply to the eyes as a compress, or bathe the eyes in an eyewash of water with 5-10 drops tincture.	If there is any infection, support with antibacterials such as echinacea taken internally.	

Aerial parts

Flowers

Leaves

Petals

Rhizome

STANDARD REMEDIES
All recipes and doses are standard unless otherwise specified; see *Making Herbal Remedies*, pp. 152-57.

AILMENT	REMEDIES	
	Herb	*Actions*
MOUTH ULCERS Painful ulcers in the mouth are often related to fungal or bacterial infection. They may be associated with excessive consumption of sugar or other foods that encourage fungal proliferation. Split or cracked lips occurring with the ulcers may indicate a vitamin deficiency. **KEY SYMPTOM** • Painful, white, raised patches, which may be very persistent.	*Commiphora molmol* MYRRH (see p. 54) *(Resin)*	Antimicrobial, astringent herb that heals wounds.
	Polygonum bistorta BISTORT (see p. 228)	Astringent, demulcent, and anti-inflammatory; also suitable for other mouth inflammations.
	Salvia officinalis Purpurescens group or *Salvia officinalis* PURPLE or GREEN SAGE (see p. 115)	Antiseptic and astringent. Also suitable for gingivitis and gum disorders.
COLD SORES Cold sores are small blisters on the face, usually around the lips. Once you are infected with the *Herpes simplex* virus, cold sores tend to recur when the immune system is weakened by infection, stress or fatigue. **KEY SYMPTOM** • Area that is painful or has a tingling sensation.	*Lavandula spp.* LAVENDER (see p. 81)	Topically antiseptic.
	Melaleuca alternifolia TEA TREE (see p. 89)	Antibiotic; stimulates the immune system.
SORE THROAT This common symptom may be associated with infection or chemical irritants. It may accompany tonsillitis, pharyngitis or laryngitis. **KEY SYMPTOMS** • Pain at the back of the mouth • Difficulty swallowing • Red, raw throat • Hoarse or croaking voice • Related fever or cold may be present or starting.	*Agrimonia eupatoria* AGRIMONY (see p. 31)	Astringent and healing for the mucous membranes.
	Alchemilla vulgaris LADY'S MANTLE (see p. 32)	Astringent; reduces inflammation; helpful for laryngitis.
	Echinacea spp. ECHINACEA (see p. 58)	Antibacterial, astringent; useful for all throat problems including tonsillitis.
	Terminalia belerica BIBHITAKI (see p. 126)	Astringent, antiseptic, and cooling; closely associated in Ayurvedic tradition with both the throat and voice.
TONSILLITIS Inflammation of the tonsils is usually associated with a bacterial or viral infection. **KEY SYMPTOMS** • Very sore throat • Difficulty swallowing • Fever • Red, enlarged tonsils, which may discharge pus. *IMPORTANT: An abscess on the tonsils (quinsy) needs professional medical attention.*	*Baptisia tinctoria* WILD INDIGO (see pp. 229)	Antimicrobial, anticatarrhal; cleanses the lymphatic system; good for persistent infections.
	Galium aparine CLEAVERS (see p. 67)	Alterative; cleanses the lymphatic system; good for all lymphatic problems including mononucleosis and adenoids.
	Gnaphthalium uliginosum MARSH CUDWEED (see pp. 229)	Anti-inflammatory; tonifies the mucous membranes; also good for laryngitis, pharyngitis and quinsy.
	Phytolacca americana POKEROOT (see p. 101)	Anticatarrhal; cleanses the lymphatic system; reduces lymphatic swellings.

How to use	*Combinations*	*Cautions*
Add 5-10 drops oil or 5 ml tincture to a glass of warm water and use as a mouthwash.	Add 5 ml sage or rosemary tincture to a mouthwash, or chew bilberries after using the mouthwash to help disguise the flavor.	Avoid in pregnancy.
For a mouthwash, use a decoction or add 5 ml tincture to a glass of water.	Add healing antibacterials like self-heal, rosemary, bilberry, or wild indigo to the mouthwash. For persistent problems, take echinacea or garlic internally.	
For a mouthwash, use a standard infusion or add 10 ml tincture to a glass of water.	Add rosemary tincture to a mouthwash, or echinacea to enhance the antibacterial action.	Avoid therapeutic doses in pregnancy.
Mix 10 drops oil in 25 ml carrier oil, and dab on to the affected area.	Use as a simple; if the sore heralds a cold, take echinacea or garlic internally.	
Mix essential oil with 10 times its volume of carrier oil, and dab on to the affected area as soon as a developing cold sore starts to tingle.	Use as a simple. If sores recur frequently, take *huang qi* to boost the immune system or take patent Siberian ginseng pills to increase stress tolerance.	
Gargle with an infusion or with 10 ml tincture diluted in a glass of warm water.	Use as a simple or add purple sage, witch hazel or rosemary tincture to the gargle.	
Gargle with an infusion or with 10 ml tincture diluted in a glass of warm water.	Add 5 ml rosemary or purple sage or up to 5 drops of cayenne tincture to the gargle for laryngitis.	Avoid in pregnancy.
Gargle with 10 ml tincture diluted in a glass of warm water, and swallow the gargle.	Use as a simple.	High doses can cause nausea and dizziness.
Take 1 tsp powder in honey for sore throats and vocal problems; use the infusion or juice as a gargle.	Use as a simple or add antimicrobials such as 5 ml echinacea infusion to the gargle to combat infection.	Avoid in pregnancy and severe exhaustion.
Take 10-20 drops tincture three times a day.	Can be combined with other antibacterials such as echinacea, dried pokeroot, or thyme, up to 5 ml tincture.	Do not exceed the stated dose; high doses may cause vomiting.
Take an infusion, or drink 10 ml fresh juice, three times a day.	Can combine with antibacterials like goldenseal (5-10 drops), echinacea (up to 10 ml) or dried pokeroot (10-20 drops) added to the juice in tincture form; support with gargles, as for sore throat (see above).	
Take an infusion or tincture and use as a gargle.	Combine with cleavers or echinacea tinctures as additional antibacterials and lymphatic cleansers.	
Take 10-20 drops tincture made from dried, not fresh, root three times a day (Fresh root is toxic.)	Can be combined with lymphatic cleansers like cleavers or cooling antibacterials like goldenseal, up to 5 ml tincture.	Do not exceed the stated dose; avoid in pregnancy.

KEY

Aerial parts

Essential oil

Fruit

Leaves

Root

Stem

Whole herb

STANDARD REMEDIES
All recipes and doses are standard unless otherwise specified; see *Making Herbal Remedies*, pp. 152-57.

SKIN & HAIR

A HERBAL APPROACH to skin problems focuses on restoring internal balance, often using cleansing or cooling herbs rather than creams that may alleviate symptoms but do little to treat the cause of the problem. The same emphasis on rebalancing is found in Ayurvedic medicine: too much *pitta* (fire) causes the blood to overheat and poison the skin, too much *vata* (wind) causes dryness and itching, while excess *kapha* (damp) leads to weeping or oozing sores. Treatment is with cooling, moistening or drying herbs and an appropriate diet. The Chinese approach associates the skin with the lungs, *wei qi* (defence energy) and body fluids. Treatments based on this philosophy have been used for childhood eczema at a London hospital. Dry, flaky eczema, which is difficult to treat using modern Western medicine, has been helped by cooling Chinese herbs that increase body fluids. Trials at the hospital have produced impressive results. Fungal or parasitic skin conditions and hair problems can signify immune or energy weakness, and may be treated with tonic herbs and immunostimulants.

See also: candidiasis, pp. 192-93; vaginal thrush, pp. 204-05; nits, pp. 218-19.

AILMENT	REMEDIES	
	Herb	*Actions*
ECZEMA Skin inflammation, which may be associated with allergies, nervous stress, or chemical or metal irritants. It can be highly localized if an irritant such as a metal watch strap is involved, but allergic eczema can affect all parts of the body. Creases of skin such as the folds inside the elbows or under the breasts are often affected. **KEY SYMPTOMS** • Red, inflamed patches • Itchiness • Oozing serum from raw patches • Crusts of serum form • Lesions may bleed in acute conditions.	*Arctium lappa* **BURDOCK** (see p. 40)	Cleansing, diuretic and laxative; good for any toxic skin condition, especially scaling eczema.
	Oenothera biennis **EVENING PRIMROSE** (see pp. 228) *(Seed oil)*	The seed oil contains essential fatty acids needed to maintain healthy tissues.
	Paeonia lactiflora **CHI SHAO YAO** (see p. 97)	Cools and stimulates blood flow; useful for "hot" conditions.
	Stellaria media **CHICKWEED** (see p. 122)	Soothing and slightly astringent; heals wounds, eases irritation and helps to heal lesions.
	Urtica dioica **STINGING NETTLE** (see p. 131)	Astringent, tonic, and circulatory stimulant; useful if eczema is associated with poor circulation.
ACNE Inflammation of the sebaceous glands in the skin, which may start with blackheads. It is especially common among teenagers. **KEY SYMPTOMS** • Inflamed pustules • Excessively oily skin • Infected cysts and scarring in severe cases.	*Allium sativum* **GARLIC** (see p. 33) *(Bulb)*	Antibacterial and antifungal; good antiseptic action for infected skin conditions.
	Brassica oleracea **CABBAGE** (see p. 46)	Antibacterial and anti-inflammatory; nutritive and healing.
	Melaleuca alternifolia **TEA TREE** (see p. 89)	Potent antibacterial for infected skin conditions.
PLANTAR WARTS & OTHER WARTS Small, hard growths in the outer layer of skin, due to a virus. They can be spread by contact and may be persistent. **KEY SYMPTOM** • Obvious growth on the skin.	*Chelidonium majus* **GREATER CELANDINE** (see pp. 228) *(Resin)*	Potent antiviral to destroy warts.
	Thuja occidentalis **ARBOR VITAE** (see pp. 228) *(Leaf tips)*	Volatile oil contains thujone, which is antiseptic and effective for many topical fungal and viral infections.

<u>CASE HISTORY</u>
Teenage acne

PATIENT: Edward, 17, a typical teenager.

HISTORY AND COMPLAINT: Edward had acne with pustules around his nose and cheeks. The problem started 18 months previously and he had also suffered from heavy catarrh and recurrent colds for the better part of a year. His diet was far from perfect, with an excess of chocolate, potato chips, and soda. He had a very sweet tooth, which his mother translated as at least two chocolate bars a day and as many cookies as he could find when he got home from school.

TREATMENT: Edward did not relish the prospect of rubbing his face with garlic each evening or washing in cabbage water, so tea tree oil in rosewater was used

as a lotion instead. Internal herbal remedies focused on clearing dampness and heat from the system, and improving immunity. Pimples around the nose suggested excess lung heat, so *huang qin* and *sang bai pi* were included with *chi shao yao*, heartsease, yellow dock, and echinacea. Edward also promised to try very hard to cut down on his consumption of chocolate.

OUTCOME: After six weeks, the acne was considerably reduced and the catarrh had disappeared. Then came exams. In between bouts of studying, Edward ate chocolate bars, and before long the pimples and catarrh were back. Fortunately, he realized his sweet tooth was a contributing factor, and after a further course of herbs he is managing to avoid excess chocolate.

How to use	*Combinations*	*Cautions*
Take a decoction or up to 4 ml tincture three times a day.	Can combine with other cleansing herbs such as yellow dock, figwort, cleavers, heartsease and red clover. Add flowers and leaves to a decoction for 1-2 minutes only.	
Take 3 g a day in capsule form (1-2 g a day for children).	Use as a simple.	
Best used in combinations; take a tincture or a decoction.	Combine with cooling, cleansing herbs such as *sheng di huang*, heartsease and *mu dan pi* to enhance the effect.	
Apply ointment or cream as required; add 1 tbsp infused oil to bath water.	Use as a simple.	
Take an infusion or tincture, or use externally in ointment or cream.	Use as a simple or add other cleansing herbs like heartsease, red clover, figwort or cleavers to the infusion or tincture.	
Rub the affected area with a cut clove.	Use as a simple. Add garlic to cooking. Limit the odor by eating parsley.	Because of the odor, apply at night.
Liquidize 250 g fresh leaves with 1 cup (250 ml) distilled witch hazel, strain, add 2 drops lemon oil and use as a lotion.	Use as a simple, but tinctures of cleavers, yellow dock and burdock can be taken as additional cleansers. Reduce sugar and acid foods in the diet.	
Add 1 ml tea tree oil to 10 ml water and use as a lotion.	Use as a simple, but cleavers, yellow dock, burdock or echinacea can be taken internally as additional cleansing or antibacterial herbs.	
Squeeze fresh sap from the stems directly on the warts; repeating at least twice a day will usually clear even long-standing warts in 2-3 weeks.	Use as a simple; dandelion stem sap can be used in a similar way.	Do not take internally, or use in pregnancy; do not put sap on surrounding skin.
Apply drops of tincture frequently to the wart or verruca; can also be made into an ointment.	Use as a simple or combine with an equal amount of tea tree oil and shake well.	Avoid in pregnancy.

KEY

Aerial parts

Essential oil

Leaves

Root

Stem

STANDARD REMEDIES
All recipes and doses are standard unless otherwise specified; see *Making Herbal Remedies, pp. 152-57.*

AILMENT	REMEDIES	
	Herb	*Actions*
PSORIASIS This is due to overproduction of skin keratinocytes, which fail to mature into normal keratin. It can be associated with immune dysfunction, and may follow streptococcal infection or skin injury. It can be linked to a tense, isolated personality, affected by stress and worry. A tendency for psoriasis often runs in families. KEY SYMPTOMS • Patches of red skin, often with silver colored scales • Cycle of remission and recurrence.	*Galium aparine* CLEAVERS (see p. 67)	Cleansing, diuretic and astringent; useful for many types of skin problem.
	Iris versicolor BLUE FLAG (see pp. 228) *(Rhizome)*	Anti-inflammatory and cleansing for both the circulatory and lymphatic systems; a favorite with physiomedicalists and stimulating for the liver.
	Rumex crispus YELLOW DOCK (see pp. 229)	Cleansing, diuretic and laxative; stimulates bile flow and clears toxins.
	Scrophularia nodosa FIGWORT (see p. 117)	Anti-inflammatory, cleansing and circulatory stimulant; good for many chronic skin conditions.
	Trifolium pratense RED CLOVER (see p. 128)	Cleansing and diuretic; useful for many skin problems including eczema.
FUNGAL INFECTIONS Ringworm, athlete's foot and other skin infections are caused by fungi such as *microsporum*, *trichophyton* and *epidermophyton*. The toes and the scalp are the most commonly affected areas. KEY SYMPTOMS • Red, very irritant patches • Scaly or peeling skin.	*Aloe vera* ALOE (see p. 34) *(Resin)*	Demulcent, cooling for irritated skin, antiparasitic; useful for scabies.
	Calendula officinalis POT MARIGOLD (see p. 47)	Antifungal and astringent; heals wounds; soothing for dry or inflamed skin.
	Commiphora molmol MYRRH (see p. 54) *(Resin)*	Antifungal, immune stimulant, astringent.
HAIR LOSS (ALOPECIA) May be total or patchy; in men, often hereditary. Mild loss can be due to vitamin deficiency. KEY SYMPTOM • Bald patches or loose hairs.	*Arnica montana* ARNICA (see pp. 228)	Stimulates blood circulation.
	Artemisia abrotanum SOUTHERNWOOD (see pp. 229)	Traditional remedy to stimulate hair growth, although there is no scientific basis for its reputation.
PREMATURE GRAYING Can be hereditary, or may be linked to stress or premature menopause. KEY SYMPTOM • Hair starts to lose its color in the 20s or 30s.	*Polygonum multiflorum* HE SHOU WU (see pp. 224-26)	Kidney tonic used in China for premature menopause and early graying.
	Salvia officinalis SAGE (see p. 115)	Traditional remedy used to restore color, possibly associated with its tonic and hormonal properties.
DANDRUFF Dandruff is small flakes of dead skin on the scalp. It may be accompanied by seborrhoeic dermatitis and may be associated with yeast infection. KEY SYMPTOMS • Obvious flakes on collars • Hair dry and brittle, or greasy with yellow flakes.	*Quillaja saponaria* SOAP BARK (see pp. 229) *(Inner bark)*	Cleansing and anti-inflammatory; rich in saponins.
	Rosmarinus officinalis ROSEMARY (see p. 112)	Astringent, antiseptic, and circulatory stimulant; also useful for psoriasis affecting the scalp.

How to use	*Combinations*	*Cautions*
Take 10 ml fresh juice or an infusion three times a day; also use externally as an ointment or cream.	Combines well with red clover to reduce over-production of cells, and with cleansing stimulants like stinging nettle or figwort. Use 3 parts cleavers to 1-2 parts other herbs.	
Use in decoction (½ tsp per cup in ½ cup doses) or tincture.	With cleansing remedies such as pokeroot and yellow dock; add valerian to a decoction if stress or anxiety are significant factors; use aloe vera sap or slippery elm powder as a topical treatment.	
Take an infusion or tincture.	Combines well with burdock as a general cleanser. Add dandelion root or figwort to help cleanse and cool the liver.	
Take an infusion or tincture.	Use with red clover or heartsease to help normalize skin growth, or with cleansing herbs like cleavers and yellow dock.	Heart stimulant, so avoid in heart-beat abnormalities (tachycardia).
Take an infusion or tincture; also use externally in cream or ointment.	Can be combined with anti-inflammatory and cleansing herbs such as cleavers, yellow dock, or 10 drops *arbor vitae* tincture.	
Apply gel from a fresh leaf directly on the affected area; ointment can also be used.	Use as a simple.	
Use as a cream or ointment, or use an infusion as a footbath or as a wash.	Add 5 ml tea tree oil to 2 cups (500 ml) infusion for a wash to enhance antifungal action.	
Add 10 drops oil or 10 ml tincture to ½ cup (100 ml) water and use as a wash; take 1 ml tincture three times a day.	Use as a simple. Externally, add an equal amount of *arbor vitae*, or add the myrrh to pot marigold cream. Internally, take echinacea capsules.	Avoid taking internally in pregnancy.
Apply as a cream or ointment to affected areas, or use well-diluted tincture as a hair rinse.	Support with nervines (see pp. 162-5) and vitamin B supplements. Drink stinging nettle and burdock infusion as a cleansing stimulant.	Do not use on broken skin; do not take internally.
Take 10-20 drops tincture up to three times a day; use an infusion as a hair rinse.	Support with nervines and add stinging nettle, rosemary, or sage to the infusion; take mineral and vitamin B supplements.	Avoid completely in pregnancy.
Take a decoction or tincture (up to 15 ml a day); commercial mixtures are available.	Use as a simple or combine with tonics like *nu zhen zi*, *shu di huang*, or buchu. Use 2 parts *he shou wu* to 1 part other herbs.	Avoid if also suffering from diarrhea.
Take an infusion; use an infusion as a hair rinse.	Can add rosemary and stinging nettle to the infusion for the rinse to help darken the hair.	Avoid therapeutic doses in pregnancy or if epileptic.
Mix 2 cups (500 ml) decoction with 200 g soft soap and use as a shampoo.	Use as a simple.	For external use only. Do not take internally.
Use an infusion as a hair rinse; macerate 15 g herb in 1 cup (250 ml) ordinary shampoo for two weeks before using.	Add stinging nettle root to the rinse as a circulatory stimulant and cleansing tonic.	

KEY

Aerial parts

Essential oil

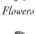
Flowers

Inner bark

Leaves

Petals

Root

Root bark

Stem

Twigs

Whole herb

STANDARD REMEDIES
All recipes and doses are standard unless otherwise specified; see *Making Herbal Remedies*, pp. 152-57.

HEART, BLOOD & CIRCULATION

ANCIENT MEDICAL TRADITIONS regarded the heart as far more than just a pump to circulate the blood. In Ayurvedic medicine, it is the seat of the soul, while according to Chinese medicine, it stores *shen* (a sense of appropriateness and right behavior). What modern Western medicine may regard as a mental or nervous disorder, Chinese medicine blames on disharmonies of *shen*, and may favor herbs such as *fu ling*, which clears "dampness" from the heart and is used as a sedative to "pacify" it. Western heart herbs boast a more conventional set of actions. Ever since foxglove (*Digitalis purpurea*) was identified as a potent heart remedy in 1768, scientists have been investigating herbal solutions. Some are still important in modern medicine. Others are suitable for home use: hawthorn and linden tea, for example, are safe enough for use in pregnancy. Herbs can also help in controlling today's *bête noire*, cholesterol: many are very effective at lowering cholesterol and helping to prevent atherosclerosis.

See also: wounds and bleeding, pp. 158-59; hemorrhoids, pp. 190-91; heavy periods, pp. 204-05.

AILMENT	REMEDIES	
	Herb	*Actions*
HIGH BLOOD PRESSURE Also called hypertension, this should be regarded as a symptom of imbalance in the body, rather than as a single disease. It may be related to atherosclerosis, heart disorders and liver problems. **KEY SYMPTOMS** • Headaches • Eye problems • Dizziness or fainting spells • High blood pressure reading on repeated examination • Diastolic reading (the lower of the two numbers in the reading) greater than 95-105 mm Hg. *IMPORTANT: Do not replace conventional medicine with herbs without consulting your practitioner.*	*Crataegus spp.* HAWTHORN (see p. 55) *(Flowering tops)*	Improves coronary circulation, strengthens heart muscle; helps stabilize blood pressure as cardiac function improves.
	Dendranthema x *grandiflorum* JU HUA (see p. 56)	Dilates the coronary arteries and increases blood flow; also clears "liver heat", which can cause hypertension.
	Stachys officinalis WOOD BETONY (see p. 121)	Circulatory tonic, relaxant, and sedative; calms the heart.
	Tilia x *europaea* LINDEN (see pp. 229)	Relaxes and heals blood vessels; helps prevent arteriosclerosis.
	Viburnum opulus GUELDER ROSE (see p. 136)	Smooth muscle relaxant for the vascular system; lowers diastolic blood pressure.
LOW BLOOD PRESSURE Also called hypotension, this is often not considered serious by doctors, but can be significant. **KEY SYMPTOMS** • General fatigue • Weak constitution • Dizziness and/or fainting spells • Palpitations. *IMPORTANT: If the systolic reading (higher number) is consistently below 110 mm Hg, seek professional help.*	*Convallaria majalis* LILY-OF-THE-VALLEY (see pp. 229)	Stimulates heart contractions and improves efficiency; useful for weak, failing and elderly hearts.
	Cytisus scoparius BROOM (see pp. 228-9)	Regulates heartbeat, steadying the arrhythmias that can be associated with low blood pressure and heart failure.
	Leonurus cardiaca MOTHERWORT (see p. 82) *(Flowering tops)*	Relaxing for palpitations and arrhythmias; also has stimulating action on the heart.
VARICOSE VEINS Stretched veins in the legs, associated with poor venous return or raised abdominal pressure, as in obesity, pregnancy or constipation. **KEY SYMPTOMS** • Enlarged, stretched veins • Pain in the legs.	*Aesculus hippocastanum* HORSE CHESTNUT (see pp. 228)	Astringent and internally strengthening to the blood vessels, possibly due to the presence of aescin.
	Melilotus officinalis KING'S CLOVER (see pp. 229)	A good venous tonic, rich in coumarin-like compounds; anticoagulant and anti-inflammatory.

CASE HISTORY
High blood pressure with menopausal symptoms

PATIENT: Sarah, 52, divorced, with a daughter in college to support. She divided her time between caring for elderly parents and work as a musician.

HISTORY AND COMPLAINT: Sarah had been diagnosed as having slightly elevated blood pressure 10 years previously. She was prescribed beta blockers but disliked taking drugs, and soon abandoned the pills for various herbal and homeopathic remedies. Eight years later, another check-up revealed glaucoma and blood pressure of 180/110 mm Hg. She also had menopausal symptoms, lower back pain, dizziness, and a tendency for tinnitus, palpitations, and hot flashes whenever she felt emotionally upset or did anything energetic. Her doctor urged a return to beta-blockers.

TREATMENT: Herbs to boost kidney energy and nourish the liver, rather than drugs to slow down her heart, were used. These included *shu di huang, shan zhu yu, mu dan pi,* and *he shou wu.* She was also given herbal tea containing *ju hua,* hawthorn and motherwort.

OUTCOME: Within a month, Sarah's hot flashes vanished, she had fewer palpitations and more energy with none of the dizzy feelings. Her blood pressure was down to 155/95 mm Hg. The herbs were continued for three months, by which time her blood pressure had stabilized at 140/85 mm Hg, so she continued with only the herbal tea. Six months later at a routine check-up, her blood pressure was still stabilized and her glaucoma had improved.

How to use	*Combinations*	*Cautions*
Take an infusion or tincture.	Can combine with linden and yarrow, or with herbs such as guelder rose to relax blood vessels, or with passion flower for stress.	
Take an infusion or tincture.	Can combine with liver herbs like *gou qi zi,* diuretics such as *fu ling* or dandelion leaf, or with sedatives, depending on the cause of hypertension.	
Take an infusion or tincture.	Can combine with linden or *fu ling* if stress is contributing to the condition; use 2 parts wood betony to 1 part other herbs.	Avoid large doses in pregnancy.
Take an infusion or up to 10 ml tincture a day.	Combine with hawthorn as a cardiac tonic, or with ginkgo if arteriosclerosis is significant.	
Take a decoction or tincture.	Combine with heart tonics such as hawthorn, or sedatives like valerian if tension is significant.	
Restricted to professional use in some countries. Maximum safe dose in UK is up to 1 ml tincture 3 times a day.	Should be prescribed with a diuretic such as dandelion leaf, or with tonic herbs like hawthorn or ginkgo, depending on the cause of the condition.	Take only as prescribed; high doses cause severe vomiting.
Take an infusion made with 15 g herb to 2 cups (500 ml) water, or up to 5 ml tincture a day.	Use with tonics such as hawthorn (or lily-of-the-valley, if prescribed by a qualified practitioner), depending on the severity of the symptoms.	Avoid in pregnancy. Do not use if new to herbs; see pp. 228-29.
Take an infusion or tincture.	Combine with rosemary and *fu ling* for both tonic and calming actions.	Avoid in pregnancy.
Take up to 2.5 ml tincture three times a day; use dilute tincture for compresses.	Use internally with liver herbs such as 10 drops of goldenseal, if constipation is a contributory cause, or dilute with witch hazel for compresses.	Peel off seed-coating if making large quantities; it can be toxic.
Use an infusion or take up to 3 ml tincture three times a day; use 5 ml tincture in 45 ml witch hazel as a lotion.	Combine with pot marigold in compresses, creams and lotions, especially if there is poor circulation and varicose eczema.	Do not use with warfarin or similar drugs, or blood-clotting may occur.

KEY

Aerial parts

Bark

Berries

Flowers

Leaves

Seeds

STANDARD REMEDIES
All recipes and doses are standard unless otherwise specified; see *Making Herbal Remedies, pp. 152-57.*

AILMENT	REMEDIES	
	Herb	*Actions*
POOR CIRCULATION This may be a sign of a more serious heart disorder, but it is often simply an inherited tendency and does not constitute a major problem. **KEY SYMPTOMS** • Exceptionally cold hands and feet • Tendency for chilblains • White or "dead" fingers (Raynaud's phenomenon).	*Capsicum frutescens* CAYENNE (see p. 50)	Heating, promotes sweating; a strong circulatory stimulant.
	Cinnamomum cassia GUI ZHI (see p. 52)	Warming, promotes sweating; encourages both blood and *qi* (energy) circulation.
	Zanthoxylum americanum PRICKLY ASH (see pp. 229)	Circulatory stimulant; promotes sweating; warming for all "cold" conditions.
	Zingiber officinalis GINGER (see p. 139)	Strong circulatory stimulant; relaxes blood vessels; promotes sweating; very warming.
PALPITATIONS & ANGINA PECTORIS Palpitations are simply an awareness of the heartbeat following shock, exercise, alcohol, or excitement. Angina pectoris is associated with narrowing of the coronary artery, restricting blood supply to the heart. **KEY SYMPTOMS** • Pain in the chest in angina • Breathlessness, panic. *IMPORTANT: Angina pectoris always requires professional treatment.*	*Alpinia galanga* GALANGAL (see p.35)	Traditional heart remedy to ease heart pains, dizziness, and fatigue, and reduce the symptoms of angina pectoris.
	Leonurus cardiaca MOTHERWORT (see p. 82)	Heart tonic and relaxant to combat feelings of panic and normalize heart beat in palpitations.
	Passiflora incarnata PASSION FLOWER (see p. 99)	Sedative and calming, heart tonic and relaxant for blood vessels.
ANEMIA (iron-deficient type) Low hemoglobin levels, which can be due to a poor diet, heavy periods or digestive disorders. **KEY SYMPTOM** • Breathlessness and/or palpitations.	*Angelica sinensis* DANG GUI (see p. 38)	Nourishes the blood and invigorates the circulation; contains vitamin B12 and folic acid, so can help prevent pernicious anemia.
	Urtica dioica STINGING NETTLE (see p. 131)	Rich in iron and other minerals and vitamins; highly nutritious.
HIGH CHOLESTEROL High levels of lipids (such as cholesterol) in the blood can lead to atherosclerosis and increase the risk of heart attack. They are associated with too much saturated fat in the diet, but may be hereditary. Cholesterol is needed for many body mechanisms, and is not intrinsically harmful. **KEY SYMPTOM** • Blood tests revealing high lipid levels.	*Allium sativum* GARLIC (see p. 33) *(Bulb)*	Reduces cholesterol levels; has been shown to reduce the risk of heart attacks and atherosclerosis.
	Avena sativa OATS (see p. 43)	Effectively reduces cholesterol levels, particularly low-density lipoproteins.
	Camellia sinensis OOLONG TEA (see p. 48)	Contains phenols, which inhibit cholesterol absorption; circulatory stimulant and tonic for blood vessels; helps to prevent atherosclerosis.
CAPILLARY FRAGILITY Weakness in blood vessel walls. **KEY SYMPTOMS** • Tendency to bruise easily • Retinal hemorrhages.	*Fagopyrum esculentum* BUCKWHEAT (see pp. 228)	Rich in rutin (tonifies and repairs arteriole walls); specific for retinal hemorrhage.
	Viola tricolor HEARTSEASE (see p. 137)	Contains flavonoids, which strengthen capillary walls.

How to use	Combinations	Cautions
Add 30-50 mg herb to 2 cups (500 ml) water for an infusion; take up to 1 ml 1:20 tincture a dose; massage with infused oil.	Take with other warming stimulant herbs, such as a decoction of angelica root, or add 1-2 g bayberry to the infusion.	Do not exceed the stated dose; avoid large doses in pregnancy.
Take a decoction or tincture.	Combines well with a little ginger, or add ginkgo or rosemary.	Avoid therapeutic doses in pregnancy.
Take a decoction of 15 g herb to 2½ cups (600 ml) water; take up to 5 ml tincture a day.	Can combine with angelica root or rosemary, or add a pinch of cinnamon powder to a decoction.	
Add up to 10 g fresh root to 2½ cups (600 ml) water for decoctions; take up to 10 drops 1:5 tincture per dose.	Combine with circulatory tonics such as ginkgo, or warming herbs like rosemary or *gui zhi*.	
Take in pills, tinctures, or a decoction; a few drops of neat tincture on the tongue may help avert an angina attack.	Use with hawthorn berries, khella, and prickly ash in decoctions and tinctures.	
Take in tinctures or infusions.	Use with hawthorn flowers and linden in infusions; add rose petals or skullcap for feelings of panic or shock causing palpitations.	Avoid in pregnancy.
Take in infusions, pills, and tinctures.	Use with hawthorn and linden as an infusion for everyday drinking in angina pectoris; add skullcap or wood betony for palpitations associated with shock or emotional upsets.	Use only low doses in pregnancy; may cause drowsiness.
Take a decoction or tincture. Many commercial preparations are available.	Can combine with *shu di huang* and *he shou wu*. Eat plenty of iron-rich foods like liver, watercress and apricots. Supplements of *aswaghanda* can also help.	Avoid regular or large doses in pregnancy.
Take 10 ml juice three times a day, or take an infusion of fresh herb.	Use as a simple, but add iron-rich foods like parsley, watercress and apricots to the diet. Supplements of *aswaghanda* can also help.	
Take 1 clove daily; take 2 g powdered garlic in capsules a day if there is a high risk of heart attack.	Use as a simple, but also limit the intake of saturated fats and high cholesterol foods.	Avoid therapeutic doses during pregnancy.
Add 25 g oatbran to breakfast cereal or oatmeal.	Use as a simple, but also limit the intake of saturated fats and high cholesterol foods.	If sensitive to gluten, see caution p. 43.
Add 1-2 tsp per cup of boiling water for an infusion.	Use as a simple. *Pu erh* is the most effective variety of oolong for reducing cholesterol.	Limit to 2 cups a day in hypertension and pregnancy.
Take an infusion or tincture.	Use with 10 ml horsetail juice per dose, or take rutin tablets daily.	
Take an infusion or tincture.	Can be combined with 10 ml horsetail juice per dose, or use yarrow or ribwort plantain.	

KEY

Aerial parts

Bark

Fruit

Grain

Leaves

Root

Twigs

STANDARD REMEDIES
All recipes and doses are standard unless otherwise specified; see *Making Herbal Remedies*, pp. 152-57.

DIGESTIVE PROBLEMS

GOOD DIGESTION is central to good health: dysfunction here not only starves the body of nutrients, but also leads to a buildup of toxins. Ayurvedic theory argues that these products are the source of the three humors, *pitta*, *vata*, and *kapha*, which, if out of balance, can account for most diseases. In Chinese medicine, the digestive organs are associated with many other organs and bodily processes, including the blood supply, energy circulation, mental activity and muscles, and imbalances here can be linked with a wide range of physical and

emotional symptoms. In the West, too, herbal medicine has long focused on digestive function. Herbs can provide an impressive array of tonics, stimulants, carminatives and relaxants to ensure healthy function. Good digestion depends, also, on the nervous system to stimulate acid or enzyme production and gut motions, and many digestive herbs act on the nervous system and can help stress related problems like colitis.

IMPORTANT: Seek professional advice for any change in bowel patterns that occurs suddenly or persists.

See also: mouth ulcers, pp. 176-77; threadworms, pp. 218-19.

AILMENT	REMEDIES	
	Herb	*Actions*
CONSTIPATION Generally a symptom of other health problems, this may be associated with poor diet, sluggish digestion or muscle tone, or may be due to nervous tension inhibiting bowel action. **KEY SYMPTOMS** • Lack of bowel motions for more than 24 hours • Low abdominal pain or cramping • Difficulty passing stools.	*Plantago psyllium/P. ovata* **PSYLLIUM/ISPAGHULA** (see p. 104)	Mucilaginous and bulking laxatives, which lubricatethe bowel; useful if stools are dry.
	Rheum palmatum **RHUBARB** (see p. 109)	Contains anthraquinones, which irritate the digestive tract, increasing gut movements.
	Viburnum opulus **GUELDER ROSE** (see p. 136)	Smooth muscle relaxant; useful if constipation is linked to visceral tension.
DIARRHEA This is often a symptom of other imbalances in the digestive system, but can also be caused by food poisoning or bacterial infection. Suspect food may be apparent in cases of food poisoning. Bacterial infection can easily be caught by other household members. **KEY SYMPTOMS** • Loose, frequent stools • Abdominal cramps.	*Agrimonia eupatoria* **AGRIMONY** (see p. 31)	Astringent and healing for any intestinal tract inflammation; especially suitable for children.
	Geranium maculatum **AMERICAN CRANESBILL** (see pp. 228)	Astringent; gentle enough for children, the elderly and the debilitated.
	Potentilla erecta **TORMENTIL** (see pp. 229)	Contains up to 20% tannins, making it very astringent and reducing the inflammation associated with diarrhea.
GASTRITIS Gastritis is inflammation of the stomach lining; if persistent, it can lead to ulceration. It may be due to dietary factors. **KEY SYMPTOMS** • Heartburn and acid reflux • Nausea with persistent vomiting in acute gastritis • Diarrhea and abdominal discomfort.	*Althaea officinalis* **MARSHMALLOW** (see p. 36)	Soothing and demulcent for irritated mucous membranes; healing for damaged tissue.
	Filipendula ulmaria **MEADOWSWEET** (see p. 63)	Anti-inflammatory; reduces stomach acid secretions and is soothing and healing for the stomach lining.
	Ulmus fulva **SLIPPERY ELM** (see pp. 229)	Demulcent; soothes irritated mucous membranes; nutritive for debilitated conditions.

CASE HISTORY
Irritable bowel syndrome

PATIENT: Louise, a secretary aged 24; an only child still living with her parents, with an active social life.

HISTORY AND COMPLAINT: Louise suffered from irritable bowel syndrome for three years, following a bout of food poisoning. Her main symptoms included diarrhea (up to five times a day) and vomiting copious phlegm after each meal. Hospital tests all proved negative, and Louise was prescribed antidepressants, antibiotics, tranquilizers, and bulking laxatives. Her diet was far from ideal, with too much cake and milk. She sucked fruit candies constantly to suppress nausea.

TREATMENT: a priority was to improve Louise's diet. She had recently cut out chocolate, and agreed to limit dairy products and carbohydrates, which were producing so much mucus that her system was flooded with phlegm. Soy milk and wholegrain products were recommended instead. Herbs to help regulate body fluids, tonify the stomach, and astringe the system were prescribed, including *ban xia*, *bai zhu*, cinnamon and agrimony. She was given *Lactobacillus acidophilus* bacteria in capsules to restore the natural gut flora. Capsules of dried ginger relieved nausea.

OUTCOME: Louise began to improve, but it took about three months before she could eat without immediately vomiting. Her stools became firmer, with motions twice a day. After six months, the herbs were phased out and dietary "lapses" are now tolerated.

How to use	*Combinations*	*Cautions*
Infuse 1 tsp seeds in a cup of boiling water, let it cool, and drink with the seeds, once or twice a day or at night.	Use either as a simple or mix one part linseed to two parts psyllium or ispaghula seeds.	
Add 10-15 g herb to 2½ cups (600 ml) water for a decoction; take 2 ml tincture up to three times a day.	Add 1-2 ml fennel or lemon balm tincture per dose to prevent griping. Enhance with mild laxatives such as butternut or yellow dock, or senna pods in more severe cases.	Avoid in pregnancy, arthritic conditions and gout.
Take a decoction or tincture.	Add laxatives like butternut, senna, or licorice, or additional relaxants like chamomile, depending on symptoms.	
Take an infusion or tincture.	Add soothing herbs like chamomile, ribwort plantain, or marshmallow to ease gut inflammation; add bilberry or bistort to enhance astringency.	
Take an infusion or 2-3 ml tincture (made from leaves) three times a day; or take a decoction made with 20 g root to 2½ cups (600 ml) water.	Add soothing herbs like marshmallow root, meadowsweet, or ribwort plantain to ease gut inflammation; add bilberry or bistort to enhance astringency.	
For a decoction, add 20 g herb to 2½ cups (600 ml) water; take 2-3 ml tincture up to three times a day.	Add soothing herbs like ribwort plantain or marshmallow root to ease gut inflammation.	
Use a maceration or tincture made from fresh herb, or use powder.	Use with meadowsweet adding a pinch of cinnamon; combine with carminatives such as fennel and peppermint infusions.	
Take an infusion; or use a tincture or fluid extract in hot water allowed to cool.	Increase astringency with 10 drops bistort or American cranesbill tincture or soothe with 10 drops licorice per dose. Can also add extra anti-inflammatories, such as pot marigold.	Avoid the herb in cases of salicylate sensitivity.
Take up to 5 g powdered bark in capsules or mixed with water, before meals.	Combine with powdered marshmallow root in capsules if desired.	

KEY

 Aerial parts

 Bark

 Leaves

 Root

 Seeds

STANDARD REMEDIES All recipes and doses are standard unless otherwise specified; see *Making Herbal Remedies, pp. 152-57.*

AILMENT	REMEDIES	
	Herb	*Actions*
PEPTIC/DUODENAL ULCERS Ulceration of mucous membranes now linked with the *Heliobacter pylori* bacterium. **KEY SYMPTOMS** • Pain in the upper abdomen, often worse at night or if hungry.	*Glycyrrhiza glabra* LICORICE (see p. 70)	Anti-inflammatory; produces a viscous mucus to protect the stomach wall and limits acid production.
	Leptospermum scoparium MANUKA (see pp. 142-43) *(Pollen)*	Studies in New Zealand suggest that manuka honey destroys *Heliobacter bacterium*.
INFLAMED GALL BLADDER Also known as cholecystitis; may be chronic or acute. **KEY SYMPTOMS** • Constant, severe pain in the upper abdomen. • Sweating and nausea.	*Berberis vulgaris* BARBERRY (see pp. 228)	Stimulates bile flow and eases liver congestion; bitter and laxative.
	Chionanthus virginicus FRINGE TREE (see pp. 228)	Stimulates bile flow and liver function; laxative and cleansing.
GALLSTONES Stones made of bile pigment and/or cholesterol obstructing the bile duct. **KEY SYMPTOMS** • Brief attacks of severe upper abdominal pain • Jaundice, indigestion, vomiting.	*Citrus limon* LEMON (see pp. 229)	Used in traditional treatments with olive oil to break down and encourage excretion of gallstones; liver tonic and restorative.
	Peumus boldo BOLDO (see pp. 228)	Stimulates bile flow and liver activity; reduces inflammation and helps protect the liver.
INDIGESTION & ACIDITY Usually due to eating too much, too quickly, missing meals or to anxiety. Antacids encourage further stomach acid secretion and can worsen the condition. **KEY SYMPTOMS** • Bloating and feelings of abdominal fullness • Heartburn or acid reflux • Stomach pain.	*Foeniculum officinale* FENNEL (see p. 64)	Carminative and anti-inflammatory; effective for cramping pains.
	Melissa officinalis LEMON BALM (see p. 90)	Carminative and relaxing; sedative action is useful for nervous stomach.
	Mentha x piperita PEPPERMINT (see p. 91)	Cooling carminative; stimulates bile flow; good for nausea and nervous stomach.
IRRITABLE BOWEL SYNDROME & COLITIS Various symptoms linked to food intolerance, anxiety or infection. **KEY SYMPTOMS** • Alternating bouts of diarrhea and constipation • "Rabbit dropping" stools • Bloating and gas • Mucus in stools.	*Matricaria recutita* GERMAN CHAMOMILE (see p. 88)	Sedative, anti-inflammatory, and carminative; good for nervous dyspepsia.
	Dioscorea villosa MEXICAN WILD YAM (see p. 57) *(Rhizome)*	Visceral relaxant, anti-spasmodic; anti-inflammatory and bile stimulant.
	Iberis amara BITTER CANDYTUFT (see pp. 228-29)	Antispasmodic, relaxant; tonifies the digestive tract; carminative.
LIVER DISORDERS In our polluted society, liver congestion is very common. It may be a pathological disorder, but often simply involves feelings of anger and frustration. **KEY SYMPTOMS** • Tendency for constipation • Abdominal bloating • Emotional instability • Small, red abdominal spots • Sore, itching eyes • Menstrual disorders.	*Bupleurum chinense* CHAI HU (see pp. 228)	Bitter liver tonic; encourages energy flow.
	Picrorrhiza kurroa KATUKA (see pp. 140-41)	Ayurvedic digestive remedy that protects the liver from several toxins and stimulates bile flow to help cleanse the gall bladder.
	Silybum marianus MILK THISTLE (see p. 120)	Encourages liver cell renewal and repair in degenerative conditions, e.g. alcoholism.

How to use	Combinations	Cautions
Take a decoction or suck juice sticks; use a tincture or fluid extract in very hot water allowed to cool.	In severe cases can add extra soothing and healing herbs, such as 10-20 drops marsh-mallow or slippery elm, or add anti-inflamm-atories such as pot marigold or meadowsweet.	Avoid in high blood pressure or if taking digoxin-based drugs.
Take 1-2 tsp manuka honey twice a day or use the flowers and leaves in infusions or the bark in decoctions.	Add other antibacterials such as echinacea, blue flag, or thyme; add soothing demulcents such as marshmallow root or licorice as decoctions.	
For a decoction, add 15 g herb to 2½ cups (600 ml) water; or take up to 8 ml tincture a day.	Combine with anti-inflammatories such as goldenseal (5 drops tincture per dose) and liver tonics such as vervain or globe artichoke.	Avoid in pregnancy.
Take a decoction in 1 tbsp doses; or take up to 5 ml tincture a day.	Combine with bitters, liver tonics or stimulants such as dandelion, milk thistle, chicory, globe artichoke, or centaury, plus anti-inflammatories such as pot marigold.	
With olive oil (see right).	Fast for a day; take 50 ml olive oil and the juice of 2 lemons in water at 6 p.m.; repeat three times during the next hour; bile sand is passed in stools over the following three days.	
Use 10-30 drops tincture per dose or ½ tsp dried leaves to 2 cups infusion, in ½-cup doses.	Traditionally combined with barberry and fringe tree for gallstones; add guelder rose or wild yam to help relieve spasmodic pain.	Avoid in pregnancy.
Take an infusion or tincture; useful as an after dinner tisane.	Use as a simple or add American cranesbill to reduce acidity, or peppermint, meadowsweet or chamomile to enhance carminative action.	Avoid high doses in pregnancy.
Take an infusion or tincture.	Add chamomile or meadowsweet as anti-inflammatories, or a little hops as a bitter and antispasmodic.	
Add 15 g dried herb to 2 cups water for an infusion; take up to 2.5 ml tincture per dose.	Use as a simple; add American cranesbill to reduce acid secretions; add marshmallow root, meadowsweet, and licorice for inflammation.	May reduce milk flow; caution if breast-feeding.
Take an infusion or tincture.	Add a few drops of peppermint or fresh ginger tincture to relieve abdominal bloating and regulate bowel activity.	Avoid excessive internal intake in pregnancy.
Add 1 tsp herb to 2 cups water for an infusion; or take as a tincture in combinations.	Add meadowsweet to soothe stomach lining; chamomile for anxiety; or a few drops fresh ginger tincture to regulate bowel activity.	Avoid in pregnancy.
Take up to 2 ml tincture per dose or an infusion made from 15 g to 2 cups water.	Add angelica root and milk thistle seed as liver tonics; or lemon balm, passion flower or chamomile as relaxants.	High doses may cause nausea.
Add 10 g herb to 2½ cups (600 ml) water for a decoction.	Combine with *bai shao yao*, *chuan xiong*, goldenseal and dandelion root to help regulate liver function.	
Take 1 g per dose as capsules of powder or mixed with ghee, or use ½ tsp crushed root for 3 doses of decoction.	Use with other bitter digestive or liver stimulants such as turmeric, barberry, *gotu kola* and cardamom.	High doses may cause abdominal cramping, diarrhea and gas.
Take an infusion; or take up to 10 ml tincture a day in hot water allowed to cool.	Use as a simple or add vervain, dandelion root, gentian or globe artichoke and 5 drops goldenseal as additional liver tonics.	Do not exceed the stated dose of essential oil.

KEY

Aerial parts

Bark

Fruit

Flowers

Leaves

Root

Root bark

Seeds

STANDARD REMEDIES All recipes and doses are standard unless otherwise specified; see *Making Herbal Remedies*, pp. 152-57.

189

AILMENT	REMEDIES	
	Herb	*Actions*
NAUSEA & VOMITING Can be due to food poisoning, infections, fever or migraines. *IMPORTANT: Projectile or prolonged vomiting requires professional medical help.*	*Syzygium aromaticum* CLOVES (see pp. 228-29) *(Flower buds)*	Stimulant and carminative; locally antiseptic.
	Zingiber officinalis GINGER (see p. 139)	Prevents vomiting; very effective for motion sickness as well as digestive upsets.
GAS & ABDOMINAL BLOATING Often associated with minor digestive or liver problems, but may indicate serious illness. **KEY SYMPTOMS** • Gas that may go up or down • Uncomfortable abdominal distention.	*Cnicus benedictus* HOLY THISTLE (see pp. 228)	Bitter digestive stimulant which encourages stomach secretions and normalizes function.
	Elettaria cardamomum CARDAMOM (see pp. 228)	Carminative and soothing for the digestive system; relieves abdominal cramps and stimulates appetite.
FOOD-POISONING & GASTROENTERITIS Gastric infection by viruses, bacteria or protozoa which may be due to pets, farm animals or environmental hazards. **KEY SYMPTOMS** • Sudden onset with abdominal pain, nausea and vomiting • Diarrhea, general malaise and weakness.	*Alchemilla xanthoclora* LADY'S MANTLE (see p. 32)	Astringent digestive tonic to reduce inflammation and discomfort.
	Matricaria recutita GERMAN CHAMOMILE (see p. 88)	Antimicrobial to combat infection; soothing and calming for the digestive system; reduces inflammation in the digestive tract.
POOR APPETITE Loss of appetite may be due to chronic illness, stress or debility, all of which should be treated. **KEY SYMPTOMS** • No interest in meals or eating • Weight loss and absence of menstruation in severe cases. *IMPORTANT: Poor appetite may suggest eating disorders such as anorexia nervosa; seek immediate professional help if this is suspected.*	*Jateorhiza calumba* CALUMBA (see pp. 228)	Bitter and stimulating for the digestive system; also helps to relieve indigestion and normalize digestive function; stimulates production of stomach acid.
	Trigonella foenum-graecum FENUGREEK (see p. 129)	Stimulating and tonifying for the whole digestive system; a traditional remedy for thin people hoping to put on weight.
HALITOSIS/BAD BREATH Poor dental hygiene is often to blame, but infections in the mouth, throat, lungs, or stomach can all contribute to bad breath. **KEY SYMPTOM** • Stale or offensive smelling breath.	*Iris versicolor* BLUE FLAG (see pp. 228)	Cleansing and stimulating for sluggish digestive, lymphatic and glandular systems.
	Levisticum officinale LOVAGE (see pp. 229)	Tonic to normalize both digestive and respiratory function, improve the appetite, ease gas, and combat bacteria; seeds also contain aromatic oils.
HEMORRHOIDS Anal varicose veins associated with poor muscle tone and often due to straining or constipation. **KEY SYMPTOMS** • Palpable hemorrhoids at anus • Bleeding on passing stools.	*Ranunculus ficaria* PILEWORT (see pp. 229)	Astringent; tonifies blood vessels and stops bleeding.
	Sophora japonica HUAI JIAO (see pp. 229)	Cooling, anti-inflammatory; lowers blood pressure; clears "liver heat", cools blood, stops bleeding; helps constipation.

How to use	*Combinations*	*Cautions*
Take an infusion; or take 1-2 drops essential oil on a sugar lump; add powder to food.	Use as a simple.	Do not exceed the stated dose of essential oil.
Take a tincture in drop doses while symptoms persist, or chew crystallized ginger.	Use as a simple or combine with black horehound, black pepper or chamomile tincture.	Use with care in early pregnancy (see pp. 206-07).
Use in infusions or tinctures.	Add lemon balm or chamomile with teas or centaury as an additional bitter; add carminatives such as a pinch of fennel seeds, black pepper, or cinnamon.	May cause vomiting in excessive doses.
Use crushed seeds in tinctures or infusions; use 2-5 drops essential oil in 5 ml carrier oil for abdominal massage; use seeds in cooking.	Use with soothing digestive remedies such as *gotu kola*, fennel, chamomile, or lemon balm in infusions; add a pinch of galangal, ginger or black pepper.	
Use in infusions or tinctures.	With milk thistle seeds and marshmallow root to soothe the digestive tract and normalize function; eat garlic or take echinacea to combat infection.	
Use in infusions.	With astringents such as agrimony or lady's mantle, soothing demulcents such as meadowsweet or marshmallow, and digestive tonics such as *gotu kola*; add a pinch of ginger or cinnamon to combat nausea.	
Use in macerations – take ¹/₂ cup 30 minutes before meals or 20-40 drops tincture in a little water before meals.	Combine with mugwort tincture for menstrual disorders or mix the maceration with agrimony, lemon balm, and chamomile infusions to soothe the digestive tract.	Avoid in pregnancy and gastric ulceration.
Take the seeds in infusions or use drops of the tincture on the tongue 30 minutes before meals.	Combine with milk thistle seeds or agrimony in infusions with a pinch of powdered ginger or galangal for additional stimulation; add chamomile, vervain, or wood betony if stress is a factor.	
Use powdered in capsules, 200 mg daily.	Combine with powdered goldenseal, licorice, and echinacea or myrrh to combat underlying infections and congestion.	
Chew a few seeds as required to freshen the breath and help normalize digestive function.	Mix with dill or fennel seeds if preferred; gargle with 5-10 drops of myrrh tincture in a glass of water to help clear any mouth or gum infections; use appropriate remedies to treat any associated disorders contributing to the problem.	
Apply ointment frequently.	Use as a simple, but take supportive liver herbs or venous tonics such as king's clover.	Do not take internally.
Take a decoction or tincture; take 400 mg powder in capsules three times a day.	Use as a simple or combine with liver tonics and digestive remedies such as dandelion root, barberry, *dang gui*, and *zhi ke*.	Avoid in pregnancy.

KEY

Aerial parts

Essential oil

Flowers

Fruit

Leaves

Root

Seeds

STANDARD REMEDIES All recipes and doses are standard unless otherwise specified; see *Making Herbal Remedies*, pp. 152-57.

ALLERGIC CONDITIONS

A HEALTHY SYSTEM copes with allergens, but if there is tension, infection or fatigue, the arrival of an allergen tips the balance and an allergic response occurs in the form of hay fever, skin rashes, or gastric upsets. Food allergies often start in infancy, when the immature gut has to cope with unknown proteins, such as cow's milk. The immune system is triggered to repel the invader, producing inflammation, mucus, and irritation. If the allergen continues to be taken, the response becomes muted with no tell-tale symptoms, merely a general weakening of the immune system. This masked allergy can manifest itself as vague arthritic pains, irritable bowel syndrome or persistent sinusitis. Herbal remedies can strengthen the respiratory and immune systems, so the allergen does not cause the characteristic response.

See also: asthma, pp. 172-73; eczema, pp. 178-79; vaginal yeast infections, pp. 204-05.

AILMENT	REMEDIES	
	Herb	*Actions*
HAY FEVER & ALLERGIC RHINITIS Generally triggered by grass or tree pollens, hay fever occurs when these are prevalent. Allergies to animal fur or house dust occur throughout the year. **KEY SYMPTOMS** • Copious nasal catarrh, sneezing • Sore, irritated eyes • Asthma-like symptoms in severe cases.	*Euphrasia officinalis* EYEBRIGHT (see pp. 228)	Decreases nasal secretions and soothes mucous membranes and conjunctiva.
	Glechoma hederacea GROUND IVY (see pp. 229)	Astringent and anticatarrhal; good for drying secretions and inflammations.
	Plantago lanceolata RIBWORT PLANTAIN (see p. 104)	Good for allergic rhinitis, toning mucous membranes and healing inflammations.
FOOD INTOLERANCE Common food allergens include cow's milk, wheat, and beef. They can cause a wide range of symptoms. Candidiasis can be related to food intolerance. Allergy to salicylates (aspirin) is common. Gluten intolerance can cause severe health problems. **KEY SYMPTOMS** • Digestive upsets • Stiffness and joint pain • Skin rashes and eczema • Respiratory problems • Persistent urinary infections, or vaginal yeast infections in candidiasis • Nervous disorders in candidiasis.	*Agrimonia eupatoria* AGRIMONY (see p. 31)	Soothes gut irritation and inflammation; heals damaged mucous membranes.
	Allium sativum GARLIC (see p. 33)　*(Bulb)*	Antifungal; useful for excess yeasts in the gut; supports recovery of gut flora.
	Calendula officinalis POT MARIGOLD (see p. 47)	Antifungal; useful for excess yeasts in the gut in candidiasis.
	Hydrastis canadensis GOLDENSEAL (see p. 74)　*(Rhizome)*	Good liver stimulant; eases gastric sensitivity; astringent and healing for mucous membranes.
HIVES (URTICARIA OR NETTLE RASH) Skin blisters and rashes caused by allergens, including foods, particularly those containing salicylates, or by contact with chemicals. The reaction is generally transient. **KEY SYMPTOM** • Irritant, red swellings on skin. *IMPORTANT: Severe reactions may lead to anaphylactic shock; seek professional help.*	*Brassica oleracea* CABBAGE (see p. 46)	Anti-inflammatory and healing; useful standby for emergencies.
	Urtica dioica STINGING NETTLE (see p. 131)	Taking nettles for nettle rash may seem a contradiction, but it can reduce itching and act as an antihistamine.
	Viola tricolor HEARTSEASE (see p. 137)	Anti-inflammatory and soothing for any skin inflammation.

CASE HISTORY
Hay fever

PATIENT: Jonathan, aged 10, was generally healthy.

HISTORY AND COMPLAINT: Jonathan suffered from hay fever every year since he was seven. He started sneezing in early spring and continued, with increasing severity, through summer. Antihistamines were proving less and less effective, and it was when the doctor suggested trying steroids that Jonathan's worried mother turned to alternative medicine.

TREATMENT: Jonathan started treatment in January with 5 ml a day of a brew containing elderflower, white horehound and ground ivy for the upper respiratory tract, with self-heal, dandelion and gentian to cool and cleanse the liver. This medication was continued until early spring. In the first year, symptoms were kept in check with eyebright and goldenseal capsules, supplemented by antihistamines in early summer when the oilseed rape crop peaked.

OUTCOME: In the first year, symptoms did not start until early summer. The next year, a similar regime reduced symptoms still further. Three years after starting treatment, the hay fever disappeared.

How to use	Combinations	Cautions
Take an infusion or tincture; or take two 200 mg capsules three times a day; bathe eyes with an eyewash containing water and 5 drops tincture.	Combine with goldenseal powder in capsules or with elderflower in an infusion or tincture. Often prescribed with *ma huang* (restricted herb in UK, Australia and New Zealand).	
Take an infusion or tincture.	Combine with anticatarrhals such as marsh cudweed, ribwort plantain and golden rod in tincture; take with chamomile in an infusion.	
Take an infusion or up to 4 ml tincture three times a day.	Add astringent anticatarrhals such as marsh cudweed or ground ivy. Take with chamomile in an infusion as an antiallergenic.	
Take an infusion or up to 4 ml tincture three times a day.	Add lemon balm and chamomile to reduce stress. Combine with soothing demulcents such as marshmallow root; take garlic or echinacea as antifungals.	
Use 1 clove a day in cooking or take two 200 mg capsules a day.	Best used as a simple, or with parsley to reduce the garlic odor.	
Take an infusion or tincture, well diluted in water.	Add antimicrobials such as echinacea, nervines such as lemon balm or anti-inflammatories and astringents such as elderflower or agrimony.	
Take two 200 mg capsules up to three times a day, or 2-4 ml doses of tincture up to three times a day.	Add powdered fenugreek or agrimony to capsules or licorice to tincture, to soothe and heal mucous membranes.	Avoid in pregnancy or high blood pressure; do not exceed the stated dose.
Apply a fresh leaf directly on to the affected part, or apply juice as a lotion.	Use as a simple. Onion can be used in the same way.	
Use in infusions, tincture or take two 200 mg capsules of powdered herb.	Use with red clover, wood betony and meadowsweet in infusions; add 20 drops *ma huang* tincture dose to reduce the allergic reaction (restricted in the UK, Australia and New Zealand).	
Take an infusion, or up to 15 ml tincture a day; also use as a wash or in an ointment or cream.	Add 1-2 drops thyme oil to 20 ml heartsease cream, or add stinging nettle to an infusion or tincture as an additional astringent.	

KEY

Aerial parts

Leaves

Petals

Root

STANDARD REMEDIES All recipes and doses are standard unless otherwise specified; see *Making Herbal Remedies, pp. 152-57.*

URINARY DISORDERS

THE KIDNEYS AND URINARY system often mirror the health of an individual: persistent cystitis sufferers know well that their symptoms increase at times of stress and fatigue. Repeated urinary infections can indicate a weak immune system. Tonic herbs and immune stimulant herbs are often needed after symptoms have eased. Herbal remedies usually include a urinary antiseptic, which often contains volatile oils that survive the digestive process, pass into the bloodstream and are excreted via the kidneys. Soothing and softening herbs are added to help reduce inflammation and repair damage to the mucous membranes, and diuretics to increase the flow of urine and flush out toxins and dead bacteria. In Chinese medicine, urinary inflammations are regarded as problems of heat and damp, and are treated with "cooling" herbs.

See also: vaginal yeast infections, pp. 204–05; incontinence, pp. 212–13; bed-wetting, pp. 218–19.

AILMENT	REMEDIES	
	Herb	*Actions*
URINARY TRACT INFECTIONS & CYSTITIS Infections of the urinary tract usually lead to cystitis in women and urethritis in men. In some cases, the kidneys are affected. KEY SYMPTOMS • Frequent, painful urination • Blood, mucus or pus in urine • Fever • Pain in the groin or mid-back. *IMPORTANT: Consult a professional practitioner if the symptoms are severe or persistent. If the infection is sexually transmitted, the case must under UK law be referred to a doctor.*	*Apium graveolens* CELERY (see p. 39)	Urinary antiseptic; cleanses uric acid from the system.
	Arctostaphylos uva-ursi BEARBERRY (see pp. 228)	Produces potent antiseptic in the kidney tubules; effective for acid urine.
	Barosma betulina BUCHU (see pp. 228)	Diuretic and urinary antiseptic; has a warming and stimulant effect on the kidneys.
	Elymus repens COUCHGRASS (see pp. 228) *(Rhizome)*	Contains mannitol (a diuretic) and mucilages to soothe mucous membranes; antibiotic.
URINARY GRAVEL Deposits of insoluble material – usually calcium salts or uric acid particles – formed in the bladder, possibly linked with changes in the acidity or alkalinity of the urine. KEY SYMPTOMS • Sensation of "grittiness" on passing urine • Blood in urine in severe cases.	*Eupatorium purpureum* GRAVELROOT (see p. 62)	Diuretic and soothing for the urinary mucous membranes; useful for all irritations.
	Juniperus communis JUNIPER (see p. 80)	Urinary antiseptic and diuretic; good for clearing acid wastes.
	Parietaria diffusa PELLITORY-OF-THE-WALL (see pp. 229)	Diuretic and demulcent; useful for pain on urination; also for kidney stones.
KIDNEY STONES Insoluble calcium or oxalates that form in the kidney, causing renal colic as they pass along the ureter to the bladder. Stones have been linked with excess calcium intake. KEY SYMPTOMS • Agonizing "loin to groin" pain due to passage of stones or gravel • Nausea and blood in the urine. *IMPORTANT: Always consult a professional practitioner.*	*Amni visnaga* KHELLA (see p. 37)	Relieves spasmodic pain by relaxing the muscles in the ureter, which helps ease the stone towards the bladder.
	Aphanes arvensis PARSLEY PIERT (see pp. 229)	Also called parsley breakstone for its ability to break down stones in the kidney or bladder; diuretic, demulcent and soothing for the urinary tract.

CASE HISTORY
Recurrent cystitis and thrush

PATIENT: Pamela, a 48 year old sales representative, married, with an adult son and a daughter of 10.

HISTORY AND COMPLAINT: Pamela had recurrent cystitis for 15 years, which was treated with regular antibiotics. Symptoms included burning when passing urine and increased frequency of urination. She was prone to yeast infections and tended to eat too much chocolate and yeast extract. Two weeks of antibiotics had had little effect on the latest flare-up of cystitis.

TREATMENT: Strictly curtailing sugar and yeast intake helped in the long-term control of yeast infections,

while medication focused on the immediate symptoms with buchu, bearberry, echinacea, cornsilk, and couchgrass. Capsules of buchu and couchgrass powder were used during the day. Tea tree suppositories were used for yeast infections, and *Lactobacillus acidophilus* capsules to restore the gut flora after the antibiotics.

OUTCOME: After six weeks, Pamela had been free of cystitis for a month. A "twinge" was treated with echinacea capsules, and she drank a weak infusion of buchu and couchgrass tea daily as a preventative. Two years later, she has only had one further bout of cystitis, again quickly treated with a similar remedy.

How to use	*Combinations*	*Cautions*
Take an infusion or up to 4 ml tincture three times a day.	Use with horsetail, cornsilk, or couchgrass to soothe inflamed mucous membranes.	Avoid in pregnancy; use untreated seeds only.
Take an infusion made with 15 g herb to 2 cups (500 ml) water, or take up to 2 ml tincture three times a day.	Combine with couchgrass and yarrow; add horsetail or pellitory-of-the-wall to heal damaged mucous membranes.	High doses may cause nausea.
Add 15 g herb to 2 cups water for an infusion, or take up to 2 ml tincture or three 200 mg capsules three times a day.	Add couchgrass and yarrow to infusion or capsules; add cornsilk if burning sensation is severe.	
Take an infusion or tincture.	Combine with buchu, bearberry, or juniper as more potent antiseptics.	
Take a decoction of 20 g herb to 2½ cups water, or up to 3 ml tincture three times a day.	Can be combined with diuretics such as parsley piert, cornsilk, couchgrass, or pellitory-of-the-wall for supportive healing action.	Use only under supervision of a professional.
Take 10 g berries infused in 2 cups water, or up to 2 ml tincture three times a day.	Add hydrangea or parsley piert to help clear stones, and add healing diuretics such as couchgrass, parsley piert, or cornsilk.	Do not take for more than 6 weeks or in pregnancy.
Take an infusion or tincture; take 20 ml doses of fresh juice.	Add buchu or bearberry for infections, or couchgrass or cornsilk to soothe and heal.	
Use in infusions or tinctures.	Use with soothing demulcents such as cornsilk or marshmallow root; add shepherd's purse to help reduce any bleeding.	Restricted herb in Australia; excessive use may cause nausea, headaches and insomnia.
Use in infusions or tinctures, up to 10 ml per dose.	Use with hydrangea, ginger, and gravelroot in tinctures; with cornsilk, pellitory-of-the-wall and khella (restricted in Australia) in infusions. Apply a hot compress of ginger to the lower abdomen if possible.	

KEY

Aerial parts

Berries

Essential oil

Leaves

Root

Seeds

STANDARD REMEDIES
All recipes and doses are standard unless otherwise specified; see *Making Herbal Remedies, pp. 152-57.*

NERVOUS DISORDERS

HOLISTIC MEDICINE FOCUSES on the needs of body, mind and spirit, and this is especially true of any condition labeled as "nerves". Physical manifestations of nervous disorders may include insomnia, palpitations, or headaches; emotional aspects include irritability, depression, anger, or guilt, while lack of determination or emptiness can typify a spiritual vacuum. Herbs can operate on the same three levels. Vervain is a good example: it is an effective liver tonic and relaxing nervine; taken in Bach flower remedy form, it is good for the perfectionist and a slightly obsessional person who tries to do too many jobs at once; on a spiritual level, it can increase understanding and psychic awareness. Herbs affect the mind and emotions in ways we are only beginning to understand. There are reports of aromatic chemicals from essential oils reaching the part of the brain that acts as a center for the emotions and has a role in memory. Small wonder, then, that scents are so evocative of past events, or that aromatic herbs can affect our emotions. In Eastern medicine, emotional imbalance is accepted as a possible cause of physical disease, and herbs are used to strengthen spiritual centers such as the *chakras*, which are located at points from the crown of the head to the base of the spine.

See also: tension headaches, pp. 166-67; neuralgia, pp. 166-67; forgetfulness or confusion in the elderly, pp. 212-13; Parkinson's disease, pp. 212-13; hyperactivity, pp. 218-19.

AILMENT	REMEDIES	
	Herb	*Actions*
ANXIETY & TENSION Excessive life stresses can lead to a variety of health problems, which are not always obviously linked to tension. **KEY SYMPTOMS** • Inability to relax • Emotional instability – tendency to cry or be irritable for no obvious reason • Headaches • Sleeplessness.	*Pulsatilla vulgans* PASQUE FLOWER (see p. 226-27)	Nervine and anodyne with sedative action; useful for nervous tension and sexual problems.
	Scutellaria lateriflora SKULLCAP (see p. 118)	Relaxant and restorative for the central nervous system; good for nervous debility.
	Stachys officinalis WOOD BETONY (see p. 121)	Sedative and calming for the nervous system; good for nervous debility, fearfulness and exhaustion.
	Tilia x *europaea* LINDEN (see p. 229)	Reduces nervous tension and helps prevent arteriosclerosis.
	Verbena officinalis VERVAIN (see p. 135)	Relaxing nervine with a tonic effect on the liver.
PANIC ATTACKS These can be associated with excessive stress, but may also be linked to food intolerance. Severe cases may need psychiatric counseling. **KEY SYMPTOMS** • Palpitations • Intense feelings of fear • Feelings of impending doom.	*Citrus aurantium* NEROLI OIL (see p. 53)	Sedative and antidepressant, traditionally used for hysteria, panic, and fearfulness; eases palpitations and cardiac spasm.
	Hyssopus officinalis HYSSOP (see p.76)	Antispasmodic and mildly analgesic, traditionally used for hysteria and some forms of epilepsy. Suitable for children.
	Piscidia erythrina JAMAICAN DOGWOOD (see p. 229)	Sedative and anodyne for severe nervous tension, insomnia or nervous migraine.
	Rosa damascena DAMASK ROSE (see pp. 110-11)	Very soothing for the nerves; antidepressant and prevents vomiting; gentle sedative.

CASE HISTORY
Lack of self-determination

PATIENT: Rosemary, 52, a recovering alcoholic in an unhappy marriage with a domineering husband.

HISTORY AND COMPLAINT: After many years of finding solace in the bottle, Rosemary started to take control of her own life again with the support of her friends, her church, and Alcoholics Anonymous. But she felt unable to leave her husband, largely because of financial considerations, and was concerned that his constant nagging would force her to start drinking again. Physical symptoms included rheumatic type pains in her legs and lower back, persistent colds, insomnia, and general lack of enthusiasm for life. A hysterectomy three years earlier had been followed by hormone replacement therapy, which she had recently stopped, leading to hot flashes and night sweats. Rosemary had also had a brief affair with a friend's husband, which left her feeling lonely and guilt-ridden.

TREATMENT: A massage oil of lavender, basil and rosemary was suggested to ease aches and pains and nervous problems, while chaste-berry and goldenseal capsules were given for menopausal symptoms. Wood betony, *gotu kola* and skullcap helped counter depression, a sense of loss and a lingering need for addiction, with *ling zhi* providing a spiritual boost and help self-determination. Herbs were taken as powders or teas, as tinctures are unsuitable for recovering alcoholics.

OUTCOME: The aches and pains disappeared within a week. Rosemary became more cheerful and her sleep improved. She began to feel that the alcohol problem was under control, and took a part-time job in a local shop, focusing her attention on outside activities. She now feels less threatened by her husband's behavior, and acknowledges that she might consider leaving him in the future. She continues to drink wood betony tea and takes *ling zhi* periodically.

How to use	*Combinations*	*Cautions*
Take up to 1 ml tincture three times a day, or add 5 g to 2½ cups water for infusion.	Can be combined with Jamaican dogwood and/or passionflower for overexcited states.	Use only the dried plant.
Take an infusion or tincture, or take powdered herb in capsules.	Use as a simple, or combine with wood betony, lavender, and lemon balm to increase calming, sedative action.	
Take an infusion or tincture, or take powdered herb in capsules.	Good as a simple, or combine with chamomile, vervain, skullcap, or lavender to enhance tonic or sedative action.	Large doses can cause vomiting. Avoid high doses in pregnancy.
Take an infusion or up to 10 ml tincture a day.	Add lemon balm and chamomile to infusion for a generally relaxing tea.	
Take an infusion or tincture.	Use as a simple, or combine with wood betony, linden, chamomile, or *gotu kola* to enhance sedative effect.	Avoid in pregnancy.
Mix 1 ml oil in 20 ml carrier oil for a massage; add 10 drops to a bath; take up to 5 ml orange flower water a day or use in cooking.	Can be combined with 5-10 drops lavender or benzoin oil to enhance calming action.	Use with caution in pregnancy.
Take an infusion or tincture; use 2-3 drops of essential oil in almond oil to massage temples and neck.	Add skullcap, passionflower, or wood betony to infusions to enhance sedative effect, if desired.	
Take a decoction or up to 5 ml tincture a day.	Add pasque flower, valerian, or hops to the tincture up to a combined total of 5 ml per dose for additional sedative action.	Do not exceed the stated dose.
Mix 2 ml rose oil in 20 ml carrier oil for a massage; add oil to baths; use rosewater as a lotion and in cooking.	Can combine with a few drops of sandalwood or lavender oil to increase calming effect.	Use only good-quality, genuine rose oil medicinally.

KEY

Aerial parts

Essential oil

Flowers

Root bark

STANDARD REMEDIES
All recipes and doses are standard unless otherwise specified; see *Making Herbal Remedies, pp. 152-57.*

AILMENT	REMEDIES	
	Herb	*Actions*
DEPRESSION Deficiency of the nervous system, traditionally associated with a surfeit of the "melancholic" humor in Galenical medicine. KEY SYMPTOMS • Misery, feeling down • Inability to concentrate • Lack of interest in the present • Withdrawn, silent demeanor • Poor digestive function with constipation.	*Avena sativa* OATS (see p. 43)	Antidepressant and restorative nerve tonic.
	Borago officinalis BORAGE (see p. 45)	Restorative for the adrenal cortex; eases depression.
	Ocimum basilicum BASIL (see p. 96)	Antidepressant and spiritually uplifting; especially effective for the lower chakras; useful to encourage earthing or "groundedness".
	Turnera diffusa DAMIANA (see p. 226-27)	Stimulating nervine; good for the male hormonal system; antidepressant.
INSOMNIA Can be associated with over-excitement, anxiety and worry, or a physical cause, such as pain, which needs treating. In Chinese medicine it can signify excessive "heart fire". KEY SYMPTOMS • Inability to fall asleep • Frequent wakefulness during the night • Restlessness, vivid dreams during sleep.	*Eschscholzia californica* CALIFORNIAN POPPY (see p. 228)	Gentle and nonaddictive hypnotic; tranquilizer and anodyne; safe for children.
	Humulus lupulus HOPS (see p. 73) *(Strobiles)*	Sedative, hypnotic and anodyne; calms excessive excitability.
	Lactuca virosa WILD LETTUCE (see p. 229)	Sedative – the latex was once known as "poor man's opium"; fresh herb is especially potent when it goes to seed; garden lettuce has a milder effect.
	Passiflora incarnata PASSIONFLOWER (see p. 99)	Sedative, hypnotic and anodyne; calms the nervous system and promotes sleep.
INABILITY TO RELAX Herbs have long been used to induce relaxation and, in traditional societies, trance-like states with altered levels of awareness. Tobacco and cannabis are still used in this way in the West. KEY SYMPTOMS • Restless, inability to sit still • Irritability, poor attention span • Constant chatter.	*Chamaemelum nobile* ROMAN CHAMOMILE (see p.88)	Sedative, carminative and antispasmodic; good for excitement and nervous stomach.
	Centella asiatica GOTU KOLA (see p. 222-23)	Relaxing and restorative for the nervous system; good for neurotic disturbances.
	Lavandula spp. LAVENDER (see p. 81)	Sedative and analgesic; antispasmodic action.
EMOTIONAL UPSETS The emotional ups and downs of life – temper tantrums, mood swings, irritability, grief – are an everyday occurrence at all ages. Specific extracts (such as Bach Flower Remedies or Bush Essences) can often help. KEY SYMPTOM • Irrational tears and anger with no apparent cause.	*Artemisia vulgaris* MUGWORT (see p. 41)	Gentle nervine; useful for menopausal tension, mild depression and stress.
	Melissa officinalis LEMON BALM (see p. 90)	Antidepressant and restorative for the nervous system.
	Valeriana officinalis VALERIAN (see p. 133)	Very potent tranquilizer; antispasmodic and mild anodyne.

How to use	*Combinations*	*Cautions*
Take a decoction or 2-3 ml fluid extract; eat as oatmeal.	Combines well with vervain in tincture, or add 10 drops lemon balm or St John's wort to the dose to enhance antidepressant action.	If sensitive to gluten, see caution p. 43.
Take 10 ml juice three times a day.	Use as a simple.	Restricted herb in Australia and New Zealand.
Eat fresh leaves; add 5 drops essential oil to bath water, or mix 1 ml in 20 ml carrier oil for massage; take up to 3 ml tincture three times a day or take an infusion.	Combine leaves with lemon balm or rose petals in an infusion; add a few drops of geranium or rose oil to massage oil to increase uplifting effects.	Do not use the oil in pregnancy.
Take up to 2.5 ml tincture three times a day, or add 20 g herb to 2 cups (500 ml) for an infusion.	Combine with oats for general depression; if anxiety is a problem, combine with St John's wort or wood betony using equal amounts of tincture up to a total of 5 ml per dose.	
Take an infusion or tincture at night.	Use as a simple or combine with passionflower, lavender, or cowslip flowers if overexcitability is a problem.	
Take up to 5 ml tincture a day, or add 10 g herb to 2 cups (500 ml) water for an infusion. Take at night.	Can be combined with additional calming herbs such as valerian or passionflower up to 5 ml tincture per dose.	Avoid in depression. Do not exceed stated dose.
Take an infusion or tincture before going to bed; the fresh leaves can also be eaten in salads.	Use as a simple, or add a few drops of cowslip flower tincture per dose if over excitability is a problem; valerian and passionflower can be added to increase tranquilizing action.	Excess can lead to insomnia and increased sexual activity; lower doses can cause sleepiness, so avoid if driving.
Take 5 ml tincture half an hour before bed, or drink a tea with 2-3 tsp herb per cup.	Add lavender and chamomile to infusion if desired.	Avoid high doses in pregnancy.
Add 2-3 drops essential oil or 2 cups (500 ml) infusion to baths; take tincture or drink chamomile tea regularly.	Use as a simple, or add lemon balm, skullcap or *gotu kola* to tincture as a restorative; combine with 2-3 drops lavender oil in baths as an additional sedative.	Avoid internal use in pregnancy. Do not exceed stated dose.
Take an infusion or tincture.	Use as a simple or mix with a little lavender or chamomile to enhance calming action.	Do not use for more than 4 weeks without a break.
Take infusion or up to 4 ml tincture per dose; massage dilute oil into temples.	Use as a simple or combine with wood betony, linden, or vervain in infusions to ease tensions and stress.	Avoid high doses in pregnancy.
Take up to 2 ml tincture three times a day, or drink a weak infusion.	Combine with wood betony, skullcap, or vervain for menopausal tension with emotional stress; combine tinctures up to a total of 5 ml per dose.	Avoid in pregnancy and when breast-feeding.
Drink fresh herb as tea, or take up to 5 ml tincture a day (more effective in low doses).	Use as a simple in tea or combine with wood betony, skullcap, or vervain tincture for sedative or restorative action.	
Take maceration, infusion or tincture; also available in 200 mg capsules or pills.	Use as a simple or add a small amount of hops if there is excitability. Support with massage using rose or lavender oils.	Can lead to over-excitedness; try a small dose first (see p. 133).

KEY

Aerial parts

Essential oil

Flowers

Leaves

Root

STANDARD REMEDIES
All recipes and doses are standard unless otherwise specified; see *Making Herbal Remedies*, pp. 152-57.

AILMENT	REMEDIES	
	Herb	*Actions*
COPING WITH STRESS Stress triggers production of adrenaline – the "flight or fight" hormone. Failure to respond physically leads to a "negative stress response" with excessive physical tension. **KEY SYMPTOMS** • Dry mouth, tendency to cry, palpitations, or panic attacks • Constant fatigue, difficulty sleeping or concentrating • Inability to relax, headaches, muscular aches and pains, stomach upsets.	*Eleutherococcus senticosus* **SIBERIAN GINSENG** (see p. 226-27)	Helps the body to cope more efficiently with stress and improves stamina. Useful as a preventative before exams, a busy time at work, or long distance air travel to combat jetlag.
	Ferula asa-foetida **ASAFOETIDA** (see p. 228) *(Resin)*	Calming and soothing to reduce nervous excitability, reduce high blood pressure and relieve stress.
	Matricaria chamomila **GERMAN CHAMOMILE** (see p. 88)	Calming and mildly sedative to encourage relaxation and also act as a tonic for the digestive system in stress-related upsets.
EXHAUSTION & FATIGUE Often dismissed as a symptom, but may be related to destructive emotions, overwork or illness. **KEY SYMPTOMS** • Difficulty getting out of bed • No energy to complete tasks • Difficulty concentrating. *IMPORTANT: Constant or excessive fatigue may be a sign of undiagnosed illness; seek professional help.*	*Panax ginseng* **KOREAN GINSENG** (see p. 98)	Energy tonic, traditionally used in China for older people and ideal to help the body adjust to changing seasons.
	Salvia officinalis Purpurescens Group or *Salvia officinalis* **PURPLE or GREEN SAGE** (see p.115)	Restorative, hormonal, and antioxidant; stimulates the nervous and digestive systems.
CHRONIC FATIGUE SYNDROME Also called post-viral syndrome or myalgic encephalomyelitis (ME), the problem has been linked to viral infection, immune weakness and psychological disturbances. **KEY SYMPTOMS** • Muscle fatigue and weakness after even minor exercise • Headaches, muscular pains, breathing problems • Difficulty concentrating.	*Astragalus membranaceous* **HUANG QI** (see p. 224-25)	Stimulating for both the immune system and energy levels; used in China as a tonic for younger people.
	Echinacea spp. **ECHINACEA** (see p. 58)	Antiviral and antifungal to combat associated infection including candidiasis.
	Withania somnifera **ASHWAGANDHA** (see p. 138)	A nutritive and rejuvenating tonic to act on both physical and mental energies.
SEASONAL AFFECTIVE DISORDER (SAD) Depression and emotional problems associated with short daylight hours. **KEY SYMPTOMS** • Seasonal depression • Insomnia, weariness.	*Hypericum perforatum* **ST JOHN'S WORT** (see p. 75) *(Flowering tops)*	Proven antidepressant increasingly used as an alternative to conventional drugs.
	Rosmarinus officinalis **ROSEMARY** (see p. 112)	Stimulating for the nervous system; antioxidant and tonifying for the digestion.
SHOCK Emotional shock is associated with sudden fears; physical shock may follow traumatic accidents. **KEY SYMPTOM** • Cold sweat, palpitations, confusion, breathlessness, shivering.	*Alpinia spp.* **GALANGAL** (see p. 35)	Warming and stimulating; especially effective for calming palpitations, irregular heartbeat and feelings of panic.
	Capsicum frutescens **CAYENNE** (see p. 50)	Stimulates blood circulation and tissues; warming, restorative and normalizing.

How to use	*Combinations*	*Cautions*
Take up to 600 mg a day for 10-14 days before the stress is due to peak.	Use as a simple or combine with reishi mushroom in capsules.	
Take up to 50 drops of tincture per dose, or up to 50 mg in pills or powders.	Use with spikenard or valerian tincture or powders to help soothe nerves.	Do not use for young children or babies.
Use in infusions.	Combine with lemon balm or wood betony in infusions; add a few jasmine flowers or *ju hua* to the mix if available.	
Best taken in periods of up to four weeks, 600 mg in capsules or pills, or up to 10 ml of tincture daily.	Use as a simple or combine with *huang qi*, ginkgo or *ashwaghanda* and a little ginger or galangal.	Avoid long-term or excessive use in pregnancy: may add to aggression in young *yang* men.
Take in an infusion, tincture or powdered in capsules (up to 1 g daily).	Use with rosemary, *gotu kola*, wood betony, hibiscus, or thyme in infusions.	Avoid high doses in pregnancy. Avoid completely in epilepsy.
Use in a tincture, decoction or powdered in capsules (up to 600 mg daily).	With ginseng and echinacea; support with evening primrose oil, zinc and vitamin C supplements and *gotu kola*, milk thistle, and cardamom in infusions.	
In a tincture, or take two 200 mg capsules daily; in decoction or infusion, depending on part used.	Combine with cleavers, milk thistle and galangal tinctures; use in infusions with *gotu kola* and in decoctions with *huang qi* or ginseng. Support with evening primrose, zinc, and vitamin C supplements.	High doses may rarely cause nausea and dizziness.
In a tincture, decoction, or use 250 mg to 1 g of powder per dose in capsules or with a little water; take up to 5 g in warm milk sweetened with a little sugar.	Add a little long pepper to enhance action; combine with ginseng and licorice in decoctions. Support with liver stimulants and 25 ml daily of cleavers juice to cleanse the lymphatic system. Eat plenty of shiitake mushrooms to help the immune system.	
In tinctures, teas or capsules.	Use with wood betony, basil, or lemon balm infusions or tinctures.	Reports suggest long-term use may be associated with cataracts.
Take the fresh or dried leaves in infusions or tinctures; use 5-10 drops of oil in bathwater.	Mix with basil, sage, and thyme for a stimulating and uplifting tea; add with 2-3 drops of rose geranium oil to baths.	
Take up to 5 drops of tincture directly on the tongue; use in a decoction.	Use the drops of tincture in a cup of skullcap infusion. Drink plenty of fluids.	
Take up to 5 drops of tincture in a little water or directly on the tongue.	Use the drops of tincture in a cup of sage or chamomile infusion. Drink plenty of fluids.	

KEY

Aerial parts

Essential oil

Flowers

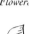
Leaves

Root

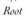

Fruit

Stem

STANDARD REMEDIES
All recipes and doses are standard unless otherwise specified; see *Making Herbal Remedies*, pp. 152-57.

GYNECOLOGICAL PROBLEMS

THE HOLISTIC APPROACH of herbal medicine is particularly relevant to the common disorders of a woman's reproductive cycle: premenstrual syndrome (PMS), period pain, menopausal problems and so on. Emotions and spiritual disharmonies can be even more significant than physical disorders. Modern Western medicine, however, all too often delivers a verdict of "no abnormalities detected" after a battery of tests, and relies on repeat prescriptions for tranquilizers, hormone replacement therapy, or even a hysterectomy. Traditional Chinese medicine closely associates the female reproductive system with the liver which, among other functions, "stores blood" and controls the flow of *qi*, or energy, around the body. Common PMS symptoms can be explained in terms of liver disharmony: irritability – the liver is associated

with anger; abdominal bloating – stagnation of *qi* in the lower abdomen; digestive upsets and sweet cravings – excess liver energy "invading the spleen" and causing deficiency and weakness. Treatment therefore often centers on herbs to stimulate and move liver energy. Modern Western herbal treatments, too, can adopt a multi-dimensional holistic approach; for example, hormone regulators like chaste-tree can be combined with uterine tonics such as motherwort or black cohosh to ease menstrual disorders. In Chinese medicine, menopausal symptoms are also explained in energy terms – as a "run-down" in kidney energy. The kidney is considered to store the body's "vital essence" or *jing*, which can be considered the body's life force – a combination of creative and reproductive energies. Menopausal syndrome can be

AILMENT	REMEDIES	
	Herb	*Actions*
PREMENSTRUAL SYNDROME (PMS) This can be associated with hormonal imbalance or stagnant *qi* levels. **KEY SYMPTOMS** • Irritability or anger • Depression and emotional upsets • Abdominal bloating • Breast swelling and tenderness • Food cravings (especially for sweet foods) • Constipation and/or diarrhea.	*Alchemilla xanthoclora* LADY'S MANTLE (see p. 32)	Regulates menstrual cycle with gentle hormonal action; astringent.
	Oenothera biennis EVENING PRIMROSE (see p. 228)	Contains γ-linolenic acid for prostaglandin production; eases breast tenderness.
	Paeonia lactiflora BAI SHAO YAO (see p. 97)	Balances liver function and soothes liver energy; nourishes blood and *yin*.
	Vitex agnus-castus CHASTE-TREE (see p. 228)	Acts on the pituitary gland to stimulate and normalize hormonal function.
PERIOD PAIN Also known as dysmenorrhea, this may be due to blood stagnation before bleeding starts, or to uterine cramps once the flow begins. **KEY SYMPTOMS** • Lower abdominal pain either before or at the start of a period • Pain spreading to thighs or legs • Abdominal bloating • Flow may be light or have excessive clots.	*Angelica polyphorma* var. *sinensis* DANG GUI (see p. 38)	Regulates menstrual function; nourishes the blood; liver *qi* stimulant.
	Caulophyllum thalictroides BLUE COHOSH (see p. 228) (Rhizome)	Antispasmodic with steroidal component that stimulates the uterus; good for pain due to blood stagnation.
	Pulsatilla vulgaris PASQUE FLOWER (see p. 226-27)	Nervine and anodyne; good for all pains involving reproductive organs.
	Viburnum prunifolium BLACK HAW (see p. 136)	Antispasmodic for uterine muscle; symptomatic remedy for cramping pain.

explained in terms of kidney energy weakness affecting both liver and heart functions (see pp. 14-15) and causing symptoms such as night sweats, hot flashes, palpitations, back pain, and irritability. Treatments therefore generally focus on kidney or liver tonics or calming heart herbs. In Ayurvedic medicine, sexual energy is seen as an aspect of the creative and spiritual forces and should be respected as such. Ayurveda also sees the reproductive organs as linked to some of the *chakras* or energy centers within the body, the root *chakra* being associated with our sense of belonging, or "groundedness". Women who are unhappy with their role in life may suffer from reproductive disorders as a physical aspect of this disharmony. A hysterectomy can also unsettle the root *chakra*, leaving some women unable to concentrate, settle or relax. They seem to have a restless, rootless quality that can be difficult to ease.

CASE HISTORY
Premenstrual syndrome

PATIENT: Lucy, a 29 year old marketing manager, found her job very stressful. She faced pressure from her mother to start a family, and from her live-in boyfriend to fulfill a domestic role.

HISTORY AND COMPLAINT: Lucy suffered from classic PMS symptoms: mood swings with extremes of irritability, abdominal bloating, and tender, swollen breasts, plus painful, heavy periods.

TREATMENT: She was advised to spend at least ten minutes relaxing every day to help her unwind, and was also given a prescription for liver *qi* stagnation, which included *chai hu, bai shao yao, bai zhu, fu ling*, peppermint, ginger and licorice.

OUTCOME: Within six weeks, Lucy's PMS was greatly reduced, with little fluid retention and much less irritability. Over the next two months, her irregular menstrual cycle returned to normal, menstrual cramps lessened and breast tenderness gradually disappeared.

How to use	*Combinations*	*Cautions*
Take a tincture or use an infusion with other herbs.	Combine with 10-20 drops black cohosh, pasque flower, mugwort, or *dang gui* tinctures per dose, or add white deadnettle or wood betony to the infusion.	Avoid in pregnancy.
Take 250-500 mg in capsules a day.	Use as a simple, but can be combined with other PMS strategies such as vitamin B supplements.	
Best used in combinations; or in a decoction of 40 g to 2 cups (500 ml) water in three doses.	Mix 10 g *bai shao yao* with 5 g each of *bai zhu, dang gui, chai hu*, licorice, *fu ling*, and 1 g ginger. Add 5 g *chen pi* for breast tenderness.	Avoid if symptoms include diarrhea.
Take 10 drops tincture in water each morning in the second half of the cycle.	Use as a simple, but can be combined with other PMS strategies such as evening primrose oil and vitamin B supplements.	High doses can cause a sensation of ants creeping over the skin.
Best used in combinations; add 30 g herb to 2 cups (500 ml) water for a decoction and take in three doses.	Combine with 5-10 g *chai hu*, mugwort, *bai shao yao*, or *chuan xiong* in a decoction. Available in many patent remedy forms in Chinese herb shops.	Avoid regular or large doses in pregnancy.
Use a tincture or decoction; best used in combinations.	Add 1-2 ml skullcap, motherwort, yarrow, false unicorn root, *mu dan pi*, or *chi shao yao* tinctures per dose.	Avoid in early pregnancy.
Take up to 20 drops tincture three times a day for symptomatic relief, or add 5 g herb to 2 cups water for an infusion.	Add 10-15 g St. John's wort to the infusion.	Use only the dried plant.
Take 20 ml tincture in water; repeat up to three times if necessary.	Use as a simple or with 20-30 drops Jamaican dogwood tincture per dose.	

KEY

Aerial parts

Berries

Seed oil

Root

Root bark

STANDARD REMEDIES
All recipes and doses are standard unless otherwise specified; see *Making Herbal Remedies, pp. 152-57.*

AILMENT	REMEDIES	
	Herb	*Actions*
HEAVY PERIODS Also known as menorrhagia, this condition often appears to have no pathological cause and herbs can help. Heavy periods increase the risk of anemia. **KEY SYMPTOMS** • Excessive bleeding • Excessive clots • Prolonged bleeding – more than seven days • Shortened menstrual cycle. *IMPORTANT: Seek professional advice if there is a sudden or unusual change in menstrual flow.*	*Artemisia vulgaris* var. *indicus* AI YE (see p. 41)	Styptic and warming herb for the meridians; useful if bleeding is prolonged.
	Calendula officinalis POT MARIGOLD (see p. 47)	Astringent with wide-ranging action for regulating menstrual cycle.
	Capsella bursa-pastoris SHEPHERD'S PURSE (see p. 49)	Astringent and antihemorrhagic herb specific for urogenital bleeding; eases root *chakra*.
	Lamium album WHITE DEADNETTLE (see p. 229)	Astringent and anti-spasmodic; regulates uterine blood flow and acts on reproductive organs.
MENOPAUSAL SYNDROME This is associated with hormonal changes and, in Chinese medicine, with kidney *qi* weakness. **KEY SYMPTOMS** • Irregular menstruation • Hot flashes and night sweats • Mood swings and depression • Vaginal dryness (eyes may also be dry) • Palpitations • Possible hypertension • Forgetfulness.	*Chamaelirium luteum* FALSE UNICORN ROOT (see p. 228) *(Rhizome)*	Stimulates ovarian hormones, and can be helpful for early menopause after hysterectomy, or to restart the system after years of contraceptives.
	Leonurus cardiaca MOTHERWORT (see p. 82)	Sedative, heart tonic and uterine stimulant; good for palpitations and anxiety.
	Polygonum multiflorum HE SHOU WU (see p. 224-25) *(Tuber)*	Kidney *qi* tonic; nourishes the blood; useful for early menopause.
	Vitex agnus-castus CHASTE-TREE (see p. 228)	Acts on the pituitary gland to stimulate and normalize hormonal function; can be helpful after hysterectomy.
VAGINAL YEAST INFECTIONS Often related to general systemic weakness, allowing opportunist yeasts to proliferate. **KEY SYMPTOMS** • Milky discharge, itching.	*Calendula officinalis* POT MARIGOLD (see p. 47)	Antifungal, astringent, and healing.
	Melaleuca alternifolia TEA TREE (see p. 89)	Effective antifungal that does not irritate the vaginal membranes.
VAGINAL ITCHING Irritation that can be associated with menopausal syndrome, psychological factors or infection. **KEY SYMPTOMS** • Itching and dryness • Possible pain on intercourse.	*Rosa damascena* DAMASK ROSE (see pp. 110-11)	Cooling, soothing, astringent, and anti-inflammatory with an uplifting effect to drive away melancholy.
	Verbena officinalis VERVAIN (see p. 135)	Gentle nervine, stimulating for liver and uterus; antidepressant and energizing.
HYSTERECTOMY Postoperative help can relieve symptoms of premature meno-pause or disordered root *chakra*. **KEY SYMPTOMS** • Menopausal syndrome • Difficulty concentrating, forgetfulness • Irritability and excitability • Lack of calm and contentment.	*Ligustrum lucidum* NU ZHEN ZI (see p. 229)	Stimulates kidney energy and alleviates symptoms of early menopause.
	Ocimum basilicum BASIL (see p.96)	Antidepressant; tonic for root *chakra*; stimulates adrenal cortex and kidney *yang*.
	Stachys officinalis WOOD BETONY (see p. 121)	Sedative, stimulant for cerebral circulation and root *chakra*; eases fears and worry.

How to use	*Combinations*	*Cautions*
Add 15 g herb to 2 cups (500 ml) water for an infusion, or take up to 2.5 ml tincture three times a day.	Add shepherd's purse, self-heal, or *bhringaraj* to tincture or infusion, or combine with *dang gui* in a decoction.	Do not use in pregnancy without professional advice.
Take an infusion or tincture.	Add 1 ml shepherd's purse, lady's mantle, or American cranesbill tincture per dose as additional astringents.	
Take an infusion or tincture.	Add 5 drops goldenseal tincture per dose or add white deadnettle to infusion.	
Take an infusion or tincture.	Combine with American cranesbill or lady's mantle.	
Take 5-10 drops tincture four to six times a day.	Use as a simple or combine with 5 drops lady's mantle, or 2-3 ml black cohosh or Mexican wild yam tincture per dose. Ease any vaginal dryness with pot marigold cream with 1-2 drops of rose oil added.	
Take an infusion or tincture.	Combine with other sedative nervines like lavender or vervain, or with sage and mugwort to ease night sweats.	Avoid in pregnancy.
Best used in combinations in a decoction of 50 g herb to 3 cups water or tonic wine.	Combine with *nu zhen zhi, gou qi zi, shu di huang* or cinnamon in a decoction.	Avoid if symptoms include diarrhea.
Take 10 drops tincture in water each morning, or take two 200 mg capsules of powdered herb.	Use as a simple or combine 15 g powder with 5 g goldenseal powder in capsules to relieve hot flashes and other symptoms.	High doses can cause a sensation of ants creeping over the skin.
Use an infusion as a douche; apply cream or use infused oil as a lotion.	Add 5 drops echinacea to the douche or take garlic internally.	
Dilute 5 ml oil in 15 ml carrier oil and put 5 drops on a tampon and insert for 4 hours; use in vaginal suppositories or cream.	Use as a simple, or combine with infused marigold oil on a tampon, or add 20 drops tea tree oil and 10 drops thyme oil to 20 g cocoa butter for 12 vaginal suppositories.	
Use rosewater as a lotion, or add 2 drops essential oil to cream.	Make a cream with 10 ml pasque flower tincture, 20 ml lady's mantle tincture and 20 ml rosewater in 50-70 ml emulsifying ointment.	Use only the best quality, genuine rose oil medicinally.
Take an infusion or up to 5 ml tincture three times a day.	Combine with lavender, oats or lady's mantle; useful for itching of nervous origin.	Avoid in pregnancy.
Take a tincture or use in combination with other herbs in a decoction.	Add tonics such as *he shou wu, wu wei zi* or reishi; add 1-2 ml rose or wood betony tincture for additional support.	
Eat 2-3 fresh leaves with salads; take a tincture or use dilute oil for a massage.	Add 2 drops rose oil to 5 ml basil oil in 45 ml carrier oil for a massage; add 10-20 drops pasque flower tincture per dose.	
Take an infusion or tincture.	Combine with lavender, vervain, or basil in tincture and infusion or add 10-20 drops chaste-tree tincture to the morning dose.	

KEY

 Aerial parts

 Berries

 Essential oil

 Flowers

 Leaves

 Petals

 Root

STANDARD REMEDIES All recipes and doses are standard unless otherwise specified; see *Making Herbal Remedies*, pp. 152-57.

PREGNANCY & CHILDBIRTH

FOR GENERATIONS OF WOMEN, herbal remedies were the only option for easing the ills of pregnancy and the trials of childbirth. Although these days we are far more cautious about using herbs during pregnancy, they still have an important role to play. They provide a safe alternative to conventional drugs, which can be harmful: butternut, for example, is a gentle laxative; nettle tea, watercress, or burdock can help anemia, while powdered slippery elm or marshmallow root will ease heartburn. Morning sickness is often best treated with a variety of remedies; women who feel sick much of the time may find that a regular repeated remedy may increase nausea. A selection of tinctures in drop doses is the best solution. The uterus can be prepared for the exertions of childbirth with tonic herbs or dilute jasmine oil massaged into the abdomen during the last three weeks. After the birth, basil and motherwort tea can help clear the placenta, and new mothers should take homeopathic *Arnica 6x* pills every 15-30 minutes for a few hours to help repair stressed tissues.

See also: cramp, pp. 164-65; backache, pp.164-65; anemia, pp. 184-85; constipation, pp. 186-87; heartburn, pp. 188-89.

AILMENT	REMEDIES	
	Herb	*Actions*
PROBLEMS WITH INFERTILITY Herbs can help improve health and readiness for conception, but they are not a magic formula for success, nor can they solve the mechanical causes of infertility, such as blocked Fallopian tubes. Professional herbal treatment can help if endometriosis, candidiasis, chronic cystitis, or ovarian cysts are interfering with conception.	*Chamaelirium luteum* **FALSE UNICORN ROOT** (see p. 228) *(Rhizome)*	Potent uterine and hormone tonic; helpful for weaknesses in the female reproductive system, including inflammations of the Fallopian tubes
	Angelica polyphorma var. *sinensis* **DANG GUI** (see p. 38)	Nourishing tonic for the reproductive system; helps to strengthen and normalize the menstrual cycle.
	Alchemilla xanthoclora **LADY'S MANTLE** (see p. 32)	Acts to regulate the menstrual cycle and normalize function.
MORNING SICKNESS Nausea and vomiting (in first three months of pregnancy), often when waking, but may last all day. Severe cases (*hyperemesis gravidarum*) may require hospital treatment because of the risk of liver disease and dehydration. **KEY SYMPTOMS** • Vomiting when waking • Feelings of nausea.	*Ballota nigra* **BLACK HOREHOUND** (see p. 228-29)	Prevents vomiting; sedative; useful for nervous dyspepsia.
	Matricaria recutita **GERMAN CHAMOMILE** (see p. 88)	Reduces feelings of nausea and calm the stomach; relaxing nervine in stressful situations.
	Zingiber officinalis **GINGER** (see p. 139)	Prevents vomiting; has been used successfully in hospital trials involving *hyperemesis gravidarum* patients.
PREPARATION FOR BIRTH Herbs have long been used to help the body prepare for childbirth by tonifying the uterine muscles.	*Mitchella repens* **SQUAW VINE** (see p. 229)	Uterine tonic and stimulant; astringent and restorative for the nervous system.
	Rubus idaeus **RASPBERRY** (see p. 113)	Tonifies the uterus.
LABOR Herbal support during labor depends on a sympathetic midwife or doctor. During the first stage, before orthodox medicine takes over, herbal infusions can help to calm the nerves, stimulate the womb and encourage regular contractions.	*Stachys officinalis* **WOOD BETONY** (see p. 121)	Stimulates the uterus to encourage contractions, while its sedative effect helps calm the mother.
	Jasminium officinale **JASMINE** (see p. 78)	Tonifying and stimulating for the uterus to encourage contractions and parturition; mildly anesthetic and sedative to calm the mother.

CASE HISTORY
Bleeding in pregnancy

PATIENT: Julie, 32, happily married with two daughters aged 2 and 4, and starting her third pregnancy.

HISTORY AND COMPLAINT: Julie suffered from continuous bleeding throughout her first two pregnancies, and spent much of the nine months confined to bed. With two active young children, she was worried that the third pregnancy would be the same – leading to severe disruption for the entire family. This time, light spotting started during the sixth week of her pregnancy. In traditional Chinese medicine, many uterine bleeding disorders can be attributed to a weakness in the *chong* (vital) and *ren* (responsibility) channels – what we in the West regard as acupuncture meridians. The *ren* channel is regarded

as being closely related to all the *yin* channels in the body, and is also called the "conception vessel", as it starts in the uterus. The *chong* channel communicates with all the other channels and also starts in the uterus. These channels are associated with childbirth, and any "coldness" and deficiency here can lead to bleeding during or after pregnancy.

TREATMENT: Herbal capsules containing *dang gui, shu di huang, ai ye, bai shao yao*, licorice, and *chuan xiong* were used to warm and nourish the deficient channels.

OUTCOME: Within two weeks, the uterine bleeding stopped. Julie continued with a normal pregnancy, and produced a healthy daughter at term.

KEY

 Aerial parts

 Flowers

 Leaves

 Root

 Essential Oil

How to use	*Combinations*	*Cautions*
Take a decoction (1 tsp per cup simmered for 20 minutes), or up to 5 ml tincture per dose.	Combine with black cohosh; add Siberian ginseng or valerian if stress is a factor.	Excess may cause nausea and vomiting.
Take a tincture, decoction, or 600 mg powdered root in capsules daily.	Use as a simple; take 10 drops of chaste tree tincture daily to help regulate hormones, if required.	Limit to 10 days from the start of each period.
Take in an infusion or tincture.	Use with red clover flowers, stinging nettles, and marigold petals (2 tsp of mix per cup) as a tonic for the female reproductive system.	Limit to 10 days from the start of each period.
Take up to 2 ml tincture in hot water up to three times a day, or sip a weak infusion.	Alternate with other remedies if symptoms persist.	
Drink one cup infusion before rising or take 5-10 drops tincture as required (up to 5 ml a day).	Best as a simple, but can alternate with lemon balm, fennel, basil, ginger, or peppermint if needed.	Do not exceed stated dose.
Take up to 1 g powdered herb in capsules per dose, or take 2-5 drops tincture (up to 1 ml a day).	Best as a simple, but alternate with other remedies as required.	Do not exceed stated dose; use with care in early pregnancy.
Take one cup infusion a day in the last two months of pregnancy.	Use as a simple or combine with raspberry leaves.	
Take one cup infusion a day in the last two months of pregnancy.	Use as a simple during pregnancy; add rose petals and wood betony to infusion during labor.	
Take regular sips of an infusion throughout the first stage of labor.	Use with rose petals, motherwort, squaw vine, and raspberry leaves.	Avoid during pregnancy except in labor.
Use 5 drops in 5 ml of almond oil as abdominal massage during labor. Use the flowers in an infusion to soak a hot compress and apply to lower abdomen.	Use with 5 drops of lavender essential oil or add 2 drops of clove or nutmeg oil; adding 1 drop sage oil may also help but can overstimulate, so use with care. Add marigold, mugwort or wood betony to the compress infusion.	An expensive oil that is often adulterated, so buy only from reliable sources.

STANDARD REMEDIES All recipes and doses are standard unless otherwise specified; see *Making Herbal Remedies, pp. 152-57.*

AILMENT	REMEDIES	
	Herb	*Actions*
PERINEAL TEARS Tears in the perineum can be painful and slow to heal. These herbs also help bruising and soreness. KEY SYMPTOM • Tears in the perineum during birth, which may require stitches.	*Hypericum perforatum* ST. JOHN'S WORT (see p. 75) *(Flowering tops)*	Anti-inflammatory, healing and astringent.
	Ranunculus ficaria PILEWORT (see p. 229)	Very astringent.
	Symphytum officinale COMFREY (see p. 123)	Healing; encourages cell growth and can help to limit scar tissue.
SORE NIPPLES Sore nipples during breast-feeding may be due to the baby's inability to latch on correctly. The whole areola (dark area around the nipple) needs to be sucked, not just the nipple. Yeast infections can also cause irritation. KEY SYMPTOM • Sore, cracked nipples.	*Calendula officinalis* POT MARIGOLD (see p. 47)	Antiseptic, antifungal, anti-inflammatory, and soothing for dry skin and yeast infections.
	Matricaria recutita GERMAN CHAMOMILE (see p. 88)	Anti-inflammatory and antimicrobial to combat possible infections and soreness.
MASTITIS & ENGORGEMENT Engorgement is most common in the first five days after birth when the milk may be far in excess of the baby's needs. Mastitis is usually caused by bacterial infection through cracked nipples or blocked milk ducts. KEY SYMPTOMS • Pain and inflammation • Lumpy, tender breasts.	*Brassica oleracea* CABBAGE (see p. 46)	Anti-inflammatory and healing; relieves both mastitis and engorgement.
	Salvia officinalis SAGE (see p. 115)	Hormonal and drying for body secretions, helping to reduce milk flow.
INSUFFICIENT MILK A poor milk supply can be related to inadequate nutrition, stress, or lack of rest – although some women are just naturally short of milk. Large babies can also prove very demanding and it may be necessary to supplement feeding from an early stage.	*Anethum graveolens* DILL (see p. 228)	Stimulates milk flow and is carminative, helping to combat colic and gas in the baby as well.
	Galega officinalis GOAT'S RUE (see p. 228)	Stimulates milk flow.
INVOLUTION OF THE UTERUS Following the birth, the uterus gradually contracts back to its pre-pregnancy shape, leading to uncomfortable after pains in the first few days. Complete involution can take two months, and is helped by breast-feeding, which releases the hormone oxytocin into the blood stream to improve lactation, so after pains are common at feed times. KEY SYMPTOM • Cramping pains, often at feeding times.	*Cimifuga racemosa* BLACK COHOSH (see p. 51)	Antispasmodic and relaxing for the uterus; mild analgesic with an aspirin-like action.
	Viburnum prunifolium BLACK HAW (see p. 136)	Specific antispasmodic for the uterus, helping to ease painful contractions; also sedative and calming for the nervous system.
	Caulophyllum thalictroides BLUE COHOSH (see p. 228) *(Rhizome)*	Oxytocic (encourages uterine contractions) to stimulate the womb; also helpful to speed labor and help combat exhaustion in childbirth.

How to use	*Combinations*	*Cautions*
Apply the infused oil or add a strong infusion to a hip bath.	Add lavender and marigold oils to infused oil, or add the dried herbs to infusion for baths.	
Apply cream to affected areas.	Combines well with witch hazel.	Do not take internally.
Apply cream, infused oil or ointment to affected areas, or add an infusion to a hip bath.	Mix 2 ml lavender oil in 20 ml infused oil base.	Can cause rapid healing: use only on clean wounds.
Apply cream to sore nipples after every feeding.	Use as a simple, or combine with squaw vine in a cream.	
Use one drop of oil in a little breast milk or wheatgerm oil to massage the nipple after feedings; use flowers in creams or a compress soaked in infusion.	Use as a simple or combine with marigold in creams and compresses.	
Place a slightly softened fresh leaf between the breast and the bra.	Use as a simple. A poultice of fresh common plantain leaves is a good alternative to cabbage. An infusion of red clover, chamomile and marigold flowers (1 tsp per cup) taken 3-4 times a day will also help.	
Drink half a cup sage infusion once or twice a day; at weaning, increase to one cup three times daily to dry up milk completely.	In engorgement, express surplus milk with a hand pump; using a warm compress soaked in lavender or chamomile infusion will help encourage milk flow.	Do not take in excess if continuing breast-feeding.
Take 3 cups of infusion daily; vary the mix with additional herbs to avoid becoming bored with the flavor.	Use with any of the herbs listed with goat's rue below. Add borage or vervain for mild depression. Take 10 drops of chaste-tree or saw palmetto tincture to stimulate hormones and tonify the mammary glands.	Strong tasting herbs may flavor the breast milk.
Add 15 g herb to 2 cups (500 ml) water for an infusion, or take up to 2 ml tincture per dose.	Can combine with other herbs, such as fennel, dill, fenugreek, vervain, borage, stinging nettles, and milk thistle, to promote milk flow.	
Take 10 drops of tincture in a little water as required up to 5 ml per day (100 drops) total.	Use with blue cohosh; add to raspberry leaf or squaw vine infusions.	Excess can cause nausea and vomiting.
Use in a decoction or tincture (up to 10 ml per dose).	Use with wild yam in decoctions or add the tincture to raspberry leaf or squaw vine infusions with a pinch of grated ginger.	
Use drops of tincture diluted in a little water on the tongue as required, or up to 1 g of powder per dose stirred into warm milk.	Use with black cohosh or mugwort in tinctures, or use betony tea sweetened with a little honey instead of milk.	Avoid in the first six months of pregnancy.

KEY

Aerial parts

Essential oil

Flowers

Leaves

Root

Petals

Root bark

STANDARD REMEDIES
All recipes and doses are standard unless otherwise specified; see *Making Herbal Remedies, pp. 152-57.*

MALE REPRODUCTIVE PROBLEMS

MEN ARE OFTEN MORE reluctant than women to seek help for health problems – doubly so with disorders that involve the reproductive system, so that prostate and testicular cancers often go undiagnosed. Regular health checks for both these ailments are essential. The prostate gland contributes to the seminal fluid and opens into the ureter, just below the bladder. Its benign enlargement, common in older men, is believed to be caused by the conversion of the male hormone testosterone into dihydrotesterone. Saw palmetto, long used for prostate problems, is now known to prevent this conversion, so can actually combat the likely underlying causes of enlargement. Physical inactivity may also trigger prostate problems, especially in the newly-retired, when creative energies and vigor may stagnate and decline. The gland's growth restricts urine flow and leads to characteristic hesitancy and dribbling, while retention of urine can result in low-grade urinary infection with lethargy and fatigue, which in turn contributes to physical inactivity and weight gain. Keeping active is important to maintain energies and vigor. In Chinese medicine, reproductive energies – also associated with creativity – reside in the kidneys. The energy supply is limited and nonrenewable. Ayurveda, too, makes the same connection between sexual and creative energies, while both

See also: low back pain, pp. 164-65; urethritis, pp. 194-95.

AILMENT	REMEDIES	
	Herb	*Actions*
IMPOTENCE/LOSS OF LIBIDO Stress, overwork, alcohol, and excess caffeine can all contribute to low libido. Physical causes include painful hemorroids.	*Tunera diffusa* var. *aphrodisiaca* DAMIANA (see p. 226-27)	Aphrodisiac and antidepressant; uplifting for the nervous system; stimulates sexual performance.
KEY SYMPTOMS • Little interest in sexual activity • Difficulty achieving or sustaining an erection • Premature ejaculation.	*Withania somnifera* ASHWAGANDHA (see p. 138)	Stimulating aphrodisiac and rejuvenative tonic to benefit the whole system and enhance sexual performance.
INFERTILITY Recent studies suggest that junk food and contaminants in the form of pesticides or polluted water contribute to a low sperm count.	*Centella asiatica* GOTU KOLA (see p. 222-23)	Rejuvenating and stimulating tonic to increase energies.
KEY SYMPTOMS • Problems with conception • Low sperm count.	*Polygonum multiflorum* HE SHOU WU (see p. 224-25)	Kidney tonic to stimulate reproductive energies.
PROSTATE PROBLEMS Prostatitis is an inflammation often associated with infection of the prostate gland; benign prostate enlargement is common in men over 50.	*Hydrangea arborescens* HYDRANGEA (see p. 229) *(Root & rhizome)*	Diuretic and soothing, helpful in prostatitis or when prostate enlargement leads to urine retention and infection.
KEY SYMPTOMS • Frequent urination, urgency at night • Pain in crotch and lower back • Dribbling and difficulty with urination • Retention of urine may be acute. *IMPORTANT: Any prostate enlargement requires professional evaluation to check for possible malignancy.*	*Lamium album* WHITE DEADNETTLE (see p. 229)	Astringent and soothing with a specific action on the reproductive system, reducing benign prostate enlargement.
	Serenoa serrulata SAW PALMETTO (see p. 226-27)	Diuretic; urinary antiseptic with specific hormonal action on the male reproductive system, reducing benign prostate enlargement.
	Urtica dioica STINGING NETTLE (see p. 131)	Extracts from root and leaves have been shown in studies to combat prostate enlargement and reduce symptoms.

theories argue that this vital energy can be damaged by excessive sexual activity. Sexual exhaustion, they argue, leads to debility, fatigue, loss of libido, and impotence. Modern Western society tends to place great emphasis on the importance of the male sex drive, and impotence is more often associated with stress, nervous tension and overwork, or occasionally physical problems needing surgery. In contrast, Eastern medicine will advise sexual abstinence as a treatment for impotence, using tonic herbs for the kidney to restore energies: *ashwagandha*, *shatavari*, *bala*, *shu di huang*, *shan yao* and *jin yin zi* are among the herbs used for male reproductive problems by strengthening kidney energies. The well-known aphrodisiac tonics of Ayurveda (pp. 222-23) are used not only to strengthen sexual energies, but also as a means of refreshing creative and spiritual energies.

CASE HISTORY
Benign prostate enlargement

PATIENT: George, 58, divorced with a younger partner, was stressed at work and hoping for early retirement.

HISTORY AND COMPLAINT: George complained of a lack of energy, fatigue, and increased frequency of urination, especially at night, coupled with hesitancy. His doctor confirmed mild benign prostate enlargement and suggested that surgery might be necessary, while offering antibiotics to combat any infection.

TREATMENT: George was given a tincture containing saw palmetto, Siberian ginseng, and hydrangea. *Ashwagandha* pills were given as a supplement with buchu and couchgrass tea used to combat infection.

OUTCOME: Within six weeks symptoms were reduced. Medication has continued, with the dosage reduced to a low maintenance level. Surgery has been averted.

How to use	Combinations	Cautions
Use in infusions, pills or tinctures.	Add a clove to each cup of infusion, or add saw palmetto, *ashwagandha* or Koran ginseng to tinctures; traditionally combined in pills with cola and saw palmetto. Take vervain tea if premature ejaculation is a problem.	
Take in milk decoction or capsules, up to 1 g per dose, or use powder in warm milk sweetened with sugar.	Use with ginseng or saw palmetto; add a pinch of long pepper to decoctions. Massage before love making can also help: use 1 drop of rose oil and 5 drops of sandalwood in 5 ml almond oil as a body massage for both partners.	
In infusions, tinctures or capsules.	With damiana in infusions; add skullcap, vervain or chamomile if stress is contributing to the problem.	
Use in decoctions, tinctures, tonic wine or capsules.	Add one clove to each cup of decoction; use in tonic wine with ginseng or *ashwagandha*.	Avoid in diarrhea associated with spleen weakness or phlegm.
Use in decoction or tinctures.	Use with bearberry, yarrow, or buchu in prostatitis; with saw palmetto and pasque flower in benign prostate enlargement.	
Take an infusion or up to 15 ml tincture a day.	Use as a simple or with cornsilk, hydrangea, or couchgrass as a healing diuretic and to enhance the action on the prostate.	
Add 10 g berries to 2 cups (500 ml) water for a decoction, or take up to 2 ml tincture three times a day.	Use as a simple or combine with hydrangea and horsetail to increase action on the prostate.	
Use in infusion, decoctions, tinctures or capsules.	Use with white deadnettle, horsetail, or marshmallow leaf; take echinacea pills if there is associated infection.	

KEY

Aerial parts

Petals

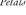

Root

Fruit

STANDARD REMEDIES All recipes and doses are standard unless otherwise specified; see *Making Herbal Remedies, pp. 152-57.*

PROBLEMS OF THE ELDERLY

FOR THOSE PEOPLE WHO REGARD the body as a machine, the problems of old age are associated with mechanical decay – joints suffer from wear and tear, leading to osteoarthritis; the digestive system rebels against a lifetime of low fiber foods and laxatives, leading to constipation or diverticulosis; and mental acuity is blunted. In Chinese medicine, the problems of old age are more likely to be associated with a rundown in vital energy: declining kidney essence – a key factor in menopausal syndrome (see pp. 204-05) – can account for the incontinence, tinnitus and deafness that affect so many old people. Strengthening tonic herbs like *he shou wu, nu zhen zi* or *bhringaraj* can often help with these problems. The Chinese also use *qi*, or energy,

weakness to explain some of the constipation problems of the elderly – a specific herb for this is *huo ma ren*, the seeds of *Cannabis sativa* or marijuana. (In the West, these are generally supplied pre-boiled, to prevent illicit cultivation.) Depending on precise symptoms, these may be prescribed in combination with herbs like apricot seeds (*xing ren*), bitter orange, *bai shao yao*, rhubarb root, or *dang gui*. Herbal tonics can also counter symptoms of mental confusion: in China, ginseng has always been popular among those wealthy enough to afford it, while in Ayurvedic medicine *Chyavan Prash* (see pp. 222-23), a mixture of around 20 herbs, sometimes with silver or gold foil added, has a similar role. Such *qi* tonics may not prevent

See also: arthritis, pp. 162-63; constipation, pp. 186-87; prostate problems, pp. 210-11; tonic herbs, pp. 222-27.

AILMENT	REMEDIES	
	Herb	*Actions*
HARDENING ARTERIES Fatty deposits in the arteries lead to restricted blood supply and increase the risk of heart attacks and strokes; in the elderly hardening of the cerebral arteries can also increase confusion. **KEY SYMPTOM** • Depending on arteries affected, there may be cold feet and hands, pallor, mental confusion, breathlessness, or heart disorders.	*Ginkgo biloba* GINKGO (see p. 69)	Improves and tonifies circulation, especially cerebral circulation; inhibits platelet activating factor.
	Vinca major GREATER PERIWINKLE (see p. 228)	Contains vincamine, which improves blood flow, and can be helpful after a stroke.
	Viscum album MISTLETOE (see p. 229)	Strengthens capillary walls; reduces inflammation and encourages repair; cardiac depressant; slows heart rate.
INCONTINENCE Involuntary urination, which may be associated with weakened pelvic floor muscles, obstruction to the bladder outflow, or lack of kidney *qi*. **KEY SYMPTOMS** • Urgent and frequent urination • Bed-wetting • Leakage with coughing or laughing.	*Astragalus membranaceus* HUANG QI (see p. 224-25)	Replenishes vital energy and helps to regulate water metabolism.
	Cupressus sempervirens CYPRESS (see p. 228)	Astringent and relaxing oil, good for all types of excess fluid production.
	Equisetum arvense HORSETAIL (see p. 60)	Healing and tonic for the urinary mucous membranes.
FORGETFULNESS OR CONFUSION This is common in old age, and can be helped by tonic herbs to strengthen the kidney *qi, yin* or *yang* energies, as appropriate (see pp. 178-79).	*Centella asiatica* GOTU KOLA (see p. 222-23)	Used in Ayurvedic medicine to promote mental calm and clarity.
	Emblica officinalis AMALAKI (see p. 222-23)	Yin tonic; widely used in Ayurvedic medicine for senility.
	Salvia officinalis "Purpurescens Group" PURPLE SAGE (see p. 115)	Traditional ingredient of many medieval longevity tonics; good *qi* tonic.

dementia, but they can certainly improve energy levels and increase alertness. Herbs can also help in distressing conditions like Parkinson's disease. Deadly nightshade, a highly toxic remedy unsuitable for home use, was the main treatment for Parkinsonism until recently. As well as reducing salivation, this antispasmodic herb helps to control tremors, and is the original source of atropine, which is still prescribed by conventional practitioners for the disease. The related plants henbane and thorn apple can also be effective, but are not for home use. Some argue that the whole plants are considerably more effective for controlling Parkinsonism than synthetic atropine or other artificially derived drugs.

Important: The metabolism of the elderly is often slow, and doses for old people may need to be lower than for adults in their prime.

CASE HISTORY
Hardening of the arteries and confusion

PATIENT: William, 88, bedridden and confused, requiring constant attention from his wife, aged 72, and home care attendants.

HISTORY AND COMPLAINT: William's wife sought treatment for him after doctors diagnosed hardening of the cerebral arteries and suggested there was nothing to be done beyond terminal care.

TREATMENT: William was given a tincture of ginkgo, wood betony, linden, *shi di huang*, and a little ginger. The normal adult dose was reduced to half to compensate for his age and frailty.

OUTCOME: William improved a little, became more lucid and started reading again; after four months he was able to go downstairs for the first time in nearly two years. Medication was continued at a reduced dose, with the addition of herbs like *dang shen, gotu kola,* and *ashwagandha.* William enjoyed his 90th birthday party and died peacefully six months later.

How to use	Combinations	Cautions
Take in pills, tinctures, or infusions of fresh leaves; numerous commercial extracts are available.	Use with garlic in capsules, or hawthorn and linden in teas and tinctures.	
Take an infusion or tincture.	Combine tincture with recommended mistletoe dose (below), or use linden and wood betony in infusion.	
Take 10-20 drops tincture three times a day.	Combine with greater periwinkle or ginkgo tinctures up to a 5 ml dose. Drink with buckwheat or linden infusion to help repair arteriole walls.	Do not use the berries, as they are toxic.
Take a decoction with other herbs, or 1-2 g doses powdered herb in capsules, or a tincture.	Combine with *dang gui, chuan xiong,* and *chi shao yao* in a decoction.	Avoid herb if condition involves excess "heat" or yin deficiency.
Add 50 drops to 25 ml almond oil and massage into the lower abdomen twice a day.	Use as a simple or add 10-25 drops niaouli to 25 ml of the diluted cypress oil massage mixture.	
Take 10 ml juice twice a day.	Use as a simple or with 2-5 ml St. John's wort or sweet sumach tincture per dose.	
Take an infusion or tincture in 5-10 ml doses.	Take as a simple or combine with *bhringaraj* in infusion or tincture.	
Eat fresh, dried (Indian gooseberry) or stewed fruit.	Generally taken in *Chyavan Prash* (a herb jelly sold in Indian markets and restaurants); with *ashwagandha* or *shatavari.*	
Take one tea cup of infusion or 10 ml tincture a day.	Use as a simple or combine with rosemary, thyme or *gotu kola.*	Can trigger fits in epileptics, who should avoid the herb.

KEY

Aerial parts

Essential oil

Fruit

Leaves

Rhizome

Twigs

STANDARD REMEDIES
All recipes and doses are standard unless otherwise specified; see *Making Herbal Remedies, pp. 152-57.*

ENDOCRINE & GLAND PROBLEMS

THE BODY HAS A number of "glands" that produce important chemicals and secretions to ensure that the system runs smoothly. The "endocrine" or "ductless gland" system includes the pituitary, thyroid, parathyroid and adrenal glands, ovaries, testes, placenta, and parts of the pancreas. These are responsible for producing a variety of hormones that are then secreted into the bloodstream, and any dysfunction in the system soon upsets body chemistry. Problems with endocrine glands can include various menstrual disorders associated with hormones produced by the pituitary glands and ovaries, obvious thyroid disorders, and diabetes, which is linked to the islets of Langerhans, endocrine cells in the pancreas. "Exocrine" or "duct glands" produce secretions via a duct on to a surface of the body. This group includes the glands that secrete saliva or sweat, and these, too, can cause health problems. The parotid glands, for example, are one of three pairs of glands that produce saliva, and inflammation leads to parotitis, common with mumps. Lymph "glands" are part of the lymphatic system, which transports various fluids around the

See also: boils pp. 168-69; weak immune system, pp. 168-69; tonsillitis, pp. 176-77; mumps, pp. 220-21; menstrual irregularities, pp. 202-03.

AILMENT	REMEDIES	
	Herb	*Actions*
LATE-ONSET DIABETES Caused by a lack of insulin, leading to high blood sugar levels. It is often associated with obesity and poor diet, and is generally non-insulin-dependent. **KEY SYMPTOMS** • Excessive thirst and urination • Mental confusion • Weight loss • Lethargy.	*Galega officinalis* **GOAT'S RUE** (see p. 228)	Enlarges the islets of Langerhans in the pancreas, which are responsible for insulin production.
	Trigonella foenum-graecum **FENUGREEK** (see p. 106)	Hypoglycemic herb – in trials, it has reduced urine sugar levels by 50%.
	Vaccinium myrtillus **BILBERRY** (see p. 109)	Hypoglycemic and increases insulin production.
THYROID PROBLEMS Over activity of the thyroid gland leads to thyrotoxicosis; under activity causes myxedema. **KEY SYMPTOMS** • Diarrhea, weight loss and hyperactivity in thyrotoxicosis. • Constipation, weight gain, and general lethargy in myxedema. *IMPORTANT: Thyroid problems should always be referred to a health-care professional.*	*Fucus vesiculosis* **BLADDERWRACK** (see p. 66)	A good source of iodine, essential for normal function of the thyroid gland; metabolic stimulant to combat lethargy in myxedema.
	Leonurus cardiaca **MOTHERWORT** (see p. 82)	Calming and normalizing for the heart in overactive thyroid problems.
	Lycopus virginicus **BUGLEWEED** (see p. 228)	Relieves palpitations and rapid heartbeat associated with overactive thyroid.
MONONUCLEOSIS Thought to be caused by the Epstein-Barr virus, this is common in young adults. Symptoms may persist for several weeks, leaving sufferers feeling debilitated. **KEY SYMPTOMS** • Enlarged and tender lymph nodes in neck, armpits and groin • Loss of appetite, lethargy • Headache, fever, sore throat. *IMPORTANT: Always consult a health-care professional; use herbal remedies to support conventional treatments.*	*Galium aparine* **CLEAVERS** (see p. 67)	Especially cleansing for the entire lymphatic system.
	Inula helenium **ELECAMPANE** (see p. 77)	Tonic and restorative; anti-microbial and expectorant to help clear any associated infections.

body. They are really nodes or small swellings that act as filters for the lymph and prevent foreign particles from entering the blood stream. They produce lymphocytes, a type of white blood cell important to the immune system. Lymph nodes often swell when there is an infection – the swollen "glands" in mono-nucleosis are enlarged lymph nodes. Herbs are useful for problems affecting glands – they influence body chemistry to normalize production of particular hormones and enzymes, and combat infections and inflammations. Traditional medicine knew little of the endocrine or lymphatic glands. Chinese and Ayurvedic treatments have no real concept of hormones or body chemistry, though there are herbs used to treat "hard swellings", which would have been associated with lymphatic problems, and are often cleansing and antimicrobial remedies.

CASE HISTORY
Late-onset diabetes mellitus

PATIENT: Henry, 72, overweight, averse to exercise.

HISTORY AND COMPLAINT: Henry had been feeling very lethargic, and complained of persistent thirst. A blood test indicated abnormally high sugar levels and suggested late-onset diabetes. Henry was given a diet plan and instructed to lose weight. Urine tests regularly showed high glucose levels.

TREATMENT: Henry disliked taking medication, so the emphasis was on diet. He ate plenty of garlic, onions, and cinnamon toast, took goat's rue and bilberry leaf tea, and doses of fenugreek powder.

OUTCOME: Within a few days, fasting urinary sugar levels were lower, with normal levels recorded occasionally after another week. His doctor was satisfied after a month, and stopped medication.

How to use	Combinations	Cautions
Take an infusion or tincture before meals.	Use as a simple or combine with stinging nettle or bilberry leaf in an infusion; add 2-4 ml sweet sumach tincture per dose. Eat a high fiber diet with plenty of garlic.	Blood sugar levels need monitoring.
Take up to 1 g powdered herb after meals, or make a decoction.	Eat a high fiber diet with plenty of garlic; add powdered cloves or cinnamon to capsules if desired.	Blood sugar levels need monitoring.
Drink an infusion before meals.	Add goat's rue or stinging nettle to infusion; eat a high fiber diet with plenty of garlic.	Blood sugar levels need monitoring.
Take in pills or capsules, up to 2 g per day; use in tinctures and infusions.	Use with parsely, damiana, and oats in tinctures and infusions; add ginseng or ginkgo to powders and capsules. Add vervain or St. John's wort if depression is a problem in myxedema.	Avoid in over-active thyroid.
Use in infusions and tinctures.	Use with half as much pasque flower and blue flag in tinctures, or with an equal amount of lemon balm in infusions.	
Use in infusions and tinctures.	With motherwort, parsley, and lemon balm in infusions to calm the system and reduce palpitations and other symptoms.	Avoid in under active thyroid and pregnancy.
Take as juiced fresh herb; process enough fresh cleavers in a food-mixer to make 2 tbsp juice when strained. Alternatively, use a tincture, an infusion or capsules.	Add the fresh juice to a cup of echinacea and blue flag decoction with a pinch of powdered dried cayenne and the juice of half a lemon; take every 3-4 hours. Take garlic supplements to combat possible infections, and drink additional red clover and marigold infusions.	
Use as a restorative to combat any lingering debility, in a decoction, tincture or syrup.	Use with wood betony infusion; add a couple of drops of wormwood or calumba tincture per cup to stimulate appetite. Take up to 600 mg Korean ginseng for up to 1 month after lymphatic swellings subside.	

KEY

Aerial parts

Leaves

Root

Seeds

STANDARD REMEDIES
All recipes and doses are standard unless otherwise specified; see *Making Herbal Remedies, pp. 152-57.*

CHILDREN'S COMPLAINTS

GENTLE HERBS can be ideal for many children's ailments: soothing and relaxing remedies like chamomile or linden can ease overexcitement and encourage sleep. In fevers, cooling herbs such as elderflower, yarrow and catmint can be freely given, while echinacea is an ideal antibiotic. For coughs try hyssop, licorice or white horehound in syrup; for persistent catarrh try replacing milk products with soy-based preparations and using herbs like ground ivy and eyebright in capsules or tinctures. Soy is a good source of calcium, so eliminating dairy products from a child's diet is unlikely to cause any deficiencies. Hyperactivity can be related to food allergy – avoid colorants (E102 and E110 in particular). Constipation needs to be treated with gentle laxatives rather than stimulating purgatives – try psyllium seeds disguised in breakfast cereal, or butternut, rather than rhubarb root or senna. Unfortunately, many herbs taste unpleasant, so persuading children to swallow them can be a problem. Babies may

See also: infections and fevers, pp. 168-69; catarrh, pp. 170-71; earache, pp. 174-75; eczema, acne and ringworm, pp. 178-81; hay fever, pp. 192-93.

AILMENT	REMEDIES	
	Herb	*Actions*
DIAPER RASH A painful, raw area of diaper rash around the anus and on the buttocks may be due to irritant stools or wet diapers; it can be related to yeast infections, especially if the mother is breast-feeding while on antibiotics. **KEY SYMPTOM** • Sore, red, painful inflammation around the anus or anywhere in the diaper area.	*Calendula officinalis* POT MARIGOLD (see p. 47)	Anti-inflammatory, anti-microbial, soothing, and astringent to encourage healing and combat infection.
	Plantago major PLANTAIN (see p. 104)	Locally healing and soothing.
	Symphytum officinale COMFREY (see p. 123)	Encourages cell regrowth; demulcent and soothing.
CRADLE CAP Cradle cap is a scaly dermatitis affecting the scalp, and is often due to overactive sweat glands; it is not serious or contagious. **KEY SYMPTOM** • Scaly crust over the scalp.	*Arctium lappa* BURDOCK (see p. 40)	Cleansing and tonifying for the sweat and oil glands of the scalp.
	Viola tricolor HEARTSEASE (see p. 137)	Soothing and anti-inflammatory; useful for a wide range of skin disorders.
COLIC Colic is caused by spasmodic contractions of the intestines associated with gas and tension, and often follows rushed or stressful feeding times. **KEY SYMPTOMS** • Pain causing small babies to scream loudly • Tense, bloated abdomen • Burping and gas.	*Foeniculum officinale* FENNEL (see p. 64)	Carminative; reduces cramping pains.
	Matricaria chamomilla GERMAN CHAMOMILE (see p. 88)	Sedative, carminative and antispasmodic; good for excitement and nervous stomach.
	Nepeta cataria CATMINT (see p. 228)	Carminative and anti-spasmodic; can encourage sleep in restless babies.
TEETHING Teething pains can affect babies from the age of 4 or 5 months.	*Chamaemelum nobile* ROMAN CHAMOMILE (see p. 88)	Sedative, carminative, antispasmodic.

be coaxed to take weak infusions of chamomile or linden from a bottle, though breast-feeding mothers can take the remedy themselves, because it will pass into their milk; this is especially useful with colic remedies like dill or fenugreek. Toddlers will generally accept powders or tinctures in half a teaspoon of honey, though capsules are ideal as soon as the child is old enough to swallow them. Empty the capsule contents into a teaspoon of honey if children cannot swallow them. Dilute tinctures given in drop doses on the tongue are acceptable, or they may be flavored with peppermint, licorice or raspberry vinegar, as appropriate. For infants or long-term use, it is best to give nonalcoholic tinctures (see p. 157).

IMPORTANT NOTE

Children's doses need to be reduced, depending on age. All doses in the tables below and overleaf are the full adult dose unless otherwise specified. For children use the following proportions:

AGE	DOSE (expressed as a fraction of an adult dose)
0 - 1 yr	one-twentieth
1 - 2 yrs	one-tenth
3 - 4 yrs	one-fifth
5 - 6 yrs	three-tenths
7 - 8 yrs	two-fifths
9 - 10 yrs	half
11 - 12 yrs	three-fifths
13 - 14 yrs	four-fifths
15 plus	full dose

How to use	*Combinations*	*Cautions*
Use the infused oil as a lotion for the affected area after each diaper change.	Add 1-2 drops of tea tree or thyme oil to 10 ml of infused oil if there is any infection.	
Apply ointment or infused oil frequently, as required; put fresh, washed, crushed leaves in the diaper at each change.	Add 1-2 drops tea tree oil to 5 ml infused oil if fungal infection develops.	
Apply ointment or infused oil frequently, as required; use a paste of powdered root as a poultice for diaper rash.	Use arrowroot powder instead of baby talcum powder when changing diapers.	Can cause rapid healing; ensure affected area is clean.
Add 5 drops tincture to a bottle for babies under 10 kg; add 10 drops tincture for babies over 10 kg.	Can combine with heartsease.	
Use an infusion as a wash on affected areas, or use cream.	Add lemon balm or ground ivy to a wash or cream. The hard crusts of cradle cap can be softened with vegetable oil left overnight.	
Give babies 5-10 drops tincture in a bottle of water or add to feedings; breast-feeding mothers should drink a cup of infusion before feedings.	As an alternative, dill can be used in the same way.	
Use homeopathic *Chamomilla 3x*: for babies, give 5-10 drops or 1-5 crushed pilules up to three times a day.	Use as a simple; breast-feeding mothers can drink chamomile tea to relax themselves and soothe the baby's colic.	Do not exceed stated dose.
Add 5-10 drops tincture to a bottle of water or to feedings, or give a dilute infusion.	Use as a simple.	
Use *Chamomilla 3x* (see above) or put 1-2 drops oil on a wet swab and apply to the gum.	Add 1 drop clove essential oil to the swab. Give a weak linden infusion by bottle.	Do not exceed stated dose of essential oil.

KEY

Aerial parts

Flowers

Root

Seeds

Essential oil

Petals

STANDARD REMEDIES
All recipes and doses are standard unless otherwise specified; see *Making Herbal Remedies, pp. 152-57.*

AILMENT	REMEDIES	
	Herb	*Actions*
GASTRIC UPSETS Bilious attacks in children can be related to a type of migraine, or may be linked to food intolerance.	*Agrimonia eupatoria* AGRIMONY (see p. 31)	Astringent and healing for stomach lining; stimulates bile flow; helpful in food allergies; ideal for diarrhea.
KEY SYMPTOMS • Sudden diarrhea and vomiting • Stomach ache.	*Geranium maculatum* AMERICAN CRANESBILL (see p. 228-29)	Astringent and tonifying for diarrhea and gastritis.
SLEEPLESSNESS Sleepless babies increase tension in the entire household. Check the room temperature and, because the problem may associated with insecurity, be very loving.	*Chamaemelum nobile* ROMAN CHAMOMILE (see p. 88)	Sedative, carminative, and antispasmodic; ideal for overexcitement.
	Eschscholzia californica CALIFORNIAN POPPY (see p. 228)	Sedative, mild hypnotic, and antispasmodic; good for overexcitement.
THREADWORM Parasitic worms are common in children, and can be due to poor hygiene. Cases are generally mild.	*Allium ursinum* RAMSONS (see p. 229)　　　　*(Bulb)*	Potent antiseptic, similar to garlic.
KEY SYMPTOMS • Anal itching • Threadlike worms in the stools.	*Brassica oleracea* CABBAGE (see p. 46)	Traditional remedy for intestinal worms; antibacterial and healing.
NITS & LICE Nits are the eggs of head lice; they are static, and found at the back of the head and nape of the neck. Lice move and are more visible.	*Azadirachta indica* NEEM (see p. 44)	Antimicrobial and antiparasitic; a strong and effective herbal insecticide.
KEY SYMPTOMS • Visible lice • Itching scalp.	*Melaleuca alternifolia* TEA TREE (see p. 89)	Effective antiseptic; also antibacterial and antifungal.
HYPERACTIVITY Excessive overactivity can be related to food intolerance, "liver fire" or excess liver *qi*.	*Prunella vulgaris* XIA KU CAO (see p. 106)　*(Flower spikes)*	Used in Chinese medicine to calm "liver fire" associated with overexcitability.
KEY SYMPTOMS • Excessive activity • Problems concentrating, clumsiness, frustration • Frequent temper tantrums • Sleeping problems, thirst.	*Thymus vulgaris* THYME (see p. 99)	Inability to concentrate has been associated with lipid imbalance; evening primrose and fish oils with thyme oil have had significant results.
BED-WETTING Can be a congenital disorder, or due to insecurity, emotional upsets or urinary tract infections.	*Arctostaphylos uva-ursi* BEARBERRY (see p. 228)	Astringent and urinary antiseptic to soothe and combat irritation and infections.
KEY SYMPTOMS • Persistent urination in bed by children over 3 years of age • May be caused by a tight foreskin in boys.	*Rhus aromatica* SWEET SUMACH (see p. 229)	Astringent and tonic for the urinary system; traditionally used for bed-wetting in childhood, although scientific evidence for efficacy is scant.
MOTION SICKNESS Nausea and vomiting related to motion, as on car trips or sea voyages, is common in childhood.	*Mentha* x *piperita* PEPPERMINT (see p. 91)	Prevents vomiting; antispasmodic.
	Zingiber officinalis GINGER (GAN JIANG) (see p. 139)	Prevents vomiting; carminative.

How to use	*Combinations*	*Cautions*
Give an infusion or tincture (see dosage chart on p. 217).	Can combine with chamomile, catmint, or lemon balm for nervous stomach; combine with a little marshmallow for inflammations.	Avoid in constipation.
Give an infusion or tincture (see dosage chart on p. 217).	Can combine with agrimony, meadowsweet, marshmallow, or chamomile to enhance action.	
For babies, add 1½-2 cups (100-500 ml) infusion or 2-3 drops essential oil to bath.	Use as a simple; breast-feeding mothers can drink chamomile tea to relax both themselves and their babies.	Do not exceed stated dose.
Give an infusion or tincture about 30 minutes before bed (see dosage chart on p. 217).	Add a little honey to make it more palatable for children; can add chamomile or a little skullcap to increase soothing action.	
Give an infusion or 10 ml juice; can also use as an enema once a week.	Use as a simple, or use garlic instead for older children.	
Give a glass of juice each morning for three days.	Can combine with carrot juice. An alternative traditional cure is to feed the child nothing but grated carrot for two days.	
Use a strong decoction as a final rinse, or infuse bark in soap-based shampoo for two weeks and use to wash hair.	Use as a simple or combine the decoction with an equal amount of almond oil and use to massage the scalp at night.	Use with caution on very young children.
Put a few drops of oil on a fine comb and comb the hair well, or add 5-10 drops to shampoo or hair rinse daily.	Use as a simple or combine with well diluted lemon oil (no more than 5 drops in 25 ml carrier oil – it can irritate).	
Give an infusion or tincture (see dosage chart on p. 217).	Combine with calming nervines such as chamomile, passionflower, St. John's wort or wood betony. Add a small amount of vervain or *bai shao yao* to soothe the liver.	
Use in prepared capsules or add 5 drops to 10 ml of evening primrose oil as a massage for lower back or abdomen. Use the dried herbs in infusions or syrups.	Use borage seed oil instead of evening primrose internally; combine the dried herbs with *xia ku cao* and vervain ; add agrimony for food allergies.	Only use oil internally under professional supervision or in licensed remedies.
In infusions, tinctures or capsules for older children who can swallow them.	Use with American cranesbill, cornsilk, and passionflower or skullcap in infusions; add valerian to tinctures.	
Give 10-15 drops tincture up to three times a day.	Combine with cornsilk or horsetail if urinary infection is suspected; combine with St. John's wort or wood betony for related nervous problems.	
Give drop doses of tincture while traveling.	Older children can be given peppermint candies.	Do not use for babies.
Give 1-2 200 mg capsules before traveling.	Best as a simple; ginger candies and cookies can be useful for younger children, or give crystallized ginger to chew.	

KEY

Aerial parts

Essential oil

Flowers

Leaves

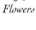
Root

Root bark

Bark

STANDARD REMEDIES All recipes and doses are standard unless otherwise specified; see *Making Herbal Remedies*, pp. 152-57.

AILMENT	REMEDIES	
	Herb	*Actions*
MUMPS A viral disease that usually affects the salivary glands in children. **KEY SYMPTOMS** • Difficulty swallowing • Enlarged salivary glands • Mild fever, irritability. *IMPORTANT: Adult sufferers should always seek professional help.*	*Calendula officinalis* POT MARIGOLD (see p. 47)	Astringent, anti-inflammatory and antiseptic to combat infection and irritation.
	Salvia officinalis SAGE (see p. 115)	Antiseptic and astringent to soothe throat discomfort.
MEASLES A contagious viral disease with an incubation period of 1-2 weeks. **KEY SYMPTOMS** • Harsh dry cough and nasal congestion • Blotchy, orange-red rash usually starts behind the ears and extends to the whole body • Bloodshot, light-sensitive eyes often followed by blepharitis. *IMPORTANT: Seek professional help as complications may occur.*	*Echinacea spp.* ECHINACEA (see p. 58)	Antibacterial and antiviral; also strengthens resistance to infections; useful for all septic or infectious conditions.
	Euphrasia officinalis EYEBRIGHT (see p. 228-29)	Antiseptic and anti-inflammatory to soothe inflamed eyes and eyelids.
	Hyssopus officinalis HYSSOP (see p. 76)	Relaxing expectorant, particularly suitable for children's coughs and respiratory infections.
CHICKEN POX (VARICELLA) In children, chicken pox is usually a mild, but contagious, infection. **KEY SYMPTOMS** • Rash that soon turns into white spots that blister and form scabs • Mild fever, sore throat, nasal congestion. *IMPORTANT: Damaging the scabs can lead to scars. In adults the same virus produces shingles.*	*Hamamelis virginianum* WITCH HAZEL (see p. 71)	Astringent and cooling to soothe irritation.
	Lonicera japonica JIN YIN HUA (see p. 85) *(Flower buds)*	Cooling for feverish conditions; antibacterial and anti-inflammatory.
	Scutellaria lateriflora SKULLCAP (see p. 118)	Sedating and calming for children irritated by fever and itching scabs.
GERMAN MEASLES (RUBELLA) A viral disease with an incubation period up to three weeks. **KEY SYMPTOMS** • Nasal congestion, swollen glands in neck and behind ears. • Irritating pink rash starting in the face and spreading downwards. *IMPORTANT: Can cause birth defects if women are affected in early pregnancy.*	*Baptisia tinctoria* WILD INDIGO (see p. 229)	Cooling, cleansing antiseptic to stimulate the immune system and combat infection.
	Melissa officinalis LEMON BALM (see p. 90)	Sedating and calming for irritated and tense children; some antiviral activity reported.
	Thymus serpyllum WILD THYME (see p. 127)	Astringent and antiseptic to ease symptoms.
WHOOPING COUGH Often starts with a mild cough and cold, with sticky mucus and distressing cough soon following. **KEY SYMPTOMS** • Cough develops over a week until it becomes convulsive. • Characteristic whoop when coughing after 14 days, often followed by vomiting • Breathlessness. *IMPORTANT: Professional help should be sought for young children.*	*Lactuca virosa* WILD LETTUCE (see p. 229)	Sedating to soothe and relax exhausted children.
	Marrubium vulgare WHITE HOREHOUND (see p. 228-29)	Combats bronchial spasms and helps clear mucus and phlegm; restorative and bitter to stimulate the digestion.
	Tussilago farara COLTSFOOT (see p. 130)	Antispasmodic and anti-tussive to ease convulsive coughing; expectorant to clear mucus and congestion.

How to use	*Combinations*	*Cautions*
In infusions.	Use with lemon balm, echinacea leaves, and yarrow in infusions: add 10 drops of pokeroot tincture or 10 ml of cleavers juice to each dose. Older children can take additional echinacea in pills or capsules.	
Use the infusion as a gargle, repeating every 30-60 minutes while symptoms are severe.	Use with thyme or rosemary in gargles, add a pinch of powdered cayenne to each dose; take with chamomile, lemon balm and betony in soothing infusions.	Do not exceed stated dose.
Give two 200-250 mg capsules of powdered root three times a day or 10 ml tincture (see dosage chart on p. 217).	Effective as a simple, or add elderflower, catmint or yarrow in feverish conditions. Add 2-5 drops fresh ginger tincture if nausea is a problem.	High doses can occasionally cause nausea and vomiting.
Use a well-strained infusion in eyebaths to soothe irritation.	Use with pot marigold or self-heal in eyebaths; sponge feverish children with a marigold or basil infusion as well.	
Give up to 10 ml tincture a day or give an infusion (see dosage chart on p. 217).	Can be combined with marshmallow leaf and ribwort plantain, or add white horehound to soothe the mucous membranes in dry, irritable coughs.	
Use the diluted tincture or a cooled decoction in a compress to sponge the body.	Use with rosewater or borage juice (restricted herb in Australia and New Zealand) or chickweed cream to ease irritation of rashes.	
Give an infusion or tincture (see dosage chart on p. 217).	Add elderflower, peppermint, catmint, or a little *lian qiao*.	
In infusions.	Use with chamomile, yarrow, lemon balm, elderflower, or boneset to combat feverish symptoms and catarrh. Give additional echinacea capsules or drops of tincture.	
Take 5-20 drops tincture or a 1/4 tsp of root per cup of decoction every two hours.	Use with an equal amount of echinacea and add 10 ml of juice to ease swollen glands.	Large doses may cause nausea and vomiting.
Use in infusions to drink or to soak a compress and sponge the child externally.	Use with hyssop, chamomile, elderflowers, or pot marigold in infusions. Add 10 ml of cleavers juice or 10 drops of pokeroot tincture to each cup to combat swollen glands.	
In infusions.	Use with chamomile, elderflowers, and sage in teas; soothe irritant rash as for chicken pox; take additional echinacea to combat infection.	
Use in infusions or tinctures.	Use with wild thyme, mullein, elecampane, white horehound, or licorice in combined infusion/decoctions, syrups or tinctures to combat and soothe convulsive coughing.	Large doses may cause drowsiness and confusion.
In infusions or syrups.	Add a pinch of ginger or cayenne to each dose or combine with catmint, echinacea leaves, and thyme in infusions. Support with chest rubs and echinacea to combat infection.	
In infusions, tinctures or syrups.	With thyme and white horehound in infusions and syrups; massage the child's chest with 5 drops of hyssop, basil or cypress oil in 5 ml of almond oil to ease congestion.	Restricted in some countries; contains pyrrolizidine alkaloids. Use only under supervision.

KEY

Aerial parts

Bark

Flowers

Petals

Root

Whole herb

Leaves

STANDARD REMEDIES All recipes and doses are standard unless otherwise specified; see *Making Herbal Remedies*, pp. 152-57.

AYURVEDIC TONICS

In Ayurveda, tonic herbs can be nutritive to strengthen the body, aphrodisiac to reinvigorate the sexual organs, and inner energies, or rejuvenative to help creativity and awareness. Nutritive tonics (*bruhana karma*) tend to be sweet in taste and are usually strengthening for *kapha* – the humor associated with earth and water, and important for weight gain – and will decrease *vata* (air) and *pitta* (fire). Aphrodisiac remedies are known as *vajikarana* (from "*vaji*", meaning a stallion) and are believed to simulate the energy and vitality of a horse, an animal renowned in Indian tradition for its sexual

activity. This focus on reproductive energy also strengthens all the body's tissues (*dhatus*). By increasing sexual energy, the *vajikarana* not only help to create new life in conception but also help to renew existing life. The rejuvenative remedies (*rasayana karma*) are among the most important in Ayurveda. These can be compared with the Taoist longevity tonics (see pp. 226-27). They help to prevent decay and aging, and enhance mental clarity and spiritual awareness, which is so important in India's "science of life". Some herbs contain all three of these different tonic properties.

RASAYANA KARMA

Rasayana means substances that enter (*ayana*) the vital essence (*rasa*). These herbal remedies penetrate and revitalize spiritual energies and enhance well-being. *Rasayanas* are sometimes called longevity tonics: in Indian tradition immortality is seen as the continued existence in a universal whole, rather than the survival of the individual. *Rasayana* tonics are also rejuvenating to renew the mind, body, and spirit and to combat aging and decay. Many are sweet to the taste, but there are also pungent, hot, spicy remedies that are particularly appropriate for *kapha* ailments. In Ayurvedic theory, *rasayanas* are believed to be rich in *soma* – a magical nectar that renews the whole being.

OTHER RASAYANA TONICS FEATURED ELSEWHERE IN THE BOOK

aloe vera	page 34	Korean ginseng	page 98
ashwagandha	page 137	long pepper	page 102
amalaki	page 222-23	myrrh	page 54
bala	page 222-23	oatstraw	page 43
bibhitaki	page 126	sesame	page 222-23
dang gui	page 36	*shatavari*	page 42
di huang	page 224-25	Solomon's seal	page 222-23
elecampane	page 77	spikenard	page 94
garlic	page 33	saw palmetto	page 226-27
guggul	page 140-41	*vamsha rochana*	page 100
haritaki	page 126	*vidari-kanda*	page 222-23
he shou wu	page 224-25	wild yam	page 57

GOTU KOLA
Centella asiatica

Indian pennywort, or *gotu kola*, is known as *brahmi* in sanskrit because it increases knowledge of *Brahman*, the supreme reality. It is one of the most important *rasayanas* in Ayurvedic medicine, helping to revitalize the brain and nervous system, combat aging and senility, and improve the memory. It is a specific tonic for *pitta*, clears excess *vata* and *kapha*, is calming (*sattvic*) and is an important aid for spiritual renewal.

🌿 PARTS USED: Aerial parts.

✋ ACTIONS: Rejuvenative tonic, cooling in fevers, immune stimulant, cleansing, bitter digestive stimulant, laxative, sedative.

⚗️🫖 HOW TO USE: Use up to 1 g powder per dose or in an infusion (¹/₂ tsp per cup); a paste made of the powder can be applied externally for eczema and skin sores.

COMBINATIONS: Use with basil as a cooling remedy in fevers and food poisoning; with rosemary or wood betony in teas when studying; or with *ashwagandha*, licorice and sandalwood for nervous irritability and mental weakness.

CAUTION: Avoid in pregnancy and epilepsy.

SAFFRON
Crocus sativus

Traditionally used in India as a blood tonic, stimulant and aphrodisiac, saffron is very restorative and in Ayurvedic medicine, it is used to strengthen feelings of devotion and compassion. It is especially good for the female reproductive system and is also one of the best anti-*pitta* herbs. The herb is known as *nagakeshara* in sanskrit; safflower (*Carthamus tinctorius*) is often used as a low-cost substitute, although it is not as effective. Saffron helps to enhance other tonic herbs, and is therefore often added to other remedies.

🌸 PARTS USED: Flower stigma.

✋ ACTIONS: Rejuvenative and aphrodisiac tonic; promotes menstruation; carminative, antispasmodic, stimulating.

🫖 HOW TO USE: Use in cooking or simmer a pinch in milk as a decoction; although expensive, a small amount goes a long way.

COMBINATIONS: Use with *shatavari* or *dang gui* as a tonic for the female reproductive organs and especially during menopause.

BHRINGARAJ
Eclipta prostata

Bhringaraj is important in both Ayurvedic and Chinese medicine (*han lian cao*) as a kidney tonic. Its Indian name actually means "ruler of the hair", and as in Chinese theory, healthy head hair is said to indicate healthy kidneys. It is used to combat aging, to rejuvenate the bones, teeth, sight, hearing, and memory, to calm the mind and encourage restful sleep. It is also rejuvenative for predominantly *pitta* people, and is a good liver tonic.

🌿 PARTS USED: Aerial parts.

✋ ACTIONS: Astringent, antibacterial; a *yin* tonic that nourishes the kidneys and liver and stops bleeding; take for kidney weakness and heavy bleeding in menstruation or after childbirth.

🫖 HOW TO USE: Take an infusion or up to 10 ml tincture a day.

COMBINATIONS: Use with *gotu kola* as a general tonic; *bhringaraj* oil is sold in India as a hair tonic to combat graying and balding.

VAJIKARANA

The aphrodisiac tonics focus on the reproductive tissues, promoting sexual vitality and strengthening or regenerating the inner organs. Although these herbs are sometimes used as aphrodisiacs, they are more important as tissue energy tonics to nurture the reproductive organs, particularly if there are problems with infertility. They also encourage the creative energies associated with reproduction and strengthen the whole body. *Vajikaranas* are divided into tonics and stimulants: tonics improve the tissues and stimulants improve functionality.

OTHER VAJIKARANA TONICS FEATURED ELSEWHERE IN THE BOOK

asafoetida	page 228-29	hibiscus	page 226-27
ashwagandha	page 138	Korean ginseng	page 98
cloves	page 228-29	long pepper	page 102
damiana	page 226-27	lotus seeds	page 95
dang gui	page 36	rose	page 110-11
di huang	page 224-25	saffron	page 222-23
fenugreek	page 129	*shatavari*	page 42
garlic	page 33	*vidari-kanda*	page 222-23
he shou wu	page 224-25	wild yam	page 57

VIDARI-KANDA
Ipomoea digitata
A member of the morning glory family, and a relative of the sweet potato (*I. batatas*), *vidari-kanda* is a versatile tonic and is sometimes known as "Indian ginseng". Related species are used in India for a wide range of ailments ranging from snake bites to leprosy.

PARTS USED: Root, leaves.

ACTIONS: Nutritive, rejuvenative and aphrodisiac tonic; stimulates milk flow; hormonal action.

HOW TO USE: Use 5 g powder in a milk decoction with ghee and honey as a daily tonic for debility and weakness in the reproductive organs.

GOKSHURA
Tribulis terrestris
Gokshura is an important remedy for urinary tract problems, including stones, cystitis, and infections. It strengthens the kidney function and is a good tonic for the reproductive system. A *sattvic* tonic, it is calming for the nervous system.

PARTS USED: Fruit.

ACTIONS: Rejuvenative and aphrodisiac tonic; diuretic, analgesic; clears urinary stones.

HOW TO USE: Use 100-250 mg powder per dose in a milk decoction to enhance its aphrodisiac action; it is included in medicated oils for scalp massage to treat baldness.

COMBINATIONS: Use with *ashwaganda* as a rejuvenating mixture, or with dry ginger as an analgesic for nerve pains.

MEDA/SOLOMON'S SEAL
Polygonatum odoratum
Solomon's seal is rare in the wild and most cultivated specimens are a cross between *P. odoratum* and *P. multiflorum*. In India, *meda*, or *mahameda*, is an ingredient in *ashtavarga* (see pp.140-1) and is a flexible all around tonic.

PARTS USED: Rhizome.

ACTIONS: Nutritive, rejuvenative , and aphrodisiac tonic; demulcent, expectorant, stops bleeding.

HOW TO USE: Use in a milk decoction or take up to 3 g powder twice a day with warm milk and ghee.

COMBINATIONS: *Meda* is one of eight members of the lily family that make up *ashtavarga*, used as a fertility tonic; it can be taken during breast-feeding and for chronic wasting disease.

BRUHANA KARMA

Bruhana karma tonics are generally heavy, oily or mucilaginous. They strengthen muscles, build tissues, increase body fluids, and are restorative in debility. They are often demulcent and soothing for mucous membranes, and tend to be calming and sedative. Because they are heavy, these tonics can be hard to digest, so warming, carminative herbs, such as galangal or cinnamon, are sometimes added. In Ayurveda their action is enhanced by taking them in milk.

OTHER BRUHANA KARMA TONICS FEATURED ELSEWHERE IN THE BOOK

dang gui	page 36	saw palmetto	page 226-27
di huang	page 224-25	*shatavari*	page 42
flax seeds	page 84	slippery elm	page 228-29
Korean ginseng	page 98	Solomon's seal	page 222-23
licorice	page 70	*vidari-kanda*	page 222-23
lotus seeds	page 95	wild yam	page 57
marshmallow	page 36		

AMALAKI
Emblica officinalis
Amalaki is both a nutritive remedy and a *rasayana* for *pitta* conditions. The herb stimulates the appetite, and its fruits are a very rich source of vitamin C (up to 3 g per fruit). *Amalaki* forms the basis of *chyavan prash* – a herbal jelly used in India as a general tonic.

PARTS USED: Fruit.

ACTIONS: Rejuvenative, nutritive and aphrodisiac tonic; laxative, astringent; stops bleeding.

HOW TO USE: Use 250-1,000 mg powder per dose, or in a decoction.

COMBINATIONS: Use with herbs such as *gokshura*, *ashwagandha*, *shatavari* and cinnamon in *chyavan prash*.

CAUTION: Avoid in diarrhea or dysentery.

TILA/SESAME
Sesamum indicum
Sesame seeds, known as *tila* in India, are rich in calcium and help to strengthen tissues and act as a rejuvenative tonic for *vata* conditions. The seeds are regarded as *sattvic*, and are used to renew spiritual energies. They are popular with yogis.

PARTS USED: Seeds.

ACTIONS: Nutritive and rejuvenative tonic; demulcent, laxative, antioxidant, antianemic.

HOW TO USE: Use up to 2 g powder per dose or a decoction of seeds; sesame oil is used externally with limewater for burns and sores, or mixed with a little camphor as a massage for migraines and vertigo.

COMBINATIONS: The seeds can be made into a confection with *shatavari*, ginger and raw sugar and eaten daily.

BALA
Sida cordifolia
Bala is a type of wild mallow and the name in sanskrit means "giving strength". It is a good heart tonic and is one of the herbs that is nutritive, rejuvenating and aphrodisiac. It is mainly used to treat *vata* disorders, often in sesame oil.

PARTS USED: Root.

ACTIONS: Rejuvenative, nutritive,and aphrodisiac tonic; demulcent, diuretic, analgesic, wound herb, stimulant.

HOW TO USE: Use in milk decoction with sugar, or take up to 1 g powder per dose. Mix with sesame oil for nerve pains and muscle cramps.

COMBINATIONS: Use with ginger or black pepper for fevers, or with basil, mullein, elecampane, and cinnamon as a lung tonic after influenza or in chronic respiratory problems.

CHINESE TONICS

Use of tonic herbs in China goes back to the early Taoists, who believed that the ideal way to achieve prosperity, longevity and immortality was to encourage "virtue". Their idea of virtue involved conforming to nature and living in harmony with all things. Herbal tonics were part of this "cultivation of the Way", helping to integrate physical and spiritual growth and encouraging the will to follow the path of virtue. Today, many of these herbs are described as "longevity tonics", although a better description is perhaps "virtue tonics".

YIN TONICS

Yin tonics are suitable for deficient *yin* syndromes that are most common in the lungs, stomach, liver, and kidneys. These remedies also help to promote body fluids, moistening tissues and having a laxative effect. They are used to help clear phlegm by making it less sticky and heavy. Modern research has shown that many popular *yin* tonic herbs tend to reduce blood pressure and cholesterol levels.

OTHER YIN TONICS FEATURED ELSEWHERE IN THE BOOK

DANG SHEN
Codonopsis pilosula
Often used as a less expensive alternative to Korean ginseng, *dang shen* is traditionally taken by nursing mothers. It is a popular ingredient in "Change of Season Soup", and is used to help the body adapt to major shifts in the weather.

PARTS USED: Root.

ACTIONS: Demulcent and expectorant acting on lung and spleen; milder and more *yin* in character then ginseng, it is good for nourishing stomach *yin*.

HOW TO USE: Take a decoction or tincture, or drink as a tonic wine.

COMBINATIONS: Use with *fu ling, bai zhu* and licorice.

SHI HU
Dendrobium officinale
Shi hu, or *suk gok* from its Korean name, is a member of the lily family used since the days of Shen Nung. It mainly affects the stomach, lungs and kidney *yin*. Modern studies have shown that it lowers body temperature and is a mild analgesic.

PARTS USED: Stems.

ACTIONS: Good for the kidneys, lungs, and stomach; increases body fluids; reputedly increases sexual vigor.

HOW TO USE: Take a tincture or decoction of 60 g herb in 3 cups water.

COMBINATIONS: With licorice as a tonic; with *sheng di huang* and *xuan shen* for low-grade fevers and heat problems.

WU WEI ZI
Schizandra chinensis
The name *wu wei zi* means "five taste seeds" and the herb is said to combine all five of the classic Chinese tastes. It has long been regarded as an aphrodisiac.

PARTS USED: Fruit.

ACTIONS: Astringent, sedative, and aphrodisiac; effective kidney and skin tonic; effective for insomnia and anxiety; good for allergic skin conditions.

HOW TO USE: Take an infusion or tincture; or take 200-250 mg powdered herb in capsules, three times a day.

COMBINATIONS: Often used with *dan shen* and *mai men dong*; with dry ginger in lung deficiency.

YANG TONICS

Yang tonics are mainly used for deficient *yang* syndromes that commonly afflict the kidney, spleen and heart. Many remedies, such as sea horses and gecko, reflect the less acceptable side of Chinese medicine, although there are also some suitable herbs.

OTHER YANG TONICS FEATURED ELSEWHERE IN THE BOOK

BU GU ZHI
Psoralea corylifolia
The name *bu gu zhi* literally means "tonify bone resin". The herb is particularly good for both kidney and spleen *yang*, and modern research has also shown it to be effective as an external remedy for alopecia, psoriasis, and vitiligo.

PARTS USED: Fruit.

ACTIONS: Strengthens kidney *yang*; diuretic, astringent, antibacterial; stops uterine bleeding.

HOW TO USE: Take a decoction.

COMBINATIONS: Combine with *wu zhu yu, wu wei zi*, nutmeg and ginger for morning diarrhea associated with kidney weakness.

CAUTION: Can cause photosensitivity of the skin.

DU ZHONG
Eucommia ulmoïdes
This was listed in Shen Nung's herbal, and first collected in the West in the 1880s. It is used for high blood pressure.

PARTS USED: Bark.

ACTIONS: Diuretic, hypotensive; reduces cholesterol levels; sedative, uterine relaxant; tonifies liver and kidney *qi*; strengthen bones and muscles.

HOW TO USE: Take in decoction, tincture, or up to 500 mg daily powdered in capsules.

COMBINATIONS: Use with *bu gu zhi* for deficient kidney *yang*, or with *gui zhi* for problems associated with cold and damp.

CAUTION: Avoid in deficient *yin*.

YIN YANG HUO
Epimedium grandiflorum
Yin yang huo translates as "licentious goat wort", and research has confirmed its aphrodisiac action – it increases sperm production and sexual desire. It focuses on kidney energy and also on the liver to help normalize menstrual activity.

PARTS USED: Aerial parts.

ACTIONS: Aphrodisiac, antibiotic; reduces blood pressure; diuretic (in low doses); tonifies the kidneys and strengthens *yang*; expels wind, cold and dampness; controls liver *yang*.

HOW TO USE: Take in tinctures or infusions.

COMBINATIONS: Use with *wu wei zi* and *gou qi zi* for weak kidney *yang*.

BLOOD TONICS

In Chinese medicine, blood and body fluids are classed as *yin*, and are often nourished by herbs that are *yin* in character. Blood deficiency can be due to anemia, although Chinese medicine also cites liver disharmony, heart weakness, or psychological factors as causes. In the East, blood tonics are used by women to regulate the menstrual cycle and as a general tonic after childbirth.

GOU QI ZI
Lycium chinense

Both fruits and root bark (*di gu pi*) are used in Chinese medicine. The root bark is listed among Shen Nong's "superior" woods as a remedy for "evil *qi*", but today the fruits are a more usual remedy.

PARTS USED: Berries.

ACTIONS: Good *yin* tonic for the kidneys; nourishes blood; cooling; stops bleeding; lowers blood sugar.

HOW TO USE: Take a decoction or tincture; eat dried berries in the same way as currants, or use in cooking and tonic wines.

COMBINATIONS: Can be combined with *ju hua* for high blood pressure associated with liver disharmony; use with *he shou wu*, *shu di huang* and *chen pi* for kidney exhaustion linked to overwork or old age; use with *wu wei zi* for general debility.

DI HUANG
Rehmannia glutinosa

Shu di huang is the prepared form of the herb, made by stir-frying the sliced tubers with wine, and used as a major blood tonic. The raw herb *sheng di huang* is colder and is sometimes cooked (without wine) to produce *gan di huang*. Both of these forms are helpful for *yin* and body fluids, as well as to clear heat.

PARTS USED: Root, raw or cooked.

ACTIONS: Demulcent, laxative; stops bleeding; also a *yin* tonic for nourishing kidney *yin*; *sheng di huang* is used as a nourishing and cooling *yin* remedy, while *shu di huang* is better for blood.

HOW TO USE: Take up to 10 ml tincture, three times a day, or up to 15 g per dose in a decoction.

COMBINATIONS: Use *shu di huang* with *shan zhu yu*, *shan yao*, *mu dan pi* and *gou qi zi* for menopausal problems; *sheng di huang* combines with *qing hao* and *mu dan pi* for *yin* deficiency.

HE SHOU WU
Polygonum multiflorum

He shou wu (also known in the West as *fo ti* from its Cantonese name) is an important blood tonic that also helps kidney and liver energy. The root is the main herb part, although the stems (*ye jiao teng*) are also used as a heart and liver tonic to calm the nerves and improve blood circulation. It is especially useful during menopause.

PARTS USED: Root.

ACTIONS: Antibacterial, heart tonic, hormonal action, raises blood sugar, laxative, liver stimulant, reduces cholesterol; used to replenish liver and kidney *jing* and nourish blood, to detoxify "fire poisons", and clear external wind.

HOW TO USE: Take as a decoction, tincture, or use in tonic wines.

COMBINATIONS: Use with ginseng and *dang gui* for chronic debility; with *xuan shen* and *lian qiao* to relieve abscesses and swellings due to "fire poisons".

QI TONICS

In China, illness is often defined in terms of energy deficiency and is treated with *qi* tonics. *Qi*, understood in the West as our inner energy level, comes in a wide variety of types. It is a mixture of energies derived from food that is eaten and air that is breathed, in addition to an inherited element. These ingredients combine in different ways to make the various sorts of *qi* that circulate in the body.

DA ZAO
Zizyphus jujube

Da zao literally means "big date" and the fruits are one of the important "harmonizers" in Chinese medicine. They are often added to prescriptions, in the same ways as licorice (*gan cao*), to help modify and blend conflicts in the actions of different ingredients. *Da zao* are also called *hong zao*, or red dates.

PARTS USED: Fruit.

ACTIONS: Energy tonic for spleen and stomach; nourishes blood; nutritive, sedative, calms the spirit; moderates toxic herbs.

HOW TO USE: Take 3-10 dates per dose in decoctions, or eat fresh.

COMBINATIONS: Use with ginseng or *dang gui* as appropriate.

HUANG QI
Astragalus membranaceous

Huang qi is an important *qi* tonic traditionally used for younger people, while ginseng is considered better for those over 40. *Huang qi* is included in Shen Nong's list of "superior" remedies, and research in recent years has confirmed its importance as an immune tonic.

PARTS USED: Root.

ACTIONS: Antispasmodic, diuretic, antibacterial; stimulates bile flow; lowers blood sugar; nervous stimulant; lowers blood pressure; immune stimulant; tonic for *qi* and blood; used to stabilize *wei qi* (defence energy); accelerates wound healing; regulates water metabolism.

HOW TO USE: Decoction or tincture.

COMBINATIONS: Use with ginseng for fatigue and general debility; with *bai zhu* for stomach weakness; with *dang gui* for deficient blood associated with prolonged bleeding; and with *fu ling* and cinnamon twigs for edema in the peripheries.

BAI ZHU
Atractylodes macrocephala

Bai zhu is one of the main *qi* tonics for spleen or stomach *qi* deficiency syndromes. The herb has been used in China since the Tang Dynasty (*c.* 650). It is included in the famous "four noble ingredients decoction" (*Si Jun Zi Tang*), an important energy giving brew containing ginseng, *fu ling* and licorice.

PARTS USED: Rhizome.

ACTIONS: Energy tonic for spleen and stomach; diuretic and carminative; helps to regulate *qi* and strengthen the lower limbs.

HOW TO USE: Take a decoction or tincture.

COMBINATIONS: Can be combined with *ban xia* and *chen pi* for stomach weakness, or with cinnamon and *fu ling* for lung problems.

WESTERN TONICS

Although tonic herbs are less common in modern Western herbal medicine, European tradition still boasts many plants that are regarded as potent energy and spiritual remedies. Much of this tradition is now lost in folklore, although the magical associations of many herbs are still apparent in surviving shamanic rituals. Numerous psychotropic herbs have been used in all cultures to raise mental awareness and alter emotional states. In North America, native medicine men smoked tobacco or took peyote (*Lophophora williamsii*) before seeking the spiritual cause of their patient's illness. In Europe, medieval witches favored henbane, deadly nightshade or mandrake to alter emotional states, while Siberian shaman used fly agaric toadstools (*Amanita muscaria*). Today, South American shaman use extracts of a vine (*Banisteriopsis caapi*), known in Columbia as *yage* and in Peru and Ecuador as *ayahuasca*, to achieve a trance-like state to aid spirit traveling and healing. Other herbs have a less dramatic effect, although old herbals are full of references to plants such as rosemary and lemon balm that "make the heart merry and glad" or "take away melancholy", while others such as *guarana* (see pp. 146-47) are cited to combat fatigue on long journeys.

MIND TONICS

Today, Western herbs tend to be labeled as "sedative" rather than "spiritual" or "emotional" remedies, but many certainly have these properties. Wood betony, for example, acts on the liver and can ease emotions such as frustration and anger, while borage can help us take a more optimistic view of life and realize that it is in our power to make essential changes. In the 1930s Dr Edward Bach "discovered" the Bach Flower Remedies that affect specific moods. Australian Bush Essences and American Quintessentials also act on the emotions.

—— OTHER HERBS TO AFFECT THE MIND —— FEATURED ELSEWHERE IN THE BOOK

basil	page 96	saffron	page. 222-23
borage	page 45	sage	page 115
gotu kola	page 140-41	sandalwood	page 140-41
jasmine	page 78	skullcap	page 118
lemon balm	page 90	spikenard	page 94
mugwort	page 41	vervain	page 135
reishi mushroom	page 144-45	wood betony	page 121
rose	page 110-11		

HIBISCUS
Hibiscus rosa-sinensis
Hibiscus flowers form the basis of *karkade*, a chilled tea traditionally served in Egypt as a restorative for travelers arriving after a long journey, and they are a popular ingredient in many modern Western herbal teas. In India, hibiscus is sacred to Ganesh, the god of wisdom, who destroys obstacles and helps realize goals. It is a good herb for promoting such determination.

❁ PARTS USED: Flowers.

🌿 ACTIONS: Stops bleeding (including excessive menstrual bleeding); eases menstrual cramps and pain associated with urinary tract inflammation; uterine stimulant; promotes menstruation; demulcent, antispasmodic, cooling in fevers.

🫖 🍵 HOW TO USE: Use in infusions or tinctures; *karkade* is made by macerating the petals in cold water, bringing the mix to the boil, straining immediately, and then sweetening and chilling; tea bags are readily available from health food shops.

COMBINATIONS: Use with rose petals for improving determination and resolution; use with raspberry leaf for menstrual problems.

CAUTION: Avoid in pregnancy.

WINTER SAVORY
Satureja montana
Winter savory is usually classified as a culinary herb and is ideal for flavoring soups and stews. Like other culinary plants, it is an effective digestive remedy, and it also shares with basil the ability to lift the spirits and stimulate the mind. It can help to clear melancholy and depression, and to improve concentration and mental activity.

🌿 PARTS USED: Aerial parts.

🌿 ACTIONS: Diaphoretic, carminative, stimulant, promotes menstruation, antispasmodic, astringent, antibacterial, stimulates pituitary gland.

🫖 🍵 HOW TO USE: Use in infusions and tinctures; the essential oil is used internally in parts of Europe but should not be used externally as it can irritate the skin.

COMBINATIONS: Use with basil in infusions and teas as a mental pick-me-up; use the oil in infusers to scent rooms.

CAUTION: Avoid in pregnancy.

PASQUE FLOWER
Pulsatilla vulgaris
Pasque flower is generally regarded in modern herbal medicine as a soothing and analgesic remedy for the reproductive organs. An important sedative, pasque flower is used by patients trying to reduce dependence on benzodiazepine tranquilizers. It is calming and restorative for the emotions and has been used effectively for obsessive syndromes in mental illness, and schizophrenia. In homeopathy, *Pulsatilla* is often prescribed as a remedy for over-dependence and indecisiveness.

🌿 PARTS USED: Aerial parts of dried plant.

🌿 ACTIONS: Nerve relaxant (especially for women), mild sedative, antibacterial, mild analgesic, antispasmodic.

🍵 ⚗️ HOW TO USE: Use 10-50 drops of 1:10 tincture per dose, three times a day; take 250 mg in capsules per dose; use prepared homeopathic remedies.

COMBINATIONS: Use with passion flower for insomnia and hyperactivity; with black cohosh and motherwort for menopausal problems; with skullcap and wood betony for emotional upset.

CAUTION: Do not use the fresh plant, which is irritant.

NERVE TONICS

In the West nervous disorders and "stress" are blamed for all kinds of ailments, and many herbs are labeled as nerve tonics, nervines, sedatives, or antidepressants. For generations herbs have been used to "lift the spirits" or "gladden the heart", but in earlier centuries these terms often referred to imbalance of the humors (see p. 10), rather than implying nervous or psychological weakness.

CARDAMOM
Elettaria cardamomum
Cardamom is a digestive stimulant used to relieve indigestion and abdominal discomfort. It also acts as an energy tonic and stimulant for the nervous system, and is traditionally believed to stimulate the mind and heart, and "bring joy". It is good for productive coughs and also eases feelings of nausea.

PARTS USED: Seeds, essential oil.

ACTIONS: Carminative, stimulating; soothing for the digestive system; appetite stimulant, expectorant, promotes sweating, antispasmodic.

HOW TO USE: Use the crushed seeds in infusions or tinctures; use 2-5 drops essential oil in 5 ml carrier oil for massage; add to bath water or take 1 drop on a sugar lump.

COMBINATIONS: Use in massage with rosemary or thyme; combine in infusions with *gotu kola* for debility and digestive weakness; use with fennel and lemon balm for nervous digestive upsets.

DAMIANA
Turnera diffusa var. *aphrodisiaca*
Damiana is a popular stimulant and aphrodisiac used to combat fatigue and promote energy. An aromatic shrub largely found in Central and South America, it acts as a tonic for the nervous system. It can help in convalescence and general debility, both as a tonic and to encourage the appetite. Damiana can also be used to treat menstrual problems, loss of libido, impotence, and prostate disorders.

PARTS USED: Leaves.

ACTIONS: Aphrodisiac, antidepressant, diuretic, nervous stimulant, digestive tonic, and stimulant for the reproductive organs.

HOW TO USE: Use in infusions and tinctures or take up to 1 g in capsules or pills daily.

COMBINATIONS: Combine with saw palmetto and kola for male sexual problems; with oats and vervain for depression; with raspberry leaf and St. John's wort for menstrual problems.

CALAMINT
Calamintha nepeta
Today, calamint is generally grown as a garden ornamental rather than as a medicinal herb, not least because, like pennyroyal (*Mentha pulegium*), it contains pulegone, which is a potent uterine stimulant. Earlier herbalists were more enthusiastic, regarding the herb as an effective remedy for a "sorrowful spirit".

PARTS USED: Whole plant, seeds.

ACTIONS: Nerve tonic, stimulant, diaphoretic, carminative, uterine stimulant.

HOW TO USE: Use in infusions or decoctions (seeds).

COMBINATIONS: Use with St. John's wort for insomnia; with lemon balm for depression and nervous tension; with fennel seeds for digestive problems.

Caution: Do not use in pregnancy.

ENERGY TONICS

The uplifting effect of a cup of tea or coffee is highly valued, but these herbs are not in the same category as ginseng or guarana. Caffeine based herbs provide only a superficial energy tonic, while herbs such as rosemary (p. 112) contain a chemical called borneol, which acts as a stimulant to the nervous system to overcome fatigue.

SIBERIAN GINSENG
Eleutherococcus senticosus
Varieties of *Eleutherococcus* have been used in traditional Chinese medicine for 2,000 years. It was "rediscovered" in the West in the 1950s and used extensively by Soviet athletes to enhance performance. It helps the body to cope with increased stress levels and improves concentration, and mental activity. It is usually regarded as gentler in action than Korean ginseng, and may be a preferred choice for women.

PARTS USED: Root.

ACTIONS: Helps to combat stress; antiviral, aphrodisiac, immune and circulatory stimulant, regulates blood pressure, lowers blood sugar levels; tonic stimulant for adrenal hormones.

HOW TO USE: Take 10 drops tincture, three times a day, or up to 1 g pills or capsules daily; it is better to take Siberian ginseng before stressful situations rather than in the heat of a crisis.

COMBINATIONS: Usually taken as a simple, but can be combined with saw palmetto or oats.

KOLA NUTS
Cola nitida
Cola contains up to 2.5 percent caffeine with traces of theobromine, making it a more effective stimulant than coffee (which contains up to around 0.3 percent caffeine). Like other caffeine sources, cola essentially provides a short-term energy boost rather than acting as a more deep-seated energy tonic. It was used in the original Coca Cola recipe, the "coca" being provided by cocaine leaves. Pills called "Forced March", containing 5 g of cola, were regularly issued to troops in the early years of the 20th century to provide an energy boost.

PARTS USED: Seeds.

ACTIONS: Diuretic, stimulant, antidepressant, astringent, tonic, nerve stimulant.

HOW TO USE: Use powdered in capsules up to 3 g per dose, or in decoctions (up to 1/2 tsp per cup).

COMBINATIONS: Use with damiana and saw palmetto for sexual problems; with skullcap for depression and nervous debility.

SAW PALMETTO
Serenoa serrulata
Saw palmetto berries originate in the southeastern United States and were popular among Native Americans as a strengthening remedy in debility. Recent research shows that saw palmetto prevents the conversion of the male hormone testosterone into dihydrotestosterone, thought to be responsible for benign prostate enlargement, and encourages its breakdown, preventing and relieving prostate problems.

PARTS USED: Fruit.

ACTIONS: Urinary antiseptic; combats benign prostate enlargement; tonic nutrient, diuretic, sedative, antispasmodic, stimulant.

HOW TO USE: Take 150 mg in pills twice a day; use 1/2 tsp per cup in decoctions.

COMBINATIONS: Use with cola and damiana as a tonic for elderly men; with Siberian ginseng as a general energy tonic; with horsetail and white deadnettle in prostatitis.

OTHER MEDICINAL HERBS

AMERICAN CRANESBILL: *Geranium maculatum*
Parts used: leaves, root.
Actions: astringent, stops external bleeding, tonic.

ARBOR VITAE: *Thuja occidentalis*
Parts used: leaf tips.
Actions: astringent, antimicrobial, expels worms, anti-inflammatory, muscle stimulant.
Caution: avoid in pregnancy.

ARNICA: *Arnica montana*
Parts used: flowers.
Actions: heals wounds, immunostimulant.
Caution: do not use on broken skin; use homeopathic *Arnica* internally only.

ASAFOETIDA: *Ferula asafoetida*
Parts used: oleo gum resin.
Actions: expectorant, carminative, antispasmodic, nerve stimulant, anti-inflammatory, anticoagulant.
Caution: do not use for infants.

BAN XIA: *Pinellia ternata*
Parts used: tuber.
Actions: antitussive, expectorant, prevents vomiting, anticatarrhal.

BARBERRY: *Berberis vulgaris*
Parts used: bark, berries, root.
Actions: cooling, antiseptic, anti-inflammatory, bitter.
Caution: avoid in pregnancy.

BAYBERRY: *Myrica cerifera*
Parts used: bark.
Actions: stimulant, astringent, promotes sweating.

BEARBERRY: *Arctostaphylos uva-ursi*
Parts used: leaves.
Actions: urinary antiseptic, astringent.
Caution: high doses may cause nausea.

BENZOIN: *Styrax benzoin*
Parts used: essential oil, gum.
Actions: expectorant, astringent, antispasmodic.

BIRCH: *Betula verrucosa*
Parts used: bark, leaves, sap.
Actions: bitter, astringent, antirheumatic.

BISTORT: *Polygonum bistorta*
Parts used: root.
Actions: astringent, stops diarrhea and bleeding, anticatarrhal.

BITTER CANDYTUFT: *Iberis amara*
Parts used: aerial parts.
Actions: antispasmodic, relaxant, tonifies the digestive tract, carminative; traditionally used for gout and rheumatism.

BLACK HOREHOUND: *Ballota nigra*
Parts used: aerial parts.
Actions: prevents vomiting, stimulant, antispasmodic.

BLUE COHOSH: *Caulophyllum thalictroides*
Parts used: rhizome.
Actions: tonic, antispasmodic, anti-inflammatory, uterine stimulant, diuretic, antirheumatic.
Caution: avoid in early pregnancy.

BLUE FLAG: *Iris versicolor*
Parts used: rhizome.
Actions: anti-inflammatory, diuretic, stimulant, cathartic.

BOGBEAN: *Menyanthes trifoliata*
Parts used: leaves.
Actions: antirheumatic, bitter, tonic.

BOLDO: *Peumus boldo*
Parts used: leaves.
Actions: liver stimulant, diuretic.

BONESET: *Eupatorium perfoliatum*
Parts used: aerial parts.
Actions: promotes sweating, relaxes peripheral blood vessels, laxative, antispasmodic, antiviral, expectorant, promotes bile flow.
Caution: high doses can cause vomiting.

BROOM: *Cytisus scoparius*
Parts used: flowering tops.
Actions: diuretic, laxative, increases blood pressure, uterine stimulant.
Caution: avoid in pregnancy or high blood pressure; prolonged use can result in liver damage.

BUCHU: *Agathosma betulina*
Parts used: leaves.
Actions: diuretic, tonic, urinary antiseptic, promotes sweating.

BUCKWHEAT: *Fagopyrum esculentum*
Parts used: leaves.
Actions: reduces blood pressure, relaxes blood vessels, repairs blood vessel walls.

BUGLEWEED: *Lycopus virginicus*
Parts used: aerial parts.
Actions: sedative, astringent, tonic, vasoconstrictor, antitussive, raises blood sugar levels, stops bleeding.
Caution: avoid in pregnancy.

CALIFORNIAN POPPY: *Eschscholzia californica*
Parts used: aerial parts.
Actions: analgesic, hypnotic, sedative.

CALUMBA: *Jateorhiza palmata*
Parts used: root.
Actions: bitter, carminative, reduces blood pressure.

CASCARA SAGRADA: *Rhamnus purshiana*
Parts used: bark.
Actions: digestive tonic, purgative.

CATMINT: *Nepeta cataria*
Parts used: aerial parts.
Actions: antispasmodic, carminative, digestive stimulant, promotes sweating, cooling.

CENTAURY: *Centaurium erythraea*
Parts used: aerial parts.
Actions: bitter, liver stimulant.

CHAI HU: *Bupleurum chinense*
Parts used: root.
Actions: energy tonic, liver stimulant, cooling, antibacterial, anti-inflammatory, analgesic, stimulates bile flow, reduces cholesterol levels.

CHASTE-TREE: *Vitex agnuscastus*
Parts used: berries.
Actions: stimulates pituitary gland and hormone production.
Caution: high doses may cause a sensation of ants creeping over the skin (formication).

CHICORY: *Cichorium intybus*
Parts used: root.
Actions: diuretic, laxative, tonic.

CLOVES: *Syzygium aromaticum*
Parts used: essential oil, flower buds.
Actions: antiseptic, anodyne, antispasmodic, carminative, stimulant, prevents vomiting.

CORNFLOWER: *Centaurea cyanus*
Parts used: flowers.
Actions: anti-inflammatory, stimulant, tonic.

CORNSILK: *Zea mays*
Parts used: stamens.
Actions: demulcent, diuretic, specifically healing for urinary mucous membranes, tonic.

COUCHGRASS: *Elymus repens*
Parts used: rhizome.
Actions: cleansing diuretic, healing, and demulcent.

CYPRESS: *Cupressus sempervirens*
Parts used: essential oil.
Actions: antiseptic, antispasmodic, diuretic, sedative.

DILL: *Anethum graveolens*
Parts used: seeds.
Actions: carminative.

DU HUO: *Angelica pubescens*
Parts used: root.
Actions: analgesic, anti-inflammatory, antirheumatic.

EVENING PRIMROSE: *Oenothera biennis*
Parts used: seed oil.
Actions: important source of γ-linolenic acid needed for prostaglandin production.

EYEBRIGHT: *Euphrasia officinalis*
Parts used: aerial parts.
Actions: antiseptic, anticatarrhal, anti-inflammatory.

FALSE UNICORN ROOT: *Chamaelirium luteum*
Parts used: rhizome.
Actions: diuretic, causes vomiting, uterine tonic.

FRINGE TREE: *Chionanthus virginicus*
Parts used: root bark.
Actions: promotes bile flow, liver stimulant, diuretic, tonic.

GERANIUM: *Pelargonium odorantissimum*
Parts used: essential oil.
Actions: antidepressant, tonic, analgesic, diuretic, sedative.

GLOBE ARTICHOKE: *Cynara scolymus*
Parts used: aerial parts.
Actions: liver tonic and restorative, promotes bile flow.

GOAT'S RUE: *Galega officinalis*
Parts used: aerial parts.
Actions: decreases blood sugar levels, insulin stimulant, promotes milk flow.

GOLDEN ROD: *Solidago virgaurea*
Parts used: aerial parts.
Actions: anticatarrhal, anti-inflammatory, healing, urinary antiseptic, sedative, reduces blood pressure, promotes sweating.

GREATER CELANDINE: *Chelidonium majus*
Parts used: aerial parts.
Actions: anti-inflammatory, liver stimulant, diuretic, cleansing.
Caution: avoid in pregnancy.

GREATER PERIWINKLE: *Vinca major*
Parts used: aerial parts.
Actions: astringent, sedative.

GROUND IVY: *Glechoma hederacea*
Parts used: leaves.
Actions: astringent, anticatarrhal.

GUMPLANT: *Grindelia camporum*
Parts used: aerial parts.
Actions: expectorant, antispasmodic, reduces heart rate.
Caution: avoid in low blood pressure; can irritate kidneys.

HERB ROBERT: *Geranium robertianum*
Parts used: leaves.
Actions: astringent, stops external bleeding.

HOLY THISTLE: *Cnicus benedictus*
Parts used: aerial parts.
Actions: bitter, antiseptic, expectorant, heals wounds.

HORSE CHESTNUT: *Aesculus hippocastanum*
Parts used: bark, seeds.
Actions: astringent, anti-inflammatory.
Caution: seed coating can be toxic.

HUAI JIAO: *Sophora japonica*
Parts used: fruit.
Actions: laxative, stops bleeding.
Caution: avoid in pregnancy.

HUAI NIU XI: *Achyranthes bidentata*
Parts used: root.
Actions: circulatory stimulant, analgesic, liver tonic.

HUANG LIAN: *Coptis chinensis*
Parts used: root.
Actions: antibacterial, analgesic, anti-inflammatory, promotes bile flow, sedative.

HUO MA REN: *Cannabis sativa*
Parts used: seeds.
Actions: stimulating laxative.

HYDRANGEA: *Hydrangea arborescens*
Parts used: rhizome/root.
Actions: diuretic, kidney stimulant, laxative.

INDIAN TOBACCO: *Lobelia inflata*
Parts used: aerial parts.
Actions: relaxant, antispasmodic, causes vomiting, expectorant, promotes sweating, antiasthmatic.
Caution: Restricted in some countries; use only under the guidance of a qualified practitioner.

IRISH MOSS: *Chondrus crispus*
Parts used: seaweed.
Actions: demulcent, expectorant, prevents vomiting, nutritive.

JAMAICAN DOGWOOD: *Piscidia erythrina*
Parts used: root bark.
Actions: anodyne, sedative.
Caution: do not exceed stated dose.

JIE GENG: *Platycodon grandiflorus*
Parts used: root.
Actions: antibacterial, antifungal, expectorant, lowers blood sugar.

KING'S CLOVER: *Melilotus officinalis*
Parts used: flowering aerial parts.
Actions: antispasmodic, anticoagulant, demulcent, diuretic.
Caution: do not use with warfarin or other blood-thinning drugs, or with any blood-clotting problem.

LEMON: *Citrus limon*
Parts used: essential oil, fruit.
Actions: antihistaminic, anti-inflammatory, diuretic, venous tonic.
Caution: ensure essential oil is well diluted before use – it can irritate the skin.

LIAN QIAO: *Forsythia suspensa*
Parts used: fruit.
Actions: antibacterial, anti-inflammatory, cooling.
Caution: avoid in diarrhea or *yin* deficiency.

LIGNUM VITAE: *Guaiacum officinalis*
Parts used: heartwood.
Actions: anti-inflammatory, antirheumatic, circulatory stimulant.

LILY-OF-THE-VALLEY: *Convallaria majalis*
Parts used: aerial parts, leaves.
Actions: heart tonic, diuretic, purgative, causes vomiting.
Caution: restricted in the UK, Australia and New Zealand; use only under the guidance of a qualified practitioner.

LINDEN: *Tilia x europaea*
Parts used: flowers.
Actions: sedating nervine, promotes sweating, relaxes blood vessels, healing for blood vessel walls.

LOVAGE: *Levisticum officinale*
Parts used: root, seeds.
Actions: carminative, promotes sweating, warming digestive tonic, expectorant, anticatarrhal.

MAI MEN DONG: *Ophiopogon japonicus*
Parts used: tuber.
Actions: promotes secretion of body fluids, tonic, sedative, antitussive, lowers blood sugar levels, antibacterial.

MARSH CUDWEED: *Gnaphthalium uliginosum*
Parts used: aerial parts.
Actions: anticatarrhal, anti-inflammatory, astringent, tonifying to mucous membranes.

MISTLETOE: *Viscum album*
Parts used: young leafy twigs.
Actions: reduces blood pressure, slows heart rate, antitumor.
Caution: do not use berries, which are toxic and restricted in the UK; avoid in pregnancy.

MOUSE-EAR HAWKWEED: *Hieracium pilosella*
Parts used: aerial parts.
Actions: anticatarrhal, antispasmodic, diuretic, expectorant, heals wounds.

NU ZHEN ZI: *Ligustrum lucidum*
Parts used: berries.
Actions: tonic, immunostimulant, diuretic.

OAK: *Quercus robur*
Parts used: bark.
Actions: strong astringent.

PARSLEY PIERT: *Aphanes arvensis*
Parts used: aerial parts.
Actions: demulcent, diuretic.

PELLITORY-OF-THE-WALL: *Parietaria diffusa*
Parts used: aerial parts.
Actions: demulcent, diuretic, soothing for urinary mucous membranes.

PILEWORT: *Ranunculus ficaria*
Parts used: root, leaves.
Actions: astringent, used for hemorrhoids.
Caution: do not take internally.

PRICKLY ASH: *Zanthoxylum americanum*
Parts used: bark.
Actions: carminative, circulatory stimulant, promotes sweating.

QUASSIA: *Picrasma excelsa*
Parts used: wood.
Actions: expels worms, bitter.

RAMSOMS: *Allium ursinum*
Parts used: aerial parts, bulbs.
Actions: decreases blood sugar levels, lowers serum cholesterol, antimicrobial.

RUE: *Ruta graveolens*
Parts used: leaves.
Actions: antispasmodic, antitussive, promotes menstrual flow, lowers blood pressure, circulatory tonic.
Caution: avoid in pregnancy.

SAFFLOWER: *Carthamus tinctorius*
Parts used: flowers.
Actions: laxative, diuretic, anti-inflammatory.

SHAN ZHU YU: *Cornus officinalis*
Parts used: fruit.
Actions: tonic, diuretic, reduces blood pressure, antimicrobial.

SLIPPERY ELM: *Ulmus fulva*
Parts used: bark.
Actions: demulcent, nutritive, astringent.

SOAP BARK: *Quillaja saponaria*
Parts used: inner bark.
Actions: detergent, expectorant, anti-inflammatory.
Caution: do not take internally.

SOUTHERNWOOD: *Artemisia abrotanum*
Parts used: aerial parts.
Actions: expels worms, antiseptic, bitter, uterine stimulant.
Caution: avoid in pregnancy.

SQUAW VINE: *Mitchella repens*
Parts used: aerial parts.
Actions: astringent, diuretic, tonic, restorative, uterine stimulant.

SWEET SUMACH: *Rhus aromatica*
Parts used: root bark.
Actions: astringent, diuretic, tonic, antidiabetic.

TORMENTIL: *Potentilla erecta*
Parts used: root.
Actions: astringent – especially for gut wall.

TRUE UNICORN ROOT: *Aletris farinosa*
Parts used: rhizome.
Actions: digestive stimulant.

WALL GERMANDER: *Teucrium chamaedrys*
Parts used: aerial parts.
Actions: anticatarrhal, antimicrobial, digestive stimulant, anti-inflammatory.
Caution: research suggests that long term use may cause liver damage; do not exceed stated dose.

WHITE BRYONY: *Bryonia alba*
Parts used: root.
Actions: antirheumatic, cathartic.

WHITE DEADNETTLE: *Lamium album*
Parts used: flowering tops.
Actions: astringent, tonic for reproductive organs, anti-spasmodic.

WHITE HOREHOUND: *Marrubium vulgare*
Parts used: aerial parts.
Actions: antispasmodic, stimulating expectorant, bitter, soothing tonic for the mucous membranes.

WILD INDIGO: *Baptisia tinctoria*
Parts used: leaves, root.
Actions: antibacterial, antiseptic, laxative, cooling.
Caution: do not exceed stated dose; excess may cause vomiting.

WILD LETTUCE: *Lactuca virosa*
Parts used: leaves.
Actions: hypnotic, sedative, decreases blood sugar levels.
Caution: may cause drowsiness; do not drive or operate machinery; excess doses may cause insomnia or decreased sex drive.

WOOD SAGE: *Teucrium scorodonia*
Parts used: aerial parts.
Actions: astringent, antirheumatic, carminative, heals wounds, promotes sweating, promotes bile flow.

WOUNDWORT: *Stachys palustris*
Parts used: aerial parts.
Actions: antispasmodic, antiseptic, heals wounds.

WU ZHU YU: *Evodia rutaecarpa*
Parts used: fruit.
Actions: analgesic, antibacterial, warming, stimulant.

XIANG FU: *Cyperus rotundus*
Parts used: tuber.
Actions: carminative, analgesic, uterine antispasmodic, encourages *qi* (energy) flow.

YELLOW DOCK: *Rumex crispus*
Parts used: root.
Actions: cleansing, promotes bile flow, strong laxative.

YELLOW JASMINE: *Gelsemium sempervirens*
Parts used: root.
Actions: analgesic, reduces blood pressure, sedative, eases neuralgia.
Caution: restricted in some countries; overdose can cause nausea and double vision.

ZE XIE: *Alisma plantago*
Parts used: rhizome.
Actions: diuretic, reduces blood pressure, antibacterial, liver cleanser.

ZHI ZI: *Gardenia jasminoides*
Parts used: fruit.
Actions: cooling, reduces blood pressure, sedative, antibacterial.

CONSULTING AN HERBALIST

MANY PEOPLE REGULARLY use herbs as safe and effective home remedies for minor ailments, but persistent or serious problems need professional help from a qualified herbal practitioner. Choosing someone with whom you feel empathy and whom you can trust can be just as important in treatment as taking the most appropriate herbs. The best way to find a practitioner is through personal recommendation from a like-minded friend. Alternatively, ask the national regulatory bodies (see p. 240) for a list of herbalists practicing in your area. You can consult an herbalist about a wide range of health problems: aches and pains, high blood pressure, urinary dysfunction, digestive ailments, menstrual disorders, asthma or bronchitis, skin complaints, nervous disorders, even chronic conditions for which herbalism is often seen as the last resort, such as rheumatoid arthritis, chronic fatigue syndrome, or emphysema.

WHO ARE THE HERBALISTS?
National practices and regulations vary around the world. In some countries – including certain states in the United States – there is a total ban on professional herbal practice, while in Japan and China free herbal treatment is available under state medical plans.

Britain is unusual in Europe in having a well-established system for training herbal practitioners, who have not necessarily obtained any other medical qualification. The National Institute of Medical Herbalists was founded in 1864. Members qualify by examination after four or five years of specialist study. Members use the initials MNIMH or FNIMH after their names. Members of the General Council and Register of Herbalists use the initials MH.

In Australia, trained herbalists become full members of the National Herbalists Association of Australia and use the initials NHAA after their names. They are classified as Health Care Professionals by the Commonwealth government.

WHAT THE HERBALIST DOES
Herbalists use a combination of traditional diagnostic techniques, history taking and simple clinical tests to reach a diagnosis. Herbal remedies will then be prescribed to match the specific mix of problems for each individual sufferer rather than using a standard selection of ready-made herbal combinations.

If a patient is already taking conventional medication the herbalist needs to know. Herbalists would certainly not recommend ceasing to take vital drugs, but any incompatibility with herbal remedies must be considered. Indeed, many patients turn to herbs because they wish to phase out pharmaceutical drugs, and a safe program of replacing them with gentler herbal remedies needs to be devised (preferably with the cooperation of the patient's regular doctor). The first consultation takes at least an hour, and subsequent ones about 20 minutes. Herbalists like to see patients soon after their first visit to check on progress, then follow this up with regular meetings every four to six weeks for three months, or more in chronic cases.

Whatever the remedy, healing is a two-way process and patients must take responsibility for their own health and actively participate in any cure.

FURTHER READING

Arvigo, R & Balick, M: *Rainforest Remedies: One Hundred Healing Herbs of Belize*, Lotus Press, Twin Lakes, Wisconsin, 1993.
Bartram, T: *Encyclopaedia of Herbal Medicine*, Grace Publishers, Christchurch, 1995.
Beinfield, H & Korngold, E: *Between Heaven and Earth: A Guide to Chinese Medicine*, Ballantine Books, New York, 1991.
Bown, D: *Encyclopaedia of Herbs and Their Uses*, Dorling Kindersley, London, 1995.
Brooke, E: *A Woman's Book of Herbs*, The Women's Press, London, 1992.
Brooker, S G, Camie, R C & Cooper, R C: *New Zealand Medicinal Plants*, Reed, Auckland, 1987.
Chmelik, S: *Chinese Herbal Secrets*, Ivy Press, Lewes, 1999.
Chevallier, A: *Encyclopaedia of Medicinal Plants*, Dorling Kindersley, London, 1996.
Davis, P: *Aromatherapy: An A-Z*, 2nd Edition, C W Daniels, Saffron Walden, 1995.
Foster, S & Yue, C: *Herbal Emissaries*, Healing Arts Press, Rochester, VT, 1992.

Frawley, D & Lad, V: *The Yoga of Herbs*, Lotus Press, Sante Fe, 1986.
Frawley, D: *Ayurvedic Healing: A Comprehensive Guide*, Passage Press, Salt Lake City, Utah, 1989.
Grieve, M: *A Modern Herbal*, Jonathan Cape, London, 1931.
Griggs, B: *Green Pharmacy*, Jill Norman & Hobhouse, London, 1981.
Gursche, S: *Healing with Herbal Juices*, Alive Books, Canada, 1993.
Hobbs, C: *Medicinal Mushrooms*, Botanica Press, Santa Cruz, 1995.
Holmes, P: *The Energetics of Western Herbs*, Artemis Press, Boulder, Colorado, 1989.
Lipp, F J: *Herbalism*, Macmillan, London, 1996.
Manniche, L: *An Ancient Egyptian Herbal*, British Musuem Publications, London, 1989.
McIntyre, A: *The Complete Floral Healer*, Gaia Books, London, 1996.
Mills, S Y: *Out of the Earth*, Viking, London, 1991.
Newell, C A, Anderson, L A &

Phillipson, J D: *Herbal Medicines*, The Pharmaceutical Press, London, 1996.
Ody, P: *The Herb Society's Home Herbal*, Dorling Kindersley, London, 1995.
Ody, P: *100 Great Natural Remedies*, Kyle Cathie, London, 1997.
Ody, P: *Herbs for a Healthy Pregnancy*, Keats Publishing, Los Angeles, 1999.
Rogers, C: *A Woman's Guide to Herbal Medicine*, Hamish Hamilton, London, 1995.
Tierra, M: *Planetary Herbology*, Lotus Press, Sante Fe, 1988.
Tisserand, R: *The Art of Aromatherapy*, C W Daniels, Saffron Walden, 1977.
Vogel, V J: *American Indian Medicine*, University of Oklahoma Press, 1970.
Weiss, R F: *Herbal Medicine*, Beaconsfield Publishers, Beaconsfield, 1988.
Whistler, W A: *Polynesian Herbal Medicine*, National Tropical Botanical Garden, Hawaii, 1992.
Wren, R C: *Potter's New Cyclopaedia of Botanical Drugs and Preparations*, C W Daniels, Saffron Walden.

GLOSSARY

ADRENAL CORTEX Part of the adrenal gland, which produces corticosteroid hormones.

ALKALOID Highly active plant constituent, containing nitrogen atoms usually in a ring-shaped molecule.

ALTERATIVE Cleansing, stimulating efficient removal of waste products.

ANALGESIC Relieves pain.

ANODYNE Eases pain.

ANTIBIOTIC Destroys or inhibits the growth of microorganisms.

ANTICOAGULANT Hinders blood clotting.

ANTIHYDROTIC Limits the production of water-based fluids including sweat.

ANTIMICROBIAL Destroys microorganisms.

ANTISPASMODIC Reduces muscle spasm and tension.

ANTITUSSIVE Inhibits the cough reflex helping to stop coughing.

APERIENT Mild laxative.

ASTRINGENT Precipitates proteins from the surface of cells or mucous membranes, producing a protective coating; has a binding and contracting effect.

AYURVEDIC Traditional system of Indian medicine, which literally means "a science of life".

BITTER Stimulates secretion of digestive juices and encourages appetite.

BLACK BILE One of the four Galenical (*q.v.*) humors (*q.v.*) associated with the earth element and considered cold and dry.

BLOOD Apart from the familiar substance, "blood" was one of the four Galenical (*q.v.*) humors (*q.v.*) associated with the air element and considered hot and damp.

BLOOD STAGNATION Concept in traditional Chinese medicine where the blood circulation is retarded or where blood vessels become blocked for any reason. Considered to interfere with the normal flow of *qi* (*q.v.*) through the body.

BULK LAXATIVE Increases the volume of feces, producing larger, softer stools.

CARDIOACTIVE Affecting heart function.

CARMINATIVE Relieves flatulence, digestive colic, and gastric discomfort.

CATHARTIC Drastic purgative (*q.v.*).

CHAKRA Center or point of spiritual power and energy in the body.

CHANNEL See *meridian*.

CHOLAGOGUE Stimulates bile flow from the gall bladder, and bile ducts into the duodenum.

CHOLERETIC Increases secretion of bile by the liver.

CHOLERIC Galenical (*q.v.*) temperament related to yellow bile (*q.v.*).

CIRCULATORY STIMULANT Increases blood flow.

COLD CONDITIONS Concept in traditional Chinese medicine associated with chills, poor circulation, thirst for hot drinks, feeling cold, fatigue, sharp pain, frequent urination or *yang* (*q.v.*) deficiency.

COLIC Spasmodic pain affecting smooth muscle, for example in the guts, gall bladder or urinary tract.

COUMARIN Active plant constituent, generally smelling of new mown hay, which has a thinning effect on the blood.

DEMULCENT Softens and soothes damaged or inflamed surfaces, such as the gastric mucous membranes.

DIURETIC Encourages urine flow.

DOCTRINE OF SIGNATURES Theory that the appearance of a plant indicates its inherent medicinal properties.

ECLECTIC System of herbal medicine developed in the United States in the 19th century.

EMETIC Causes vomiting.

EMOLLIENT Softens and soothes the skin.

ESSENTIAL OIL Commercially available volatile oil extracted from plants by steam distillation and containing a mixture of active constituents; highly aromatic.

EXPECTORANT Encourages the loosening and removal of phlegm from the respiratory tract.

FEBRIFUGE Reduces fever.

GALENICAL Traditional system of Western medicine based on the four humors (*q.v.*) theory of Ancient Greece.

GLYCOSIDE Active plant constituent containing one or more sugar groups.

HOT CONDITIONS Concept in traditional Chinese medicine associated with fevers, increased metabolic rate, thirst for cold drinks, increased heat sensitivity, irritability, burning pains, thick catarrh or *yin* (*q.v.*) deficiency.

HUMOR Theoretical body fluid important in Galenical (*q.v.*) and Ayurvedic (*q.v.*) medicine.

HYPERTENSION High blood pressure.

HYPOTENSION Low blood pressure.

IMMUNOSTIMULANT Enhances and increases the body's immune (defence) mechanism.

JING The "vital essence" of traditional Chinese medicine responsible for creative and reproductive energies, and stored in the kidneys.

KAPHA Ayurvedic (*q.v.*) humor (*q.v.*) associated with dampness or phlegm (*q.v.*).

LAXATIVE Encourages bowel movements.

MELANCHOLIC Galenical (*q.v.*) state related to black bile (*q.v.*).

MERIDIAN In Chinese medicine, a conduit which can be compared to an imaginary line (or channel) linking points on the body's surface with internal organs in which *qi* (*q.v.*) flows. Traditional Chinese medicine defines 14 main channels and eight extra channels. The surface points are used in acupuncture.

MUCILAGE Complex sugar molecules that are soft and slippery and protect mucous membranes and inflamed tissues.

NARCOTIC Causes stupor and numbness.

NERVINE Affects the nervous system – may be stimulating, sedating or relaxing.

NEURALGIA Pain along a nerve.

PERIPHERAL CIRCULATION Blood supply to limbs, skin, and muscles (including heart muscle).

PHLEGM In modern Western medicine similar to catarrh or sputum; Galenical (*q.v.*) humor (*q.v.*) associated with the water element and considered cold and damp; *kapha* (*q.v.*); associated with spleen deficiency in traditional Chinese medicine.

PHLEGMATIC Galenical (*q.v.*) state related to phlegm (*q.v.*).

PHYSIOMEDICALISM System of herbal medicine developed in the United States in the 19th century.

PITTA Ayurvedic (*q.v.*) humor (*q.v.*) associated with fire or bile.

PROSTAGLANDINS Hormone-like substances that have a wide range of functions, including acting as chemical messengers and causing uterine contractions.

PURGATIVE Drastic laxative.

QI (CH'I) In Chinese medicine the body's vital energy.

RUBEFACIENT Stimulates blood flow to the skin, causing local reddening.

SANGUINE Galenical (*q.v.*) state related to blood (*q.v.*).

SAPONINS Active plant constituents, similar to soap, producing a lather in water; can irritate the digestive tract; expectorant; some chemically resemble steroidal hormones.

SEDATIVE Soothing and calming.

SIMPLE A single herb used on its own.

STEROIDS Group of chemicals with a characteristic multi-ring molecular structure. Naturally occurring steroids include the sex hormones and hydrocortisone.

STYPTIC Stops external bleeding.

SYSTEMIC Affecting the entire body.

TANNIN Active plant constituents which combine with proteins; originally derived from plants used for tanning leather; astringent (*q.v.*).

TERPENE Complex active plant constituents with a carbon ring structure, generally highly aromatic and included in essential oil (*q.v.*).

TONIC Restoring, nourishing and supporting for the entire body.

TONIFY Strengthen and restore.

TOPICAL Local administration of herbal remedy, e.g. to the skin or eye; effect herb has in local treatment.

VASOCONSTRICTOR Reduces the diameter of blood vessels.

VASODILATOR Increases the diameter of blood vessels.

VATA Ayurvedic (*q.v.*) humor (*q.v.*) associated with wind or air.

VENOUS RETURN Blood flow from the extremities through the veins back to the heart.

VULNERARY Heals wounds.

WEI QI Concept in Chinese medicine of defence energy, comparable with the immune system.

YANG Aspect of being equated with male energy – dry, hot, ascending, exterior.

YELLOW BILE Galenical (*q.v.*) humor (*q.v.*) associated with the fire element and considered hot and dry; *pitta* (*q.v.*).

YIN Aspect of being equated with female energy – damp, cold, descending, interior.

INDEX

USEFUL ADDRESSES

UNITED STATES

ASSOCIATIONS AND ORGANIZATIONS

American Botanical Council, P.O. Box 144345, Austin, TX 78714-4345 (512) 926-4900 www.herbalgram.org.
American Herbal Products, 8484 Georgia Avenue, Suite 370, Silver Springs, MD 20910 (301) 588-1171 www.ahpa.org.
National Health Federation, P.O. Box 688, Monrovia, CA 91017 (626) 357-2181.
The American Herbalists' Guild, P.O. Box 70, Roosevelt, UT 84066 (435) 722-8483 www.healthy.net/herbalists.
The Growing and Marketing Network, P.O. Box 245, Silver Springs, PA 17575 (717) 393-3295 www.herbnet.com.
The Herb Research Foundation, 1007 Pearl Street, Suite 200, Boulder, CO 80302 (303) 449-2265.

TRAINING COURSES

California School of Herbal Studies, P.O. Box 39, Forrestville, CA. 95436 (707) 887-7457.
East West Herbal Correspondence Course, P.O. Box 275, Ben Lomond, CA 95005 (800) 717-5010 www.PlanetHerbs. com.

HERBAL SUPPLIERS

Aphrodisia, 264 Bleecker Street, New York, NY 10014 (212) 989-6440.
Lotus Light, P.O. Box 1008, Silver Lake, WI 53170 (414) 889-8501.
May Way Trading Chinese Herb Company, 1338 Mandela Parkway, Oakland, CA 94607 (510) 208-3113.
Tai Sang Trading Chinese Herb Company, 1018 Stockton, San Francisco, CA 94108 (415) 981-5364.

ESSENTIAL OIL SUPPLIERS

Kiehls Pharmacy, 109 Third Avenue, New York, NY 10009 (212) 677-3171 (mail orders accepted).
The Body Shop By Mail, 800-Bodyshop.

EQUIPMENT SUPPLIERS

WINE PRESSES
Milan Home Wine and Beer, 659 54th Street, Brooklyn, NY 11220 (212) 226-4780.
Kedco Wine Storage Systems, 564 Smith St., Farmingdale, NY 11735 (516) 454-7800.

PUBLICATIONS AND PERIODICALS

Business of Herbs, P.O. Box 245, Silver Springs, PA 7575-0245.
HerbalGram, P.O. Box 144345, Austin, TX 78714-4345.
The Herb Companion, 201 East Fourth Street, Loveland, CO 80537.
The Herb Companion Wishbook and Resource Guide, 201 East Fourth Street, Loveland, CO 80537.
The Herb Quarterly, P.O. Box 548H6, Boiling Springs, PA 17007.
Journal of Herbs, Spices, and Medicinal Plants, Haworth Press, 10 Alice Street, Binghamton, NY 13904-1580.
Medical Herbalism, P.O. Box 33080, Portland, OR 97233.
Northwind Farm's Herb Resource Directory, c/o Northwind Farm Publications, RR 2 P.O. Box 2246, Shevlin, MN 56676-9535.

CANADA

ASSOCIATIONS AND ORGANIZATIONS

Association of British Columbia, 22-12391 Bridgeport Road, Richmond, B.C. V6V 1JA (604) 278-6220 www.users.uniserve.com/aabc.
International College of Traditional Chinese Medicine, 3011847 West Broadway, Vancouver, B.C. V6M 461 (604) 731-2926.
Ontario Herbalists' Association, 7 Alpine Avenue, Toronto, ONT M6P 3R6 (416) 536-1509.

HERBAL SUPPLIERS

Eastern Currents Distributing Ltd, 200A 3540 West 41st Avenue, Vancover, B.C. V6N 3E6 (800) 667-6866.

PUBLICATIONS

The Canadian Journal of Herbalism, 11 Winthrop Place, Stoney Creek, ONT L8G 3M3.

ACKNOWLEDGMENTS

Dorling Kindersley would like to thank Rosie Pearson and Claire Le Bas for their editorial help, as well as Louise Abbot, Diana Craig and Carolyn Ryden; Helen Gatward for picture research; Nicholas Jackson for DTP; Tracey Clarke, Sarah Ponder, and Gill Shaw for assisting with design; Sarah Ashun for assisting Steve Gorton at photography; Hilary Guy for styling pages 8-9; Diana Mitchell for finding herbs; Sue Bosanko for the index; Iris and Victor Hill, Lauren and Mark Holyoake, Colin Neville, Molly and Ken Neville, and Niki Sarluis for their kind help in finding and providing herbs; Brenda Cole, Eric Clarement, and Julee Binder for assistance with the North American edition.
The following companies and individuals also provided herbs and herbal preparations: Andrew Wickens and Marion Brown of Iden Croft Herbs; East-West Herbs Ltd; Hollington Nurseries; Arne Herbs; Tony Carter of The Herbal Apothecary; Fiona Crumley of the Chelsea Physic Garden; Christopher Hedley; Allen Coombes of The Sir Harold Hillier Gardens and Arboretum; Sally Gardens.

ILLUSTRATORS
Colette Cheng: 14,15,16; Tina Hill: 10, 14-15, 27; Gillie Newman: 32, 34, 37, 44, 46, 50, 52, 53, 54, 56, 57, 61, 64, 65, 67, 69, 74, 75, 78, 79, 81, 82, 84, 85, 88, 92, 98, 113; Sarah Ponder: symbols throughout book.

KEY TO PICTURE POSITIONS
t = top; c = center; b = bottom;
l = left; r = right

PICTURE CREDITS
All photography by Steve Gorton except for: Bodleian Library (L.1.5. MED): 19br; The British Library: 13tr; Corbis UK Ltd/ Gianni Dagli: 146tc, /Penny Tweedie 142tc; Dorling Kindersley Picture Library/Glasgow Museums: 140tc; ET Archive (*Les Champignons du Voyage* by Pierre Lacombe, Exhibition Asniere/Seine 1991: 144tc; The Mansell Collection: 11cr, 19tr, 23tr; Mary Evans Picture Library: 11br, 17tr, 20bl, 20cl, 22bl; Book of Tibetan Medicine: Teaching Material Produced by the Traditional Medical School in Lhasa, Tibet: 13br; Salus-Haus: 23br; Science Photo Library: 18bl; University of Durham Oriental Museum: 12b; Wellcome Institute Library, London: 21tr; Werner Forman Archive: 11tr; Martin Cameron: 118-124; Martin Norris 126-127 except for: Peter Anderson: 126cr, 127bl.